www.harcourt-international.com

Bringing you products from all Harcourt Health Sciences companies including Baillière Tindall, Churchill Livingstone, Mosby and W.B. Saunders

- ▶ **Browse** for latest information on new books, journals and electronic products

- ▶ **Search** for information on over 20 000 published titles with full product information including tables of contents and sample chapters

- ▶ **Keep up to date** with our extensive publishing programme in your field by registering with eAlert or requesting postal updates

- ▶ **Secure online ordering** with prompt delivery, as well as full contact details to order by phone, fax or post

- ▶ **News** of special features and promotions

If you are based in the following countries, please visit the country-specific site to receive full details of product availability and local ordering information

USA: www.harcourthealth.com

Canada: www.harcourtcanada.com

Australia: www.harcourt.com.au

D0243692

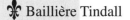

✾ Baillière Tindall   ⛵ CHURCHILL LIVINGSTONE   ...RS

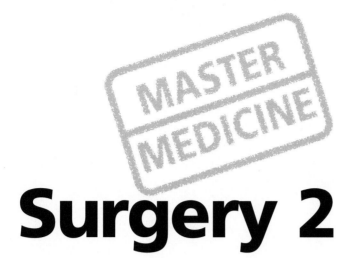

Surgery 2

Commissioning Editor: Laurence Hunter
Project Development Manager: Barbara Simmons
Project Controller: Nancy Arnott
Designers: Judith Wright, George Ajayi

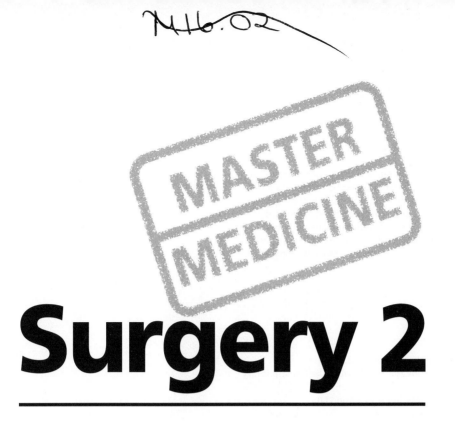

Surgery 2

A core text with self-assessment covering orthopaedics, ear, nose and throat surgery, and ophthalmology

Edited by

JOHN A. DENT

MMedEd MD FRCS (Ed)
Senior Lecturer in Orthopaedic and Trauma Surgery
Ninewells Hospital and Medical School
Dundee

SECOND EDITION

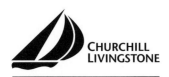

CHURCHILL
LIVINGSTONE

Edinburgh   London   New York   Philadelphia   Sydney   Toronto   2002

CHURCHILL LIVINGSTONE
An imprint of Harcourt Publishers Limited

© Harcourt Publishers Limited 2002

 is a registered trademark of Harcourt Publishers Limited

First edition 1997
Second edition 2002

ISBN 0443 07089X

British Library Cataloguing in Publication Data
A catalogue record for this book is available from the British Library

Library of Congress Cataloging in Publication Data
A catalog record for this book is available from the Library of Congress

Medical knowledge is constantly changing. As new information becomes available, changes in treatment, procedures, equipment and the use of drugs become necessary. The editor, contributors and the publishers have, as far as it is possible, taken care to ensure that the information given in this text is accurate and up to date. However, readers are strongly advised to confirm that the information, especially with regard to drug usage, complies with the latest legislation and standards of practice.

The
publisher's
policy is to use
**paper manufactured
from sustainable forests**

Printed in Spain

Contributors

Andrew Blaikie MB ChB BSc Med Sci (Path) MRCOphth
Specialist Registrar in Ophthalmology, Ninewells Hospital,
Dundee

Robin L. Blair FRCS(Ed) FRCS(C) FACS
Consultant Otolaryngologist, University of Dundee,
Dundee

John A. Dent MMedEd MD FRCS(Ed)
Senior Lecturer in Orthopaedic and Trauma Surgery,
Ninewells Hospital and Medical School, Dundee

Quentin Gardiner FRCS(Eng & Ed) FRCS(ORL)
Consultant Otolaryngologist and Honorary Senior Clinical
Teacher, Department of Otolaryngology, University of
Dundee, Dundee

Caroline J. MacEwen MB ChB MD FRCS FRCOphth
Consultant Ophthalmologist, Ninewells Hospital, Dundee

Contents

Using this book

'What do I need to know about the surgical specialties?'
'Do I know the right things?'
'Can I remember the key points in the management of…?'

These are the sort of questions which haunt us as exams approach but by then, unfortunately, there is seldom time to go back to extensive textbooks or sketchy lecture notes for the answers.

This is just the time when this new revision textbook comes in useful. In it you will find the 'core' information you require presented in a concise and systematic fashion, which highlights the key facts you should know about any topic in a way that will help you remember them. But rather than simply giving you lots of facts to memorise, the principles of diagnosis and management are explained so that it becomes easier for you to work out the answers for yourself. The book does not aim to offer a complete 'syllabus'. It is impossible to draw boundaries around medical knowledge and learning as this is really a continuous process carried out throughout your medical career. With this in mind, you should aim to develop the ability to discern knowledge which you *need to know* from that which it is *nice to know*.

The aims of this introductory chapter are:

- to help plan your learning
- to show you how to use this book to increase your understanding as well as knowledge
- to realise how self-assessment can make learning easier and more enjoyable.

Layout and contents

The main part of the text describes topics considered to be of 'core' importance to the major subject areas. Within each chapter, essential information is presented in a set order with explanations and logical 'links' between topics. Where relevant, key facts about basic sciences, aetiology and pathological features are outlined. Where it is possible the clinical features are described under the key headings of 'Listen', 'Look', 'Feel' and 'Move'. Differential diagnosis and an approach to investigation are then described. Finally, the principles of management and the prognosis are presented. It is recognised that at the level of an undergraduate or newly qualified doctor a detailed understanding is not required; instead the ability to set out principles is all that is expected.

You will need to be sure that you are reaching the required standards, so in the final section of each chapter there are opportunities for you to check your knowledge and understanding. This self-assessment is in the form of multiple choice questions (MCQs), extended matching items questions (EMIs), constructed response questions (CRQs), objective structured clinical examination questions (OSCEs) and viva questions. All of these are centred around common clinical problems, which are important in judging your performance as a doctor. Detailed answers are given. These answers will also contain some information and explanations that you will not find elsewhere, so you must do the assessment to get the most out of this book!

Using this book

If you are using this book as part of your exam preparations, I suggest that your first task should be to map out on a sheet of paper three lists dividing the major subjects (corresponding to the chapter headings) into your strong, reasonable and weak areas. This will give you a rough outline of your revision schedule, which you must then fit in with the time available. Clearly, if your exams are looming large you will have to be ruthless in the time allocated to your strong areas. The major subjects should be further classified into individual topics. Encouragement to store information and to test your ongoing improvement is by the use of the self-assessment sections — you must not just read passively. It is important to keep checking your current level of knowledge, both strengths and weaknesses. This should be assessed objectively — self-rating in the absence of testing can be misleading. You may consider yourself strong in a particular area whereas it is more a reflection on how much you enjoy and are stimulated by the subject. Conversely, you may be stronger in a subject than you would expect simply because the topic does not appeal to you.

It is a good idea to discuss topics and problems with colleagues/friends; the areas which you understand least well will soon become apparent when you try to explain them to someone else.

Approaching the examinations

The discipline of learning is closely linked to preparation for examinations. Many of us opt for a process of superficial learning that is directed towards retention of facts and recall under exam conditions because full understanding is often not required. It is much better if you try to acquire a deeper knowledge and understanding, combining the necessity of passing exams with longer-term needs.

First, you need to know how you will be examined. Does the examination involve clinical assessment such as history taking and clinical examination? If you are sitting a written examination, what are the length and types of question? How many must you answer and how much choice will you have?

Now you have to choose what sources you are going to use for your learning and revision. Textbooks come in different forms. At one extreme, there is the large reference book. This type of book should be avoided at this stage of revision and only used (if at all) for reference, when answers to questions cannot be found in smaller books. At the other end of the spectrum is the condensed 'lecture note' format, which often relies heavily on lists. Facts of this nature on their own are difficult to remember if they are not supported by understanding. In the middle of the range are the medium-sized textbooks. These are often of the most use whether you are approaching final university examinations or the first part of professional examinations. My advice is to choose one of the several medium-sized books on offer on the basis of which you find the most readable. The best approach is to combine your lecture notes, textbooks (appropriate to the level of study) and past examination papers as a framework for your preparation.

Armed with information about the format of the exams, a rough syllabus, your own lecture notes and some books that you feel comfortable in using, your next step is to map out the time available for preparation. You must be realistic, allow time for breaks and work *steadily*, not cramming. If you do attempt to cram, you have to realise that only a certain amount of information can be retained in your short-term memory, so as the classification of one condition moves in, the treatment of another moves out! Cramming simply retains facts. If the examination requires understanding you will be in trouble.

It is often a good idea to begin by outlining the topics to be covered and then attempt to summarise your knowledge about each in note form. In this way your existing knowledge will be activated and any gaps will become apparent. Self-assessment also helps determine the time to be allocated to each subject for exam preparation. If you are consistently scoring excellent marks in a particular subject, it is not cost effective to spend a lot of time trying to achieve the 'perfect' mark.

In an essay it is many times easier to obtain the first mark (try writing your name) than the last. You should also try to decide on the amount of time assigned to each subject based on the likelihood of it appearing in the exam! Commonest things are usually commonest!

The main types of examination

Multiple choice questions (MCQs)

Unless very sophisticated, MCQs test your recall of information. The aim is to gain the maximum marks from the knowledge that you can remember. The stem statement must be read with great care highlighting the 'little' words such as *only, rarely, usually, never* and *always*. Overlooking negatives, such as *not, unusual* and *unsuccessful* often cause marks to be lost. *May occur* has an entirely different connotation to *characteristic*. The latter may mean a feature which should be there and the absence of which would make you question the correctness of the diagnosis.

Remember to check the marking method before starting. Most multiple choice papers employ a negative system in which marks are lost for incorrect answers. The temptation is to adopt a cautious approach answering a relatively small number of questions. However, this can lead to problems as we all make simple mistakes or even disagree vehemently with the answer in the computer! Caution may lead you to answer too few questions to obtain a pass after the marks have been deducted for incorrect answers.

Extended matching item questions (EMIs)

EMIs begin by stating the theme to which they relate. Usually 10 possible answers are then listed. A number of questions in the form of statements or clinical scenarios folows and you have to select the correct or most appropriate answer from the previous list. There should be only one correct answer for each of these questions, but unlike MCQs, it is more difficult to guess the right one.

Slide picture questions

Pattern recognition is the first step in a picture quiz. This should be coupled with a systematic approach looking for, and listing, abnormalities. For example the general appearance of the skeleton as well as the local appearance of the individual bones and any soft tissue shadows can be examined in any X-ray. Make an attempt to describe what you see even if you are in doubt. Use any additional statements or data which accompany the X-rays as they give a clue to the answer required.

Constructed response questions (CRQs)

A more sophisticated form of exam question is an evolving case history with information being presented sequentially and you being asked to give a response at each stage. CRQs are constructed so that a wrong response in the first part of the questions does not mean that no more marks can be obtained from the subsequent parts. Each part should stand on its own. Patient management problems are designed to test the recall and application of knowledge through an understanding of the principles involved.

Objective structured clinical examination questions (OSCEs)

The objective structured clinical examination (OSCE) is now extensively used to examine clinical competencies. The questions may relate to a patient, a simulated patient, a mannikin or to a clinical photograph, radiograph, pathology specimen or laboratory report. Good questions test clinical skills, practical procedures and clinical reasoning rather than factual recall.

Vivas

Examples of viva questions are given together with notes on their answers. The viva examination can be a nerve-wracking experience. You are normally faced with two examiners who may react with irritation, boredom or indifference to what you say. You may feel that the viva has gone well and yet you fail, or more commonly, you think that the exam has gone terribly because of the apparent attitude of the examiners.

Your main aim during the viva should be to control the examiners' questioning so they constantly ask you about things you know. Despite what is often said, you can prepare for this form of exam. Questions are liable to take one of a small number of forms centred around subjects that cannot be examined in a traditional clinical exam.

During the viva there are certain techniques which help in making a favourable impression. When discussing patient management, it is better to say 'I would do this' rather than 'the book says this'. You should try and strike a balance between saying too little and too much. It is important to try not to go off the topic. Aim to keep your answers short and to the point. It is worthwhile pausing for a few seconds to collect your thoughts before launching into an answer. Do not be afraid to say 'I don't know'; most examiners will want to change tack to see what you do know about.

Conclusions

You should amend your framework for using this book according to your own needs and the examinations you are facing. Whatever approach you adopt, your aim should be for an understanding of the principles involved rather than rote learning of a large number of poorly connected facts.

SECTION 1
Orthopaedics

1 Musculoskeletal trauma

Chapter overview

This chapter highlights the importance of a reliable, uniform approach to assessing the management of the multiply injured patient. The Advanced Trauma Life Support (ATLS) approach, emphasising airway and cervical spine control, breathing, circulation, dysfunction (neurological disorder), and exposure and environmental control, is recommended.

The general principles of management of fractures, compartment syndrome and spinal injury are described.

A systematic approach to describing fracture patterns and malalignment is given and the general advantages and disadvantages of various ways of treating fractures are discussed.

1.1 Clinical examination

Learning objectives

You should:

- be familiar with the ATLS system's approach to the management of major trauma
- be able to describe a systematic approach to the management of open fractures
- recognise the clinical features which suggest that compartment syndrome may be developing.

To prevent the arrival of a patient with multiple injuries being accompanied by much ill-coordinated activity, a uniform approach such as that advocated by the Advanced Trauma Life Support (ATLS) System is recommended. This routine method of efficiently managing such patients facilitates the delivery of life-saving measures and should become second nature to the medical and nursing staff who may be called upon to attend patients with musculoskeletal trauma.

After initial assessment of injuries and appropriate resuscitation, the importance of a 'second-look' examination should be emphasised because it is at this stage that additional incidental injuries will be discovered.

During every patient interaction, the clinical skills of 'listen', 'look', 'feel' and 'move' should be followed.

Emergency treatment

The first few hours after injury is the time in which life can be saved if emergency measures are effectively applied. This emergency treatment of the multiply injured patient is best achieved if the members of the resuscitation team follow the ATLS principles:

- **a**irway and cervical spine control
- **b**reathing
- **c**irculation.

Followed by:

- dysfunction (neurological disorder)
- exposure/environmental control.

Airway and cervical spine control

The airway should be cleared of any obstructions such as dentures or vomit and in the comatose patient the tongue should be prevented from blocking the pharynx by holding the jaw forwards. An oropharyngeal or nasopharyngeal tube is often necessary but endotracheal intubation, cricothyroidotomy (Fig. 1) or a tracheostomy may be required if the upper airway is obstructed. The cervical spine must be manually steadied until it can be immobilised with a rigid cervical collar or sandbags to either side of the head and a stout piece of sticky tape across the forehead.

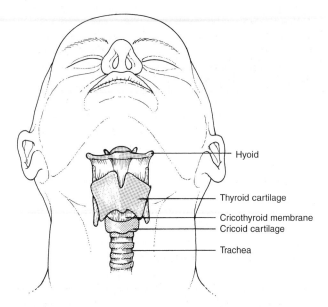

Fig. 1 A cricothyroidotomy can be made through the cricothyroid membrane between the cricoid and thyroid cartilages.

Breathing

Observe chest expansion, spontaneous ventilation and any abnormal movements of the chest wall, such as paradoxical movement, flail segment or a penetrating wound. Percuss and auscultate the chest to detect pneumothorax or haemothorax and to assess air entry. Palpate the trachea for deviation away from the affected side in tension pneumothorax.

Circulation

Bleeding should be controlled by pressure dressings and elevation. Improvised tourniquets are too dangerous. A fast-flowing intravenous infusion should be instituted in a large peripheral vein; if necessary, a cut-down on a peripheral vein is required. A volume challenge with an intravenous crystalloid is the initial treatment of hypotension. Later cross-matched blood may be required. Passing a urinary catheter allows accurate monitoring of fluid balance and relieves the agitation caused by bladder distension.

Disorder (neurological disorder)

A rapid but thorough examination for evidence of head injury is carried out. The Glasgow Coma Scale is commonly used. This records the patient's motor, verbal and eye movement responses to stimulation. Evidence of spinal cord or peripheral nerve injury can be sought at this stage.

Exposure/environmental control

The entire patient must be exposed for thorough examination to exclude the presence of any additional injuries.

The extent and depth of burns can be charted at this stage. Do not forget to examine the perineum and the back. Once this is done, steps must be taken to keep the patient warm. Recording of vital signs should be commenced.

Radiographic examination

Radiographs of chest, pelvis and lateral cervical spine are always required. Radiographs of other regions can be delayed until resuscitation is completed.

Open fractures

Open fractures require urgent treatment if bacterial invasion of the wound is to be avoided. Open fractures are classified according to their degree of contamination and soft tissue damage.

Management

Management can be divided into several steps:

- initial management in A & E dept
  — photograph, broad-spectrum intravenous antibiotics, iodine dressing
- wound excision
  — irrigation: high-pressure irrigation of the wound with saline is the initial step
  — debridement: all devitalised tissue, especially muscle, is excised and dirt washed from the wound
- reduction
  — the bony fragments are aligned into normal position
- stabilisation
  — stabilisation of a fracture may be achieved by external or internal techniques. Once the wound has been cleaned surgically and the fracture reduced, an appropriate method of fixation must be selected. If a radical debridement has been carried out, many orthopaedic surgeons would select rigid internal fixation of the fracture and primary skin cover using a local or a free flap as necessary. An external fixator (Fig. 2) is useful if

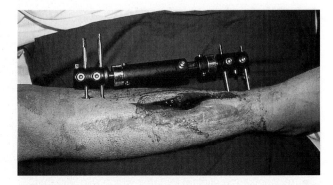

Fig. 2 External fixator used to stabilise an open tibial fracture without hindering access to the wound.

the wound is to be left open or a 'second look' operation to excise more dead tissue is anticipated in 24 hours' time.

Complications

Complications can be divided into categories (see p. 16). Those particularly associated with open fractures include:

- wound infection
- chronic osteitis
- non-union.

Compartment syndrome

Bleeding from a comminuted closed fracture of a long bone may increase the pressure in the adjacent fascial compartments. In the leg, there are four compartments (Fig. 3) and in the forearm two compartments. Bleeding from the bone and swelling of damaged muscle within these compartments increase pressure on the artery and nerve passing through them and result in progressive muscle and nerve ischaemia.

Clinical features

- **Listen** — pain more severe than would be expected from the injury alone
- **Look** — tense swollen limb
- **Feel** — altered sensation and diminished distal pulses will eventually be present
- **Move** — resistance to passive stretching of the muscle bellies in the involved compartment.

Diagnosis

A pressure transducer can be introduced to monitor pressure within the compartment but clinical features remain the most important in making the diagnosis.

Management

If the removal of circumferential dressings is ineffective, an urgent fasciotomy is required to relieve the raised compartment pressure. In the lower leg, this can be achieved by a partial fibulectomy. In the forearm, the flexor and extensor compartments must be decompressed separately. The skin wound can be left open to be closed or covered with a split thickness skin graft a few days later when the swelling has subsided.

Complications

- Volkmann's ischaemic contracture
- persisting nerve damage.

Second-look examination

After initial emergency assessment, it is important to carry out a second-look examination to identify any additional injuries.

1.2 Fracture types

Learning objectives

You should:

- understand the importance of the history in determining the type and extent of the fracture and the soft tissue injury sustained and know how this may relate to the management and the outcome

- be able to describe a fracture in terms of its pattern and type of malalignment.

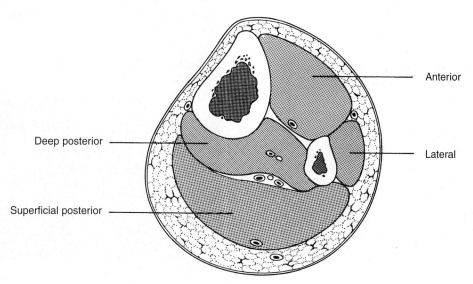

Fig. 3 Fascial compartments in the leg.

Anterior

Lateral

Deep posterior

Superficial posterior

The most important observation to make about a fracture is whether it is open or closed. In closed fractures, the skin is intact, but in open fractures there are varying degrees of severity of skin damage and contamination (see above). It is easy to think of the bone injury in isolation, especially when looking at a radiograph, but it must be remembered that the soft tissues will also have been damaged by the injuring force. An accurate history will tell something about the mechanism of the injury and about the amount of energy absorbed by the bone and soft tissues from the injuring force. The radiograph will show the pattern of the resulting fracture. Both the history and the radiograph will help in making a decision on the probable stability of the fracture and the extent of damage to be expected in the surrounding soft tissues.

Mechanism of injury

Direct violence

When direct violence is applied to a bone, the overlying skin and soft tissues are likely to be broken and damaged. A small force to a localised area, such as from a blow with a stick to the forearm, will bruise or break the overlying skin and cause a transverse fracture usually of the ulna (Fig. 4).

A large force to a large area, such as from being hit by a car bumper, will produce a comminuted fracture with extensive soft tissue damage, crushing and devitalisation. A large force to a small area from a missile injury will produce severe damage to bone and soft tissues in a localised area.

Indirect violence

The injuring force is applied to the limb at a distance from where the fracture occurs. Examples are a twisting injury to the tibia (Fig. 5), often caused when the foot is jammed (for instance in a football tackle) while the body twists and falls to the side. The fracture is less likely to be open than one caused by direct violence, but the soft tissue envelope is more likely to be extensively stripped from the bone.

When angulatory forces are directed to the limb, a transverse fracture results, which may have intact periosteum on the compression side but a tear in the periosteal sleeve on the distraction side.

Other mechanisms of injury include stress fractures from repetitive forces being applied to the bone, as seen in the 'march fracture' of the second metatarsal.

Fracture patterns

Transverse fractures. These arise when angulatory forces are applied to the limb, for instance by levering it over a fulcrum (e.g. the leg caught between the rungs during a fall from a stepladder) or a fall on the outstretched hand. Direct blows to an isolated area of the bone can also cause a transverse fracture.

Spiral fractures. Twisting forces create spiral fractures (e.g. the foot blocked in a football tackle while the player falls to the side).

Comminuted fractures. These are high-energy fractures and are inherently unstable (e.g. the leg hit by a car bumper).

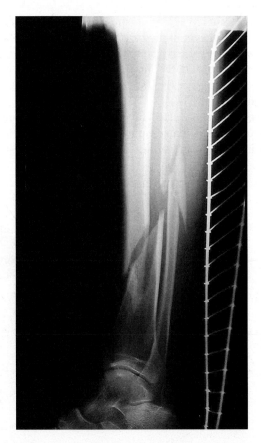

Fig. 5 Spiral fracture of the tibia and fibula.

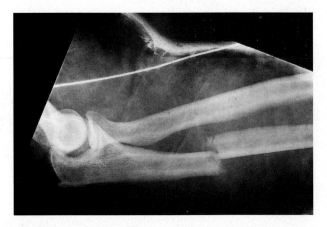

Fig. 4 Transverse fracture of the middle third of the ulna following a direct blow on the forearm.

Crush fractures. These occur as a result of longitudinal (axial) forces and are seen in areas of cancellous bone, such as the tibial condyles and vertebrae (e.g. a patient who falls from a height and lands on the feet may fracture the calcaneum and vertebrae) (Fig. 6).

Oblique fractures. These are caused by a combination of twisting, angulation and compression forces.

Greenstick fractures. These transverse fractures occur in children as a result of angulatory forces (Fig. 7). One cortex is broken but the cortex on the compression side is bent.

Malalignment

A fracture may be:

- displaced
- angulated
- shortened
- rotated.

Displacement. In a displaced fracture, the distal fragment is displaced in a sagittal or coronal plane relative to the proximal fragment but without any angulation (Fig. 8). The overall alignment of the limb is satisfactory. If the fracture is stable then healing will proceed without residual deformity as the fracture remodels.

Angulation. The distal fragment may be angulated forwards or backwards, laterally or medially (Fig. 9). Only a few degrees of lateral or medial (valgus or varus) angulation are acceptable. No remodelling will take place in this plane but it will if the angulation is in an antero-posterior plane.

Shortening. In a completely displaced fracture, the bone fragments will override each other and the limb will shorten (Fig. 10). Shortening also occurs in comminuted fractures where there is impaction of the articular surface into the metaphysis.

Rotation. The distal fragment of a fracture may be rotated on the proximal fragment. A radiograph showing the full length of the injured limb will make it easier to recognise this deformity (Fig. 11).

1.3 Methods of treatment

Learning objectives

You should:

- be able to describe methods of non-operative treatment of fractures and list their advantages and disadvantages

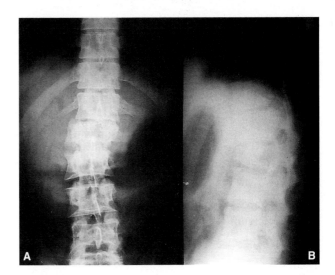

Fig. 6 A. Crush fracture of the body of the first lumbar vertebra. **B.** View of the same injury showing the displacement associated with the crush fracture.

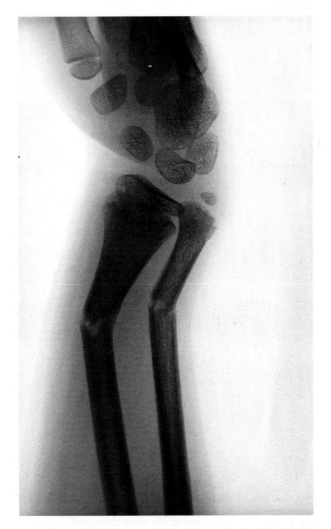

Fig. 7 Greenstick fractures of the radius and ulna in a child.

- be able to describe methods of internal fixation of fractures and list their advantages and disadvantages
- be able to describe the advantages and disadvantages of external fixation
- begin to be able to balance these approaches to the management of any particular fracture in a particular patient.

Fracture stabilisation may be achieved by external or internal techniques:

External

- traction
- splint (plaster cast)
- functional brace
- external fixator.

Internal

- intermedullary rod
- plates
- screws
- wires.

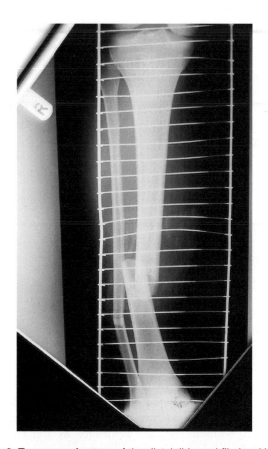

Fig. 9 Transverse fracture of the distal tibia and fibula with marked varus angulation at the fracture site.

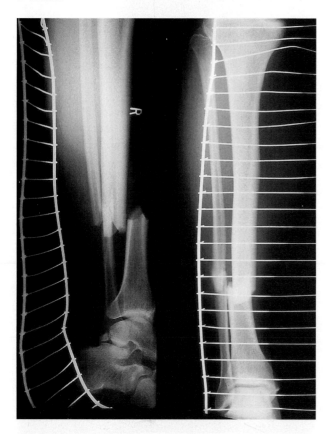

Fig. 8 Transverse fractures of the distal tibia and fibula with 100% displacement but with no angulatory deformity.

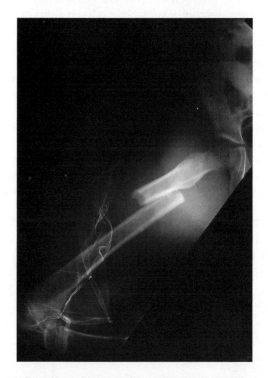

Fig. 10 Transverse fracture of the upper third of the femur in a child with considerable shortening at the fracture site due to overriding of the bone ends.

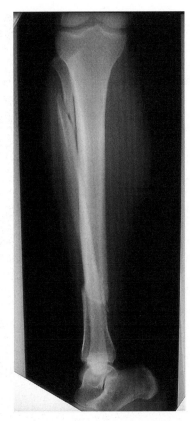

Fig. 11 Rotary deformity of a fracture of the distal tibia and proximal fibula. The radiograph shows an antero-posterior view of the knee with a lateral view of the ankle!

Traction

Traction is used to overcome muscle spasm and so allow the bone fragments to realign in the soft tissue envelope.

Skin traction to a maximum of 5 kg can be applied to the leg by fastening the weights to adhesive strapping around the limb. This is used only as a temporary measure in adults but is used for definitive treatment of femoral fractures in young children.

In skeletal traction, weights are applied to the limb via a pin passed through the tibial tuberosity for traction on the femur or through the os calcis for traction on the tibia. The limb can be nursed in a Thomas splint and the traction cords tied to its end. This is fixed traction. Alternatively, the patient can lie free in bed with the fracture supported in a cradle while traction applied distally is provided by weights which hang to the floor round a pulley at the foot of the bed. This is balanced traction (Fig. 12).

Advantages

- simple to erect
- safe to use.

Disadvantages

- prolonged immobilisation with associated problems of pressure sores, osteoporosis, muscle wasting and joint stiffness
- distraction of the fracture.

Plaster casts

Plaster of Paris immobilisation is the most common type of splintage to hold a fracture after it has been manipulated into a satisfactory position. Three-point fixation is required to prevent subsequent loss of the position achieved.

Advantages

- easy to use
- cheap
- readily available.

Disadvantages

- rigid fixation is not possible so the bone fragments can slip
- pressure sores beneath the plaster
- stiff joints
- peripheral swelling.

Functional brace

A close-fitting plaster cuff that maintains the girth of the limb will prevent shortening at the fracture site (Fig. 13). By preventing the limb from widening, the length of the limb and hence the position of the fracture are maintained. For some fractures, hinges can be placed at the elbow or knee joints to allow motion at the joint while the fracture heals.

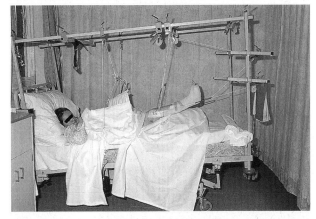

Fig. 12 Balanced traction. The femoral fracture is nursed in the canvas cradle while traction is applied distally via the tibial tuberosity.

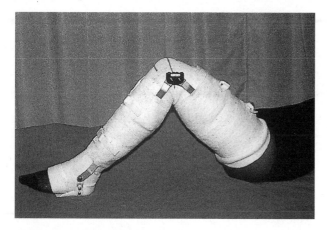

Fig. 13 Femoral fracture controlled by a functional brace. The hinges at the knee and ankle allow early rehabilitation of the joints.

Advantages

- allows joint movement
- prevents muscle stiffness and wasting.

Disadvantages

- accurate fitting is required.

External fixation

Threaded pins are drilled into the bone on either side of the fracture and fixed via universal joints to a rigid bar near the skin surface. In the Ilqizarov method, multiple 'spokes' transfix the proximal and distal fragments between circular or semicircular frames.

Advantages

- quick and easy to apply
- allows access to wounds and observation of the skin surface
- allows subsequent manipulation and repositioning of the fragments.

Disadvantages

- pin track infection
- increased risk of infection if intramedullary fixation is subsequently used
- delayed union if the fixation is too rigid.

Internal fixation

Internal fixation can be achieved by various mechanisms:

- screws
- plates
- intramedullary rods
- wire.

Screws. Lag screws are used to secure fragments of bone together, such as avulsion fractures of the medial malleolus.

Plates. A dynamic compression plate (DCP) is used to secure long-bone fractures, such as forearm fractures. The direct compression design produces compression at the fracture site. This prevents callus formation but holds the bone ends close enough together to achieve direct bone healing (Fig. 14).

Intramedullary nail. These are used for tibial and femoral fractures. The cortex is reamed under radiographic control. The nail is locked into the bone by transverse bolts above and below the fracture, which controls the rotation and length of the bone.

Wire. Tension band wire may be used to secure avulsion fractures of the patella and olecranon.

Advantages

- anatomical reduction
- early active mobilisation.

Disadvantages

- infection
- wound breakdown
- non-union
- delayed union
- considerable expertise is required for successful use of these techniques
- the fixation device produces a stress riser, which may lead to subsequent fractures
- osteoporosis
- cutting out.

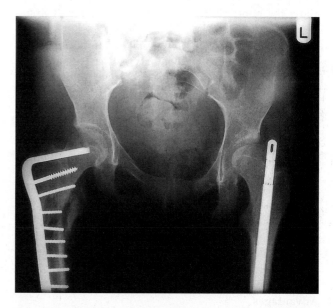

Fig. 14 Complex bilateral fractures of the femoral treated by an angled blade plate on the right and by an intramedullary rod on the left.

Internal fixation gives the best chance of early re-habilitation and return to normal life and is especially useful for problem patients and problem fractures. Problem patients include those with:

- multiple injuries
- prolonged unconsciousness.

Problem fractures include:

- intra-articular fractures
- unstable fractures
- pathological fractures.

1.4 Long bone fractures

Learning objectives

You should:

- be able to recognise the clinical appearances of a long bone fracture
- list two complications which may be associated with this injury and its treatment.

Clinical features

The characteristic features of a fracture of any long bone are:

- **Listen** — a history of trauma
  — pain
  — bruising
- **Look** — deformity
  — swelling
- **Feel** — diminished pulses and altered sensation may be present
- **Move** — loss of function
  — crepitus.

In addition there may be local bruising and examination of the periphery may show diminished pulses and areas of altered sensation.

The most important fact to establish is whether the fracture is open or closed. The presence of a skin wound which communicates with the fracture means that the fracture is open and the risk of infection is increased. Gustillo's classification of open fractures describes:

- Type I: the skin is merely punctured but the wound is clean and the skin and soft tissues are not crushed.
- Type II : the wound is larger, contaminated and there is more soft tissue damage.

- Type III: extensive periosteal stripping, muscle crushing and contamination. Type III open fractures have been further classified into three subcategories depending on the degree of soft tissue damage, contamination and vascular injury.

Diagnosis

Diagnosis is usually made clinically but radiological examination is required to confirm the configuration of the fracture and plan future treatment.

Management

Non-operative management

- plaster cast
- traction
- functional brace.

Operative management

- internal fixation
- external fixation, see page 14.

Complications

Complications can be considered as the following categories:

- early
- late
- local
- systemic — adult respiratory distress syndrome, fat embolus, pulmonary embolus
- bony — chronic osteitis, non-union, delayed union, malunion
- soft tissue — wound breakdown and infection, heterotopic calcification, compartment syndrome.

1.5 Spinal injuries

Learning objectives

You should:

- know when to suspect that a spinal injury may be present and how to supply emergency spinal stabilisation

- know how to examine the patient to determine the level of spinal injury
- know the principles of long-term management and the late complications of spinal injury.

Spinal injuries usually occur in falls from a height or in road traffic accidents. They must always be suspected if a patient has suffered multiple, high-energy injuries and especially if there has been a blow to the head.

Cervical spine

The bony injury to the cervical spine may be complicated by damage to the cervical cord.

Clinical features

- **Listen** — there may be a history of a fall from a height or other type of deceleration injury
- **Look** — abdominal respiration without thoracic expansion
- **Feel** — numbness to touch sensation in all dermatomes below the level of the injury
- **Move** — the patient is unable to move the arms or legs voluntarily.

Diagnosis

X-ray of the cervical spine shows the level of the injury, which may be a subluxation, a dislocation or a fracture (Fig. 15). The extent of the bony injury can be further defined by CT scan and the soft tissue injury by MRI or CT myelography.

Management

Patients with cervical cord injury
Emergency treatment involves urethral catheterisation, intravenous infusion to maintain circulating volume and skull traction to attempt reduction of the dislocated cervical spine. After several days, the permanent level of quadriplegia becomes apparent. Expert nursing care is required to avoid bed sores, chest infection, urinary tract infection, constipation and demoralisation.

Reconstructive surgery can sometimes restore some function to the hand and elbow by tendon transfers from functioning muscles.

Complications

- renal calculi
- urinary tract infection
- pressure sores
- impotence.

Thoraco-lumbar spine

High-velocity injuries can cause fractures of the thoracic or lumbar spine without neurological damage, but in cases of fracture dislocation, the spinal cord is often damaged, resulting in paraplegia.

Clinical features

- **Listen** — history of a fall or road traffic accident
- **Look** — there is swelling and bruising over the spine at the site of the injury
- **Feel** — local tenderness
- **Move** — loss of voluntary movement below the spinal level of the injury

Bladder function is impaired causing urinary retention.

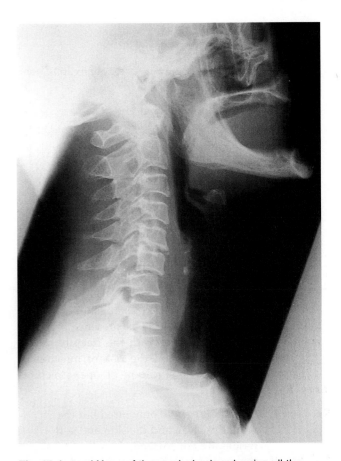

Fig. 15 Lateral X-ray of the cervical spine showing all the cervical vertebrae. There is a subluxation of C6 on C7.

Diagnosis

Radiological examination confirms the level of the spinal injury and shows the configuration of the fracture. As before, computerised tomography (CT), and MRI will show the extent of cord and nerve root compression by the bony fragments.

Management

Particular care is required to prevent further damage to the cord and to avoid bed sores. Urethral catheterisation is required. The permanent level of the neurological deficit becomes apparent over a short period of time.

Surgical stabilisation of the bony injury may be appropriate for local pain relief, but it does not reverse the neurological damage.

Patients will require a wheelchair for mobility, but with enthusiastic support a great deal of independence can be enjoyed.

Complications

- renal calculi
- urinary tract infection
- pressure sores
- impotence.

Self-assessment: questions

Multiple choice questions

1. Functional cast-bracing of a femoral shaft fracture:
   a. Should not be applied before 10 weeks after the injury
   b. Allows early knee flexion
   c. Allows weight bearing
   d. Should be ischial-bearing
   e. Has the recognised complication of inducing quadriceps wasting

2. In the conservative treatment of fractures:
   a. Joint stiffness is associated with plaster cast immobilisation only when this has been applied too tightly
   b. In a patient with a forearm fracture treated in plaster, pain on passive extension of the fingers is caused by impingement of flexor muscles at the fracture site
   c. Malalignment of 5° in a tibial fracture in any plane is acceptable
   d. Functional bracing is a recognised treatment of tibial shaft fractures after the first 3 to 4 weeks
   e. A recognised method of treatment of complex intra-articular fractures is traction and active mobilisation of the affected joint

Extended matching items questions (EMIs)

1. Theme: Complications of fractures

A non-union
B heterotopic calcification
C muscle impingement on the fracture fragments
D delayed union
E reflex sympathetic dystrophy
F compartment syndrome
G overriding of the bone ends at the fracture site
H angulation at the fracture site of >15°
I rotary malalignment
J infected non-union

Select the complication from the list above which most accurately matches the condition described below:

1. A child with a forearm fracture treated in plaster complains of pain when the fingers are passively extended.

2. An undisplaced spiral tibial fracture in an adult treated conservatively by functional bracing is still painful for weight-bearing at 12 weeks.

3. Three months after treatment of a fracture of both bones of the forearm in plaster, a 12-year-old complains of lack of full pronation despite having had extensive physiotherapy.

2. Theme: Treatment of fractures

A functional bracing
B balanced traction
C intermedullary fixation
D plate and screw fixation
E tension band wire
F fixed skin traction
G plaster of Paris cast
H external fixator
I overhead traction
J interfragmentary screws

From the list above identify the most suitable method for treating the fractures described below:

1. A fracture of both bones of the forearm in an adult.

2. A displaced fracture of the olecanon.

3. A femoral shaft fracture in a 3 year old.

Constructed response questions (CRQs)

CRQ 1

> A 20-year-old man has been thrown from his motor-cycle in a collision with your car. He is lying on his back motionless at the roadside.

a. What is the first thing that you should do?
b. What is the next important thing to do for the victim?
c. The patient is conscious but has bleeding wounds over both shins; the legs below this level are obviously out of alignment. What should you assess next?
d. Subsequent examination in hospital reveals open, comminuted fractures of the upper third of both tibia and fibula. What would be a suitable method of managing these injuries for this patient?

CRQ 2

The ward nurse calls you to a patient complaining of pain beneath his plaster. He has had a closed fracture of the tibia manipulated and an above-knee cast applied earlier in the day. When you observe the patient, he has swollen, purplish toes and does not like to move them.

a. What do you think is the cause of the patient's symptoms?
b. What clinical manoeuvre could you carry out to reinforce this diagnosis?
c. What simple measure would you take next?
d. Despite this measure the patient's symptoms are unaltered. Describe the pathological process which is taking place.
e. If you do nothing now what will develop?
f. What should your next line of management be?

Objective structured clinical examination questions (OSCEs)

OSCE 1

a. Study the picture of an X-ray of a femoral shaft fracture (Fig. 16). How would you describe the fracture pattern and malalignment?

b. What can you usually not tell from the X-ray?
c. The fracture is to be treated in a functional brace. What are the advantages of this?
d. How long do you think it would take the fracture to heal?

OSCE 2

Study the photograph of an X-ray of the cervical spine from a patient in a high velocity accident (Fig. 17).

a. At which cervical vertebrae level has there been an injury?
b. What symptoms would you expect the patient to be complaining of:
   i. in the neck?
   ii. in the arms?
c. You are uncertain whether the spinal column is stable. How could this be visualised more accurately?
d. What conservative management could be used? What other definitive treatment can you suggest?

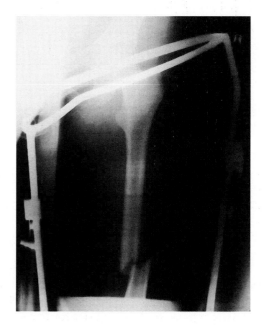

Fig. 16

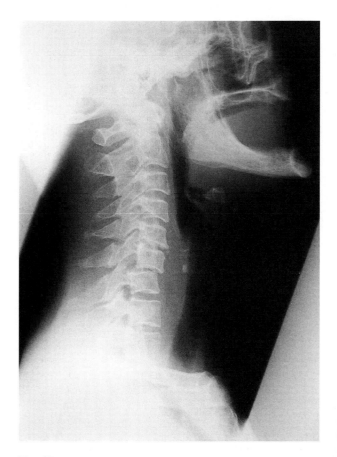

Fig. 17

Viva questions

1. List the advantages and disadvantages of internal fixation of fractures and illustrate your answer by reference to a bimalleolar fracture of the ankle.

2. How would you manage a grade two open fracture of the tibia?

Self-assessment: answers

Multiple choice answers

1. a. **False.** A favourable femoral shaft fracture which has been treated conservatively in traction for 4 to 6 weeks should then be suitable for application of a functional brace.
   b. **True.**
   c. **True.**
   d. **True.** This design allows load sharing between the orthosis and the fractured femur.
   e. **False.** Muscles are able to exercise in the functional brace so that wasting is avoided.

2. a. **False.** Joint stiffness is associated with immobility, not ischaemia from a tightly applied cast.
   b. **False.** The presence of pain on passive extension of the fingers suggests ischemia of the flexor muscle bellies and an impending compartment syndrome.
   c. **True.** This minor degree of malalignment is acceptable. More angulation is acceptable in the antero-posterior plane as remodelling can be expected, but greater degrees of varus or valgus malalignment will not remodel.
   d. **True.** The above-knee plaster can be changed to a patella tendon-bearing cast, which is a type of functional brace, at 3 to 4 weeks after the injury.
   e. **True.** In cases where there are local or general contraindications to operation, then traction and active mobilisation will help realign complex intra-articular fractures and allow remoulding of the articular surfaces.

EMI answers

1. Theme: Complications of fractures

1. f. Pain on passive extension of the digits is a classical finding of compartment syndrome.
2. d. You would expect the fracture to be united by 12 weeks. The fact that it is still painful suggests delayed union (See Perkins' classification of fracture healing times).
3. i. Rotary malalignment is a risk of a displaced forearm fracture. Non-anatomical reduction limits supination and pronation.

2. Theme: Treatment of fractures

1. d. Anatomical reduction with DCP plate fixation or LCDC plate (low contact direct compression plate) is the treatment of choice for a fracture in an adult.

2. e. A displaced fracture of the olecranon requires to be held in place. Tension band wire is a recommended way of doing this.
3. f. Fixed traction using elastoplast attached to the skin provides satisfactory control of this fracture.

CRQ answers

CRQ 1

a. Take measures to ensure the safety of yourself and the victim both from other vehicles and from petrol fire at the site of the accident.
b. Check airway and cervical spine control.
c. Peripheral pulses distal to the site of injury.
d. Wound excision and debridement
   External fixation.

CRQ 2

a. Compartment syndrome.
b. Pain on passive dorsi-flexion of the toes.
c. Split the plaster down to the skin.
d. Swelling or bleeding within a fascial compartment causing flexor muscle compression and nerve ischaemia.
e. Continuing pain with progression to loss of peripheral sensation and circulation.
f. Surgical decompression of the fascial compartments in the leg.

OSCE answers

OSCE 1

a. This is a transfer fracture. There is a 50% displacement but no angulation or shortening.
b. Whether the fracture is open or closed.
c. It allows knee flexion and weight bearing while controlling the position of the fracture by the plaster cuff.
d. 12–18 weeks.

OSCE 2

a. Forward subluxation of C6 on C7.
b. The patient may complain of localised mechanical neck pain due to soft tissue and joint injury in this area. In the arms, the patient may have pain, tingling or numbness in the C7 dermatome on the ulnar side of the hand and forearm.

c. CT scan or MRI scan.

d. The patient's neck can be stabilised in a rigid cervical collar with metal supports between the occiput support and breast plate. Surgical treatment would be formal reduction of the dislocated vertebrae with posterior stabilisation using plates or white loops.

Viva answers

1. The advantages of internal fixation are anatomical reduction and the ability to carry out early active mobilisation of the joint. The disadvantages include infection, wound breakdown, delayed union and implant failure. In a bimalleolar fracture of the ankle, the use of a neutralisation plate on the lateral malleolus and a lagged malleolur screw on the medial malleolus will restore the configuration of the ankle mortis and allow early active mobilisation of the joint, which will aid healing of the articular cartilage.

2. An open fracture of the tibia should be managed by wound irrigation, debridement and prophylactic antibiotics. Irrigation with copious volumes of saline is necessary. The wound edges should be excised and the wound cleaned. Any devitalised tissue should be excised. A prophylactic course of appropriate antibiotics should be instituted. In a more severe fracture, a second-look operation should be planned 24 hours later.

2 Fractures in the elderly

Chapter overview

Osteoporosis in the ageing skeleton is a frequent cause of fractures especially in postmenopausal females. Several common fractures are discussed:– Colles' fracture, fractured neck of humerus, femoral neck fractures and vertebral body fractures. Pathological fractures through secondary deposits anywhere in the skeleton should also be remembered, however, especially if the fracture has occurred with minimal trauma. A search for the primary cause is then important.

Finally, treatment in this age group must be focused on the most appropriate means of regaining function, mobility and independence.

2.1 Clinical examination

Learning objectives

You should:

- practice how best to communicate with an elderly patient who may be deaf, demented or otherwise debilitated

- remember the sequence for examination of 'look', 'feel' and 'move'

- remember that a patient with one osteoporosis-related fracture may soon develop another fracture elsewhere

- remember that pathological fractures from malignancy are most common in older age groups.

The full clinical examination of an elderly patient is often difficult. History taking may be complicated by deafness, dementia or debility, so the physical examination must be sufficiently extensive to identify the presence of other medical or surgical conditions.

The physical examination of the injured part involves the usual sequence of 'look, feel and move', but in the presence of a suspected pathological fracture, general physical examination must include the neck, breasts, chest, abdomen and rectum.

Osteoporosis

Osteoporosis in the ageing skeleton is a primary cause of the increased frequency of fractures in the elderly.

Osteoporosis is not necessarily a result of increasing age, but it is associated with a decreased level of mobility, which may be associated with older age groups. Lack of stress on the bones and dietary deficiency contribute to osteoporosis but the most important cause in elderly females is postmenopausal hormone change. Unsteadiness on the feet for whatever reason and syncopal attacks lead to an increased likelihood of the patient suffering a fracture from a simple fall at home.

2.2 Distal radius fractures

Learning objectives

You should:

- be able to recognise a Colles' fracture clinically

- remember the importance of a true lateral radiograph in assessing the direction and degree of angulation

● know that high velocity fractures in younger people will be unlikely to behave as satisfactorily with plaster immobilisation alone as low velocity fractures of the same area in older people.

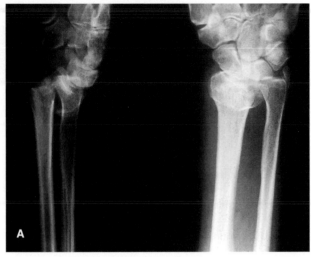

The Colles' fracture is the classical injury seen in the postmenopausal female, usually in the seventh decade of life. The fracture may be comminuted and may extend into the radio-carpal joint, the inferior radio-ulnar joint or both.

Clinical features

● **Listen** — there is usually a history of a fall on the outstretched hand
● **Look** — the distal fragment of the radius and the attached carpal bones are usually displaced posteriorly to create the characteristic 'dinner fork' deformity of the wrist (Fig. 18). There is often swelling and bruising. Radial deviation and supination of the distal fragment may also be present.
● **Feel** — tenderness
    — the median nerve may be compressed, producing altered sensation in the radial three and a half digits
● **Move** — the patient is reluctant to move the wrist
    — crepitus may be apparent.

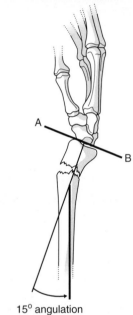

B 15° angulation

Fig. 19 A. Lateral and antero-posterior radiograph of a Colles' fracture, showing the posterior displacement of the distal radial fragment and shortening of the radius. **B**. Method of measuring the degree of angulation present at the fracture site.

Diagnosis

An antero-posterior and a true lateral radiograph of the wrist are required to confirm the diagnosis (Fig. 19A). There is often impaction at the fracture site as the distal fragment is displaced proximally. This produces shortening of the radius, and the ulna now appears relatively long.

Management

The casualty officer dealing with this injury needs to decide whether the fracture requires to be reduced. To do this the amount of displacement at the fracture site must be assessed to see if it is acceptable and can be simply splinted, or whether an anatomical position should be sought by means of manipulation under anaesthesia.

If the fracture is not manipulated or 'reduced', the fracture will still unite but in an abnormal position. Moderate degrees of displacement may be acceptable, but more severe malunion will cause limitation of wrist

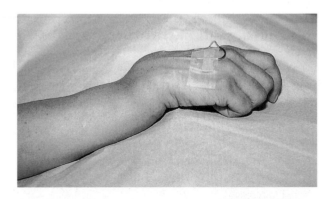

Fig. 18 Classical dinner fork deformity of a Colles' fracture.

function, especially flexion and supination. Figure 19B shows the method of measuring the degree of angulation present at the fracture site between the two fragments. The line AB has been drawn across the articular surface of the radius on the lateral radiograph. A perpendicular line to this transects the line drawn along the long axis of the proximal fragment of the radius; usually 15° of angulation is acceptable. Angulation greater than this is usually corrected by manipulation.

Manipulation of the fracture requires reversal of the direction of the deforming force that produced the original injury. After manipulating a fracture into an acceptable position, there are several ways available to hold it until the fracture has united.

Usually a Colles' fracture can be held in place with a plaster of Paris cast. This holds the wrist in the reduced position of flexion, ulnar deviation and pronation. This position is exactly the opposite from the displaced position of the Colles' fracture.

A minor degree of malunion is acceptable as the functional result may be unimpaired. In some cases, the fracture may be very unstable when manipulated and consequently difficult to hold in correct position in relation to the ulna by plaster of Paris alone. In such cases percutaneous pins or an external fixator may be used to splint the fracture until union is achieved. The external fixator can be applied to the second metacarpal and the proximal radius (Fig. 20).

Very rarely, open reduction and internal fixation of a Colles' fracture is required. A buttress plate on the radius and a bone graft may be necessary to hold this position.

After 4–6 weeks' immobilisation, the wrist will become stiff and a period of physiotherapy is often required to regain a full range of mobilisation. The patient is required to attempt active dorsiflexion, palmar flexion and supination/pronation exercises and also to exercise the elbow and shoulder.

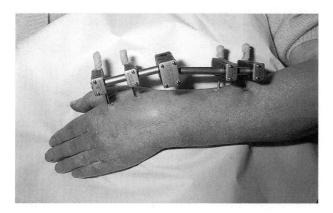

Fig. 20 Comminuted fracture of the distal radius in a younger patient stabilised by an external fixator which holds the radius at its correct length and position.

Complications

Complications can be divided into those occurring early and late:

- early complications
  — median nerve compression
- late complications
  — malunion
  — elbow and wrist stiffness
  — frozen shoulder
  — spontaneous rupture of extensor pollicis longus
  — reflex sympathetic dystrophy (Sudek's atrophy).

2.3 Upper humerus fractures

Learning objectives

You should:

- be able to distinguish extracapsular fractures of the surgical neck from intracapsular fractures involving the tuberosities and/or anatomical neck of the humerus

- be able to recognise the complications of axillary nerve or brachial artery damage

- be aware of the importance of early mobilisation in rehabilitating soft tissues and preventing shoulder stiffness.

A history of a fall on the outstretched hand in a woman in her 70s is a common presentation of a fracture of the upper humerus.

Classification

- intracapsular fractures occur at the anatomical neck with avulsion of one or both tuberosities
- extracapsular fractures occur at the surgical neck, the narrowest portion of the proximal humerus.

The blood supply to the humeral head may be disrupted in intracapsular fractures because of its separation from the greater and lesser tuberosities (and their soft tissue attachments) and because of the fracture in the shaft below it. The head is liable to undergo avascular necrosis in the same way as that seen in subcapital fractures of the head of the femur (see p. 27).

Clinical features

There is bruising and swelling over the shoulder with loss of abduction because of pain. Axillary nerve damage may be present and must be searched for by eliciting an area of decreased sensation in the 'badge patch' area at the point of the shoulder.

Diagnosis

An antero-posterior and lateral or axial radiograph of the shoulder are required. The bone fragments may be impacted into each other or widely displaced. The greater and lesser tuberosities may form separate fragments and the humeral head may appear to have 'capsized' in the joint (Fig. 21A). Coexisting dislocation of the shoulder joint occurs rarely.

Management

Intracapsular fractures with marked displacement of the fragments may lead to avascular necrosis of the head. In these cases, a hemiarthroplasty is used (Fig. 21B). The stem of the prosthesis is fitted down the shaft of the humerus and the rotator cuff and greater and lesser tuberosities secured around its head. Early mobilisation of the shoulder is important to prevent the joint becoming stiff.

Impacted fractures of the surgical neck of the humerus are usually rested for a few days in a collar and cuff sling and pendulum exercises begun early in order to avoid shoulder stiffness.

Complications

Complications can involve:

● Early — axillary nerve palsy
● Late   — frozen shoulder
             — malrotation.

2.4 Femoral neck fractures

Learning objectives

You should:

● be able to recognise the classical clinical appearances of external rotation and shortening

● be able to distinguish an extracapsular fracture from an intracapsular fracture on radiological examination

● anticipate when avasacular necrosis of the femoral head may be expected to occur

● appreciate the importance to the patient of early postoperative mobilisation and rehabilitation.

A fracture of the femoral neck is the most common fracture seen in the elderly female and usually occurs in the eighth and ninth decade of life. The cause is usually a simple fall at home but it may be associated with another medical problem, such as a stroke, hypotensive crisis or poor vision. Whatever the cause, the result may be the ultimate loss of independence, especially for someone who was previously just managing to live alone safely.

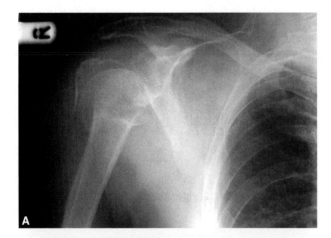

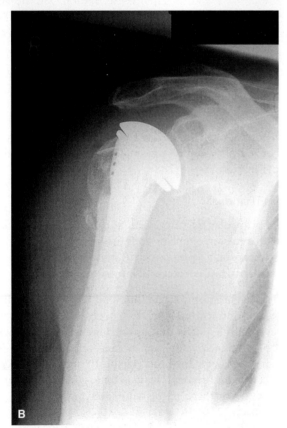

Fig. 21 A. Four-part fracture of the humerus in a 65-year-old man. The articular surface of the humerus is rotated away from the glenoid. **B**. Fracture seen in Figure 21A treated by excision of the humeral head and insertion of a hemiarthroplasty.

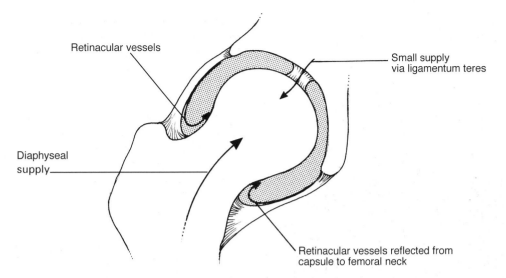

Fig. 22 Blood supply to the femoral head.

Classification

- intracapsular fractures occur within the capsule and may be transcervical or subcapital
- extracapsular fractures occur outside the capsule and may be sited through the base of the femoral neck (basal) or through the trochanters (intertrochanteric).

Why is it so important to differentiate intracapsular fractures from extracapsular fractures? Figure 22 shows the blood supply to the femoral head, which comes through the diaphyseal vessels along the femoral neck, via the foveal artery to a small area of the articular surface and, most importantly, via the retinacular vessels, which are reflected from the capsule along the femoral neck to enter the head around its margin. If these vessels are damaged by a significantly displaced subcapital fracture then avascular necrosis of the femoral head will result.

Clinical features

- **Listen** — a usual history of the event is that of a frail elderly woman who has fallen at home and been found by neighbours after she has been lying on the floor all night. Apart from pain at the hip, the patient is often confused and may be suffering from hypothermia.
- **Look** — the affected leg is shortened and externally rotated.
- **Feel** — tenderness over the greater trocanter
- **Move** — pain on attempting movement of the hip.

A variety of medical problems are often present.

Intracapsular fractures

Diagnosis

An antero-posterior and lateral radiograph of the femoral neck are required (Fig. 23). If the line of the cortex of the medial side of the femoral shaft is traced

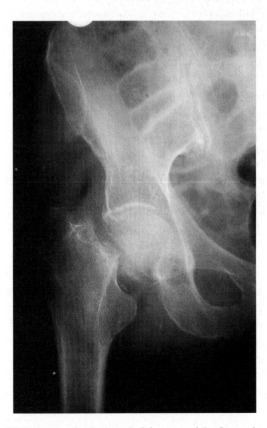

Fig. 23 Intracapsular (subcapital) fracture of the femoral neck.

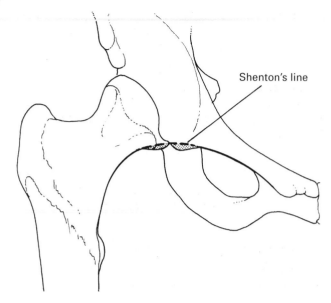

Fig. 24 Normal appearance of Shenton's line. Compare this with the radiograph of the fracture of the femoral neck in Figure 23.

upwards towards the pelvis, it can be seen how this line continues along the inferior side of the neck of the femur until it comes to a sudden stop at the fracture site. The fracture in this case is intracapsular and in particular a subcapital fracture. If the fracture were not there, the line traced along the medial side of the shaft of the femur and the inferior side of the femoral neck would continue in a smooth curve along the inferior side of the superior pubic ramus (Shenton's line). A break in continuity of this line helps to find a fracture in the femoral neck (Fig 24).

Management
Initial management includes rehydration, pain relief (often by skin traction to the affected leg) and treatment of underlying medical conditions.

An undisplaced subcapital fracture can be satisfactorily fixed with lag screws but the natural history of a displaced subcapital fracture is eventually avascular necrosis of the femoral head. However, this predicted sequel is pre-empted by prosthetic replacement of the femoral head at the time of injury. A bipolar hemiarthroplasty is used in active patients but in the more debilitated a simple hemiarthroplasty is often used.

Complications
Avascular necrosis of the femoral head is the main complication arising from an intracapsular fracture. Other complications may occur after hemiarthroplasty:

- dislocation

- erosion of acetabular floor
- need for revision surgery.

Extracapsular fractures

In Figure 25, you can see how the fracture line passes obliquely through the greater trochanter at the top left of the picture across towards the lesser trochanter. This is an extracapsular fracture. This fracture is distal to the capsule and is sited through the trochanters at the base of the femoral neck.

Management
General medical management is required initially as before.

Extracapsular fractures will unite without treatment, but malunion will be present unless external rotation and shortening are corrected. Traction could be used to prevent this, but the prolonged period of bed rest involved would give rise to many other complications which together would probably be fatal. For this reason the fracture is usually treated by closed reduction and fixed with an internal fixation device such as the

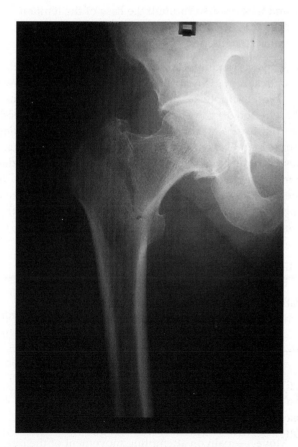

Fig. 25 Extracapsular (intertrochanteric) fracture of the femoral neck.

dynamic hip screw. The barrel and sliding screw portion are positioned in the neck and head of the femur with radiographic screening using an image-intensifier. The plate is then secured to the upper femoral shaft by screws.

The patient can begin weight-bearing within 2 or 3 days of surgery allowing the screw to retract into the barrel as the fracture impacts. With this device, the patient has the best chance of regaining mobility and independence and of returning home.

Complications
Complications of prolonged bed rest include:

- pressure sores
- hypostatic pneumonia
- urinary tract infection
- disuse osteoporosis
- deep venous thrombosis
- pulmonary embolus.

Complications of internal fixation include:

- general complications of surgery
- implant failure
  — cutting out
  — breaking
- fracture through the porotic bone at the end of the plate.

2.5 Vertebral body fractures

Learning objectives

You should:

- be able to recognise these fractures on a lateral radiograph

- remember that, although osteoporosis is a common cause, secondary deposit in the vertebral bodies should be looked for.

Patients with osteoporosis may suffer spontaneous vertical compression fractures of the vertical bodies. The thoracic vertebrae are most commonly affected but the lumbar vertebrae may also be involved.

Clinical features
An elderly woman gives a history of sudden onset of back pain after merely stooping or lifting a light object. Often there is a history of multiple similar events and, as a result, an increasing kyphosis becomes apparent in the thoraco-lumbar spine.

Characteristically, there are no neurological deficits in the limbs as there is no impingement of the spinal cord or nerve roots. The fractures are stable.

Diagnosis
Crush fractures of vertebrae characteristically form wedge shapes compressed anteriorly when seen on the lateral radiograph (Fig. 26).

Management
Symptoms are relieved by a short period of bed rest. Mobilisation should be recommenced as soon as possible.

Complications

- increasing kyphosis
- pressure sores over the prominent spinous processes.

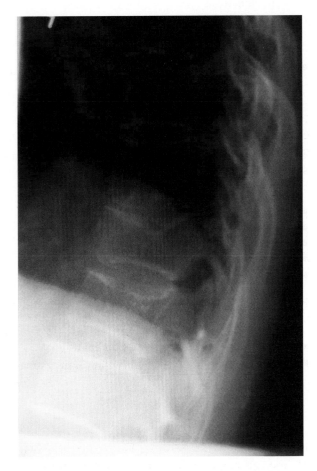

Fig. 26 Both wedge-shaped and bi-concave compression fractures are seen in the lower thoracic vertebrae in this woman with osteoporosis.

2.6 Pathological fractures

Learning objectives

You should:

- be able to list the common primary tumours which metastasise to bone

- recognise features in the history which may suggest a pathological fracture

- remember that treatment may be required for hypercalcaemia, dehydration and the primary pathology as well as for the fracture.

Pathological fractures occur through areas of abnormally weak bone.

Classification

Bone may be weak because of:

- generalised disease
  — myelomatosis
  — osteoporosis
  — osteomalacia and rickets
  — Paget's disease
- local disease
  — metastatic tumour
  — primary tumour
  — fibrous dysplasia
  — bone cysts.

The most common tumour seen in the skeleton is a metastasis from a primary tumour elsewhere. Usual sites of the primary are:

- bronchus
- breast
- prostate
- thyroid
- kidney.

Clinical features

The key features of a pathological fracture are:

- pain at the site, which pre-dates the injury
- a fracture caused by minimal trauma.

Diagnosis

Pathological fractures are characteristically transverse and may be widely displaced (Fig. 27).

Management

The local management of pathological fractures of long bones is best with clozed intramedullary nailing without opening the fracture, reaming or curettage. Postoperative radiotherapy controls pain and any micrometastases. The general management includes further investigation to find an occult primary tumour and to control it.

Complications

- hypercalcaemia
- dehydration
- occult primary
- second deposit elsewhere.

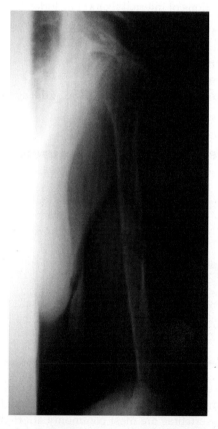

Fig. 27 Pathological fracture in the humerus in a patient with a primary breast carcinoma.

Self-assessment: questions

Multiple choice questions

1. Recognised complications of Colles' fracture include:
   a. Median nerve compression
   b. Loss of full supination
   c. Loss of dorsiflexion
   d. Reflex sympathetic dystrophy
   e. Avascular necrosis of the lunate

2. The following complications are associated with a fracture of the surgical neck of the humerus:
   a. Avascular necrosis of the humeral head
   b. Non-union of the greater tuberosity
   c. Axillary nerve damage
   d. Loss of abduction
   e. Non-union

Extended matching items questions (EMIs)

1. Theme: Fracture complications

A muscle wasting
B malunion
C delayed union
D reflex sympathetic dystrophy
E perioperative morbidity
F avascular necrosis
G implant failure
H nerve compression
I loss of abduction
J non-union

For the complications listed above select the one most commonly associated with the injuries below:

1. Colles' fracture.
2. Intracapsular fracture of the humerus.
3. Extracapsular fracture of the femoral neck.

2. Theme: Fracture descriptions

A a transverse fracture through a previously painful area
B undisplaced Colles' fracture
C multiple vertebral crash fractures
D fracture of the surgical neck of humerus
E subcapital femoral neck fracture
F displaced Colles' fracture
G fractured greater tuberosity
H vertebral body fracture
I lytic area in a vertebral body on radiograph
J extracapsular femoral neck fracture

Which of the descriptions listed above most commonly matches the statements below:

1. This is a pathological fracture.
2. There is a substantial risk of avascular necrosis.
3. Further general investigations are needed.

Constructed response questions (CRQs)

CRQ 1

An 86-year-old woman is found lying on her kitchen floor. She is unable to bear weight on her right leg. She appears to have been lying overnight but has no other injuries.

a. What clinical features would confirm a diagnosis of a fractured femur?
b. What other general medical problems are likely to be present in this particular case?
c. X-ray examination shows a fracture extending from the greater trochanter to the lesser trochanter. What type of fracture is this?
d. How is this injury usually managed?
e. List four postoperative complications associated with this line of management.

CRQ 2

An emaciated 65-year-old woman with a lifetime history of smoking and a recent non-productive cough, presents with a sudden exacerbation of back pain. She has had discomfort in the same area for some months, but while bending to pick something from the floor today experienced a sharp, severe and persisting pain in this region.

a. What do you expect to find on physical examination of her back?
b. AP and lateral radiographs are taken. What would you particularly look for?
c. What is the site of the likely cause of these features?
d. Outline aspects of the management now required.

Objective structured clinical examination questions (OSCEs)

OSCE 1

Look at the photograph of the X-ray of the Colles' fracture (Fig. 28).

a. What deformity does the distal fragment show?
b. Looking at the AP X-ray, what does this show has happened to the radius?
c. In this type of injury the patient may complain of pins and needles in the radial three digits. Why should this be?
d. Manipulation and plaster of Paris immobilisation are the usual ways of treating this injury in an elderly patient. List four complications.

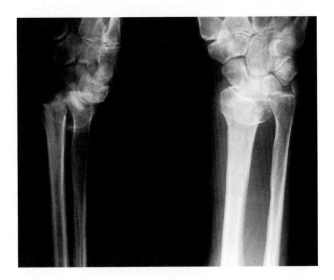

Fig. 28

OSCE 2

Study the photograph of an X-ray of a fracture of the upper humerus in a 60-year-old woman (Fig. 29).

a. The fracture has divided the humerus into three large portions. What are they?
b. Is this then an intracapsular fracture, an extracapsular fracture, or both?

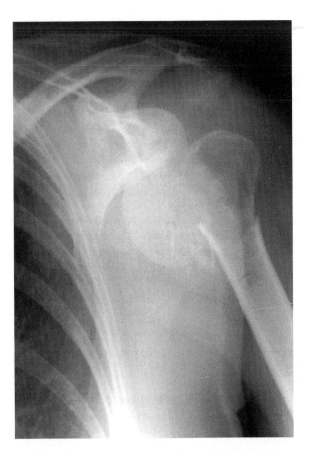

Fig. 29 Radiograph of a fracture of the upper humerus in a 60-year-old woman.

c. The rotator cuff muscles are attached to which of these portions?
d. What is the risk to the humeral head in this fracture?
e. If the axillary nerve has been damaged by the fracture, how could this be detected?

Viva questions

1. List three possible ways in which a Colles' fracture can be immobilised after reduction has successfully been achieved.

2. What types of bone disorders may give rise to a pathological fracture of the femoral neck?

Self-assessment: answers

Multiple choice answers

1. a. **True.** Median nerve compression is sometimes seen as a complication of a displaced Colles' fracture. Bony fragments or haematoma compress the median nerve in the carpal tunnel. It is not seen in the majority of cases in elderly patients. However, if compression is suspected, carpal tunnel decompression should be carried out early.
   b. **True.** Full supination may be lost as a result of malunion of a Colles' fracture. The distal fragment is displaced into pronation and unless corrected will not rotate normally into full supination as the distal radio-ulnar joint moves.
   c. **False.** The distal fragment in a Colles' fracture is displaced dorsally so loss of dorsiflexion is not seen in cases of malunion. However, palmar flexion may be lost as the normal arc of motion of the wrist joint is displaced dorsally. After reduction of a Colles' fracture, there may be residual stiffness of the wrist, causing some loss of dorsiflexion.
   d. **True.** Although some stiffness, pain and swelling may persist after treatment of a Colles' fracture, a full-blown reflex sympathetic dystrophy is rare. In these cases there is pain, swelling, stiffness in the hand and wrist, which is sweaty and cold.
   e. **False.** Avascular necrosis of the lunate (Keinbock's disease) is an uncommon condition affecting the lunate. It occurs spontaneously. The aetiology is unclear.

2. a. **False.** A fracture of the surgical neck of the humerus does not interrupt the blood supply to the humeral head. Avascular necrosis is not, therefore, seen.
   b. **False.** A fracture of the surgical neck is below the tuberosities.
   c. **True.** The axillary nerve winds round the neck of the humerus to supply the deltoid muscle and a small area of skin over its insertion onto the humerus.
   d. **True.** Damage to the axillary nerve associated with the fracture results in paralysis of the deltoid and loss of abduction.
   e. **False.** Fractures of the surgical neck of the humerus unite readily.

EMI answers

1. Theme: Fracture complications

1. B. Malunion. In the elderly population, displacement of the fracture even after manipulation is a common complication. It is probably under-diagnosed but hardly ever requires a particular treatment as the functional range of movement it allows is adequate for the patient's lifestyle. Mild forms of reflex sympathy dystrophy are less common but probably occur more often than is recognised.
2. I. Loss of abduction fractures involving the tuberosity of the humerus will prevent abduction by dysfunctioning the rotator cuff muscles especially supraspinatus. Malunion of a greater tuberosity fracture will mechanically limit abduction.
3. E. Perioperative morbidity. Although the fractures may be fixed there is a high instance of perioperative morbidity after an extracapsular fracture.

2. Theme: fracture descriptions

1. A. The deposit in the bone has been a source of pain before the fracture occurs. Fractures are usually transverse with minimum trauma.
2. E. Loss of blood supply to the femoral head from a displaced subcapital fracture may lead to avascular necrosis.
3. I. Isolated lytic area in a vertebral body on a radiograph requires further investigation to determine its nature. It is probably best considered a secondary deposit until proved otherwise.

CRQ answers

CRQ 1

a. Local pain and deformity
   Shortened leg
   External rotation.
b. Hypothermia.
c. Extracapsular/intertrochanteric fracture.
d. Internal fixation under X-ray control using a dynamic hip screw or a nail and plate.
e. Chest infection
   Deep vein thrombosis
   Wound break down
   Loss of mobility.

CRQ 2

a. Localised tenderness and swelling at the site of the pain with prominence of the spinus process suggest an underlying kyphosis.
b. Wedge fracture of a vertebrae at the site. Evidence of bone destruction nearby suggesting a metastatic tumour deposit.
c. Bronchogenic carcinoma.
d. Bed rest until comfortable with analgesics and mobilisation
Radiotherapy to the secondary deposits
Investigation to find the site of the primary tumour and start appropriate therapy
Investigations for hypercalcaemia and dehydration.

OSCE answers

OSCE 1

a. Dorsal angulation.
b. Impaction and shortening.
c. Median nerve compression from the deformity and associated swelling.
d. Loss of reduction
Stiffness
Swelling
Reflex sympathetic dystrophy
Loss of full range of movement.

OSCE 2

a. Humeral head, greater tuberosity, humeral shaft.
b. There are aspects of both an intracapsular and extracapsular fracture present in this injury.
c. Greater tuberosity.
d. Avascular necrosis.
e. Numbness in the 'badge-patch' area at the point of the shoulder.

Viva answers

1. A variety of methods of splinting a Colles' fracture are available. Minimally displaced and stable fractures are usually treated in a below-elbow plaster cast. Unstable and comminuted fractures may require stabilisation with percutaneous wires or with an external fixator.

2. Osteoporosis is the most common.
   In Paget's disease the bone appears deformed, enlarged and without its normal medullary architecture.
   In myelomatosis the cortex appears scalloped and multiple lucent areas are seen throughout the medullary cavity.
   Metastatic carcinoma is usually characterised by pre-existing bone pain and a lucent area on X-ray.

3 Fractures in children

Chapter overview

Fractures in children may have specific radiological appearances which make them different from fractures seen in adults. In addition, fractures involving the growing ends of long bones have their own specific classification (Salter–Harris classification) and methods of management.

Finally, underlying bone pathology such as dysplasia or tumour must not be forgotten; and in suspicious circumstances remember that non-accidental injury may be present.

Fractures around the elbow, especially supracondylar fracture, may cause significant vascular or neurological damage requiring prompt emergency treatment.

3.1 Clinical examination

Learning objectives

You should:

- know how to adapt your history taking and examination technique to the injured child
- be able to describe greenstick fractures and classify epiphyseal injuries
- be able to describe the management of these conditions.

A gentle and friendly approach is always required when examining children. Care must be taken not to cause any additional pain. Fracture sites must always be palpated very gently and any movement likely to cause pain carried out cautiously and slowly. An initial temporary splint or sling is comforting and after this has been applied it is usually possible to check the presence of peripheral circulation and sensation without causing more discomfort. On examining injuries around the elbow, much information can be gained by comparing the injured with the non-injured site, paying particular attention to the carrying angle. A radiograph of the uninjured elbow can be useful, but the parents' permission to X-ray the uninjured side must always be sought and the reason explained.

When interviewing the family of a child with a skeletal tumour, or in whom you suspect non-accidental injury, great sensitivity must be exercised to avoid causing unnecessary grief or hostility.

Fracture patterns

Because the growing bone has not yet fully ossified, skeletal injuries are different from those seen in adults. The bones are less brittle (more plastic) than those of adults. A moderate force will cause a child's bone to buckle on the compression side. With more force the distraction side of the bone will fracture causing the classical 'greenstick' fracture (Fig. 30A). The growth plate of the bone (the physis) has not yet fused and can be seen between the epiphysis and the metaphysis (Fig. 30B). Through this area particular injuries have been described.

Physeal injuries. These injuries take place through the calcifying layer of chondrocytes in the growth plate or physis. Salter and Harris described various types of physeal injury (Fig. 31).

Slipped lower radial epiphysis

Clinical features
A fall on the outstretched hand in a child is the common presentation of this injury. Dorsal swelling and deformity are obvious.

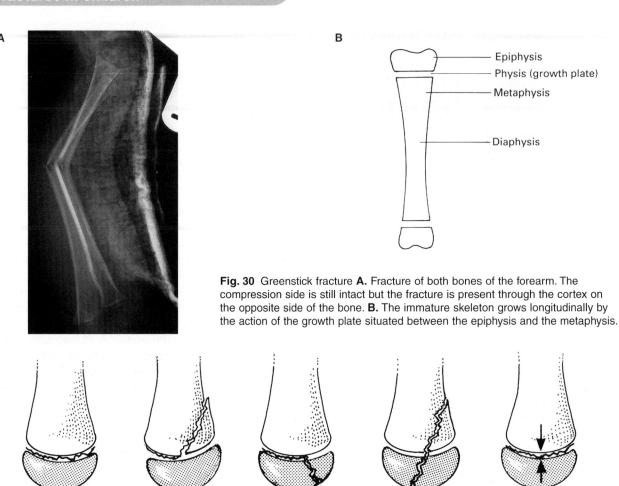

Fig. 30 Greenstick fracture **A.** Fracture of both bones of the forearm. The compression side is still intact but the fracture is present through the cortex on the opposite side of the bone. **B.** The immature skeleton grows longitudinally by the action of the growth plate situated between the epiphysis and the metaphysis.

(B: Epiphysis — Physis (growth plate) — Metaphysis — Diaphysis)

Fig. 31 Salter and Harris classification of physeal injuries. I — The injury has separated the epiphysis from the metaphysis through the growth plate. II — The injury passes through a corner of the metaphysis. This is the most common injury. III — The injury passes through the epiphysis itself. IV — The fracture line crosses the physis from epiphysis to metaphysis. This type of injury can result in premature fusion of the epiphysis to the metaphysis. V — There has been a compression force on the physis. The radiograph appears normal.

Diagnosis

Careful examination of a lateral radiograph is necessary to detect posterior displacement of the epiphysis and to identify any associated fracture in the metaphysis or epiphysis.

Management

Gentle, accurate manipulation under anaesthesia is required to reduce the fracture and avoid damaging the blood supply to the epiphysis. Open reduction is occasionally indicated but if internal fixation is required only fine wires should be placed across the physis as mechanical disturbance may cause premature fusion of the epiphysis and growth arrest.

Complications

- premature epiphyseal growth arrest
- median nerve compression.

Slipped upper femoral epiphysis (SUFE)

Clinical features

Patients are usually boys. Classically two types of patient present with this condition. One is an athletic adolescent with sudden onset of hip pain often occurring at sports. The other is characteristically hypogonadal and overweight with a gradual history of pain usually involving both hips.

- **Listen** — pain is often referred to the knee.
- **Look** — the leg is externally rotated and appears short (Fig. 32).
- **Feel** — local tenderness
- **Move** — internal rotation is resisted.

Diagnosis

Careful examination of an antero-posterior radiograph and comparison with the opposite side, if this is not

3.2 Forearm fractures

Learning objectives

You should:

- be able to recognise a forearm fracture
- understand the principles of management
- be able to recognise the complications that may occur.

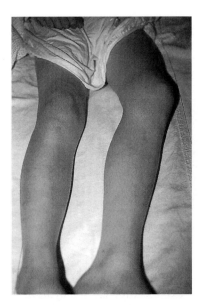

Fig. 32 This 15-year-old presented with sudden pain in the left hip after a sporting event; the leg is externally rotated and shortened.

affected, shows the displacement of the femoral head. Lateral radiographs and other specially angled views will show the extent of the posterior slip of the head on the neck more clearly (Fig. 33).

Management

Manipulation of the slipped epiphysis runs the risk of causing avascular necrosis of the head. Pinning of the capital epiphysis in the slipped position is, therefore, favoured. In cases of severe slip, an osteotomy of the femoral neck can be planned later.

Complications

- avascular necrosis
- chondrolysis, which later causes osteoarthritis.

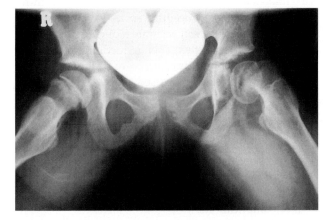

Fig. 33 The radiograph of the pelvis shows the capital epiphysis has slipped off the femoral neck on the left side. On the right side there is a suggestion of an early slip.

Because of their structural immaturity, children's bones are more plastic than adult bones. Consequently, when subjected to bending forces such as those occurring in a fall on the outstretched hand, they suffer plastic deformation rather than a break.

In some cases, the bone only buckles on the compression side (torus fracture). In other cases, the cortex breaks on the distraction side of the bone and bends on the compression side (greenstick fracture, see Fig. 30A).

Clinical features

Fractures of both the bones of the forearm is a common injury in children. Falls from a height or from a bicycle are often the cause.

- **Listen** — the injured limb is painful.
- **Look** — the fracture site is swollen, bruised and deformed.
- **Feel** — peripheral circulation and sensation may be compromised by compression of the neurovascular bundles by the displaced fracture or the resulting swelling (Fig. 30A).
- **Move** — movement is restricted and rotational deformity may be apparent.

Diagnosis

Two radiographs at right angles to each other are required to assess fully the extent of the fracture. The amount of displacement, angulation or rotation at the fracture site can be assessed. Complete displacement at the fracture site results in overriding of the bones' ends, causing shortening.

Management

Manipulation under anaesthetic is required to correct the deformity. The fracture is immobilised in the reduced position by an above-elbow plaster cast.

During the following few days, the limb must be carefully observed for signs of acute compartment compression, which may develop as a result of the injury or of the manipulation. Pain in the forearm aggravated by passive extension of the fingers suggests that the muscle bellies are compressed within their fascial compartments. Peripheral sensation and circulation may be impaired. Emergency treatment consists of releasing all constricting dressings. If this does not relieve the symptoms, an extensive surgical decompression of the two forearm compartments by incision of the skin and deep fascia is required. These wounds are left open for 2 to 3 days before attempting delayed primary closure or covering with a split thickness skin graft.

Complications

- acute compartment syndrome
- median nerve compression
- malunion, causing loss of rotation.

3.3 Elbow fractures

Learning objectives

You should:

- be able to recognise a supracondylar fracture and institute emergency treatment

- know how to manage any early complications of this injury

- become familiar with the normal pattern of ossification at the elbow so that you can distinguish secondary centres of ossification from fractures.

Supracondylar fractures

This injury is an orthopaedic emergency as a delay in treatment may cause irreversible forearm ischaemia by pressure on the brachial artery. The median nerve also may be compressed or injured.

Clinical features
- **Listen** — a fall from a bicycle or a swing onto the outstretched hand in a young child is the usual presentation.
- **Look** — there is deformity and bruising at the elbow and a tense swelling develops quickly (Fig. 34).
- **Feel** — the radial pulse must be palpated and if weak or absent the elbow should be gently extended to minimise any kinking of the brachial artery in the ante cubital fossa. Symptoms and signs of medial

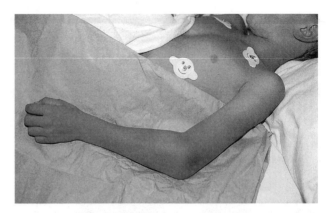

Fig. 34 Supracondylar fracture of the elbow of an 8-year-old boy.

nerve compression may be apparent in the hand, and rarely the ulna and radial nerves may be affected too.
- **Move** — all elbow movements are resisted.

Diagnosis
An antero-posterior radiograph shows varus or valgus angulation at the fracture site but a lateral view looks the most dramatic especially in a completely displaced fracture (Fig. 35A). The distal fragment is displaced or angulated posteriorly in nearly all cases.

Management
It is usually possible to correct the displacement by manipulation under anaesthetic. The reduced position is checked by axial and lateral radiographs. The reduced position is maintained by elbow flexion (usually more than 90°), which locks the distal fragment in place by tensioning the triceps aponeurosis posteriorly. However, to allow immobilisation in less flexion, Kirschner-wire fixation may be used. These are introduced by an open procedure so as to visualise and protect the ulnar nerve. If accurate reduction is not possible by closed means, then open reduction is required to visualise the fracture. Kirschner-wire fixation (Fig. 35B) in an anatomical position is used again.

Complications
- early complications:
  — acute occlusion of the brachial artery
  — median nerve damage
  — compartment syndrome
- later complications:
  — Volkmann's ischaemic contracture
  — myositis ossificans
  — malunion.

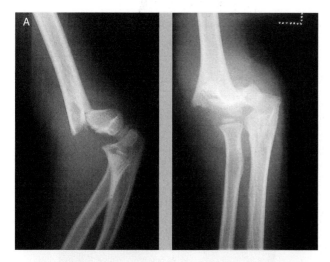

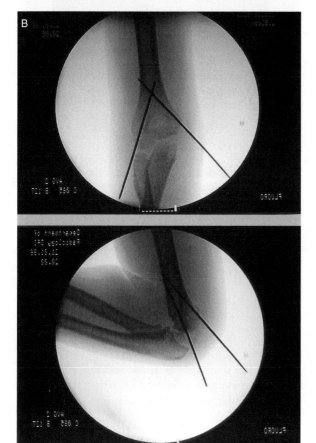

Fig. 35 Supracondylar fracture. **A.** Radiograph showing gross displacement at the fracture site. The associated kinking and compression of the brachial artery and median nerve can be imagined as they pass anterior to the bone fragments.
B. Kirschner wires used to secure a supracondylar fracture in the reduced position.

Fractured lateral condylar mass

Avulsion fractures of the lateral aspect of the humerus may produce a displaced fragment that may be rotated, and therefore, will be impossible to correct by closed manipulation (Fig. 36A).

Diagnosis
The radiograph may be difficult to interpret if there is no familiarity with the normal pattern of the centres of secondary ossification around the elbow. A comparison radiograph of the uninjured elbow is often helpful.

Management
Accurate reduction by operative exposure and securing the fragment with a suture or Kirschner wire produces a secure anatomical position (Fig. 36B).

Complications

- non-union
- development of valgus deformity as a result of premature growth arrest
- tardy ulnar palsy.

Medial epicondylar avulsion

A valgus injury to the elbow may avulse the medial epicondyle (Fig. 36C). Sometimes it is only slightly displaced but on other occasions it is widely separated and becomes trapped in the joint space.

Diagnosis
Careful comparison of the radiograph with that of the non-injured elbow makes it easier to recognise the displaced epicondyle.

Management
Anatomical reduction usually requires an open procedure with fixation of the avulsed epicondyle by a Kirschner wire.

Complications

- pressure on the ulnar nerve
- premature epiphyseal growth arrest causing varus deformity of the elbow with growth.

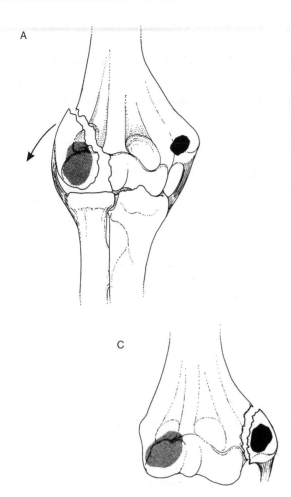

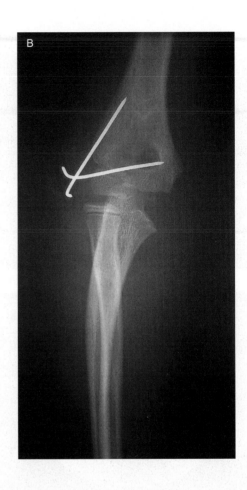

Fig. 36 Fracture of the lateral condylar mass. **A.** Diagram showing the mechanism of rotation and displacement caused by the fracture. **B.** Kirschner-wire fixation of the fracture seen in (A). **C.** A fracture of the medial epicondyle may displace so that the fragment lies within the joint.

3.4 Femoral fractures

Learning objectives

You should:

- know the principles of resuscitation and management of femoral fractures in different age groups.

Clinical features

Direct trauma, often from being knocked down by a vehicle, accounts for the majority of femoral fractures in children. On examination, the affected leg is shorter, swollen and externally rotated. There may be considerable blood loss into the tissues.

Diagnosis

Although the diagnosis is apparent clinically, a radiograph is necessary to assess the fracture pattern and the degree of displacement and angulation.

Management

Prompt fluid replacement is required to avoid cardiovascular collapse, but care must be exercised in young children to avoid circulatory overload. Fractures in young children can be managed in gallows traction for 3 to 4 weeks until healing occurs (Fig. 37), but older children require skin traction, usually on a Thomas splint.

Complications

- shock
- nerve or vessel injury

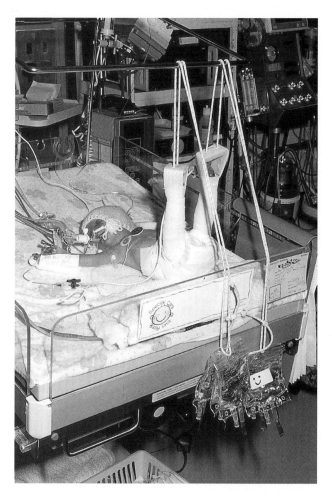

Fig. 37 Gallows traction being used to manage a femoral fracture in a neonate.

- malunion
- leg length discrepancy.

3.5 Dysplasia, tumour and non-accidental injury

Learning objectives

You should:

- know when to suspect that a fracture may be caused by one of these

- be able to recognise some of the specific radiological features of each.

Fractures in children in the absence of significant injury raises the possibility of bone dysplasia, tumour or non-accidental injury. If a fracture is not apparent on the radiograph in the painful area, it must be scrutinised carefully to look for any periosteal elevation. This is seen as a thin calcified line above the cortex and is caused by elevation of the periosteum by:

- blood from a crack in the cortex
- a subperiosteal haematoma
- pus
- tumour.

Dysplasia

Fibrous dysplasia. The bone is soft and weak with extensive areas of fibrous tissue. Fractures and deformity develop.

Osteogenesis imperfecta. There is often a positive family history, but occasionally a case occurs as a result of a new mutation. A spectrum of severity can occur from multiple fractures, causing deformity and stunted growth, to mild cases with only discoloured sclerae or joint laxity.

Management

- simple immobilisation of fractures
- prevention of more fractures
- early discharge after hospital treatment.

Complications

- decreased growth
- progressive deformity
- multiple fractures.

Tumour

Bone tumours may be benign or malignant.

Bone cyst. A bone cyst is an apparent space in the medullary cavity surrounded by thinned cortex containing solid, uncalcified material. Radiographically the appearance suggests a tumour. However, it is benign and may resolve spontaneously if a fracture occurs through it.

Other tumours:

- enchondroma
- aneurysmal bone cyst
- multiple exostoses, diaphyseal aclasis (Fig. 38)
- malignant bone tumours (occur rarely).

Non-accidental injury

This must be suspected in any child if there seems to be parental indifference to the injury and if no reasonable explanation for the fracture is given. Particular vigilance is necessary with very young children who are unable to

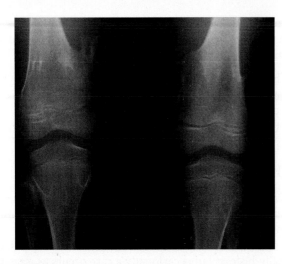

Fig. 38 Multiple exostoses around the knees of a 6-year-old child. They characteristically appear to grow away from the epiphysis.

speak for themselves. Other features that support this diagnosis are:

- fractures at a variety of stages of healing
- soft tissue injuries
- depressed attitude of the child
- indifferent or aggressive attitude of the parents.

Management

- admit to hospital
- skeletal survey
- paediatrician
- social worker.

Self-assessment: questions

Multiple choice questions

1. A boy aged 12 presents with pain and a limp in the right leg of 2 months' duration. Likely diagnosis includes:
   a. Late presentation of congenital dislocated hip
   b. Transient synovitis of the hip
   c. Perthes' disease
   d. Acute septic arthritis
   e. Slipped femoral epiphysis

2. When managing fractures in children:
   a. The presence of multiple fractures of different ages is suggestive of non-accidental injury (NAI)
   b. The presence of pain on passive extension of the toes after a closed tibial fracture is due to impingement of the muscle bellies at the fracture site
   c. Failure to achieve a satisfactory reduction of a fracture at the elbow warrants open reduction and internal fixation
   d. Conservative treatment is used less frequently than internal fixation for the stabilisation of femoral shaft fractures
   e. The initial treatment of impending compartment syndrome would be the release of all constricting plaster bandages

Extended matching items questions (EMIs)

1. Theme: Diagnoses
A   transient synovitis of hip
B   Perthes' disease
C   femoral shaft fracture
D   slipped upper femoral epiphysis
E   acute septic arthritis
F   late presentation of CDH
G   bone dysplasia
H   primary malignant bone tumour
I   tibial fracture
J   ligamentous injury

Match the most appropriate diagnosis from the list above to each of the clinical histories below:

1. A prolonged history of painful limp with loss of internal rotation of the hip in an obese 14-year-old boy.
2. Persistent pain around the knee of an 11-year-old with no history of trauma but abnormal bony appearance on X-ray.

3. Pain in the mid-thigh of a cyclist following collision with a car.

2. Theme: Complications
A   myositis ossificans
B   ischaemic contracture
C   varus deformity developing with growth
D   loss of full flexion
E   valgus deformity developing with growth
F   initial bone length discrepancy
G   vascular injury
H   acute ulnar nerve dysfunction
I   risk of avascular necrosis
J   loss of full extension

Which of the complications listed above is most likely to be associated with the conditions below:

1. An overriding transverse femoral shaft fracture in a 4-year-old boy.
2. Fracture of the lateral condylar mass involving the growth plate.
3. Severe displacement or over-aggressive manipulation of a slipped femoral epiphysis.

Constructed response questions (CRQs)

CRQ 1

An 8-year-old boy presents to the Accident and Emergency department with a history of having fallen from a swing and hurt his elbow.

a. You are the casualty officer on duty. What would you expect to find on physical examination?
b. He is holding the elbow flexed in a sling. What additional damage may this be causing beyond the fracture site?
c. What would you do to remedy this situation?
d. You suspect a supracondylar fracture of the humerus. What X-rays would you request?
e. What is the name given to the condition caused by prolonged vascular occlusion with this injury?

CRQ 2

An athletic 12-year-old boy presents after school sports with an injury to his hip following a high jump. You suspect a slipped upper femoral epiphysis.

a. What would you expect to find on physical examination of the hip?
b. What X-ray view would you request?
c. You decide to suggest surgery. What two methods of treatment are appropriate depending on the degree of severity?
d. What are the complications of aggressive manipulation?
e. Why might an X-ray of the pelvis showing both hips be relevant in this case?

Objective structured clinical examination questions (OSCEs)

OSCE 1

Study the photograph of the X-ray of an elbow of an 8-year-old (Fig. 39).

a. What condition does this show?
b. What are the principles of treating this injury?
c. What is a long-term complication of this injury?
d. What is the effect of this on the ulnar nerve?

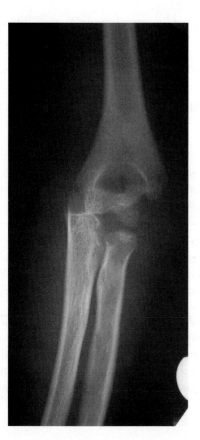

Fig. 39

OSCE 2

Study the photograph of the X-ray of a child's wrist (Fig. 40).

a. What injury does it show?
b. In the lateral X-ray is the distal fragment displaced in a dorsal or palmar direction?
c. Name a classification for this injury.
d. How is this treated?

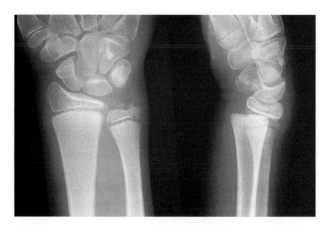

Fig. 40

Viva questions

1. Discuss the conditions that should be considered by the incidental finding of periosteal elevation on the radiograph of a child's tibia.

2. How would you manage a child who you suspect is a victim of non-accidental injury?

Self-assessment: answers

Multiple choice answers

1. a. **False.** A case of congenital dislocation of the hip (CDH) missed on routine screening in infancy would have presented early in childhood when the patient began walking. It is unlikely that the first presentation of CDH would be as late as the age of 12.
   b. **False.** Transient synovitis of the hip has a short duration and usually resolves within 3 to 4 days.
   c. **True.** Perthes' disease develops spontaneously, causing pain and limp that may persist for episodes of several weeks. Symptoms are relieved by rest but recurrent relapses are characteristic until the area of avascular necrosis heals.
   d. **False.** Acute septic arthritis is characterised by acute severe pain in the hip and loss of movement.
   e. **True.** A gradual slip of the upper femoral epiphysis presents with a prolonged history of pain and loss of movement. The condition is associated with hormonal imbalance in the adolescent. Acute slips have a shorter history and may be associated with direct trauma.

2. a. **False.** The child may have bone dysplasia such as osteogenesis imperfecta. Other features such as bruising are required to make the diagnosis of NAI.
   b. **False.** The presence of pain on passive extension of the toes in this case is caused by ischaemia of the muscle bellies and not by impingement at the fracture site. The findings suggest compartment syndrome.
   c. **True.** In general, operative techniques and anaesthetic procedures are now so safe and reliable that it is in the patient's best interests to change the fracture management to open reduction and internal fixation if a satisfactory position cannot readily be achieved or held by conservative measures.
   d. **False.** Conservative treatment is the usual method of splinting femoral shaft fractures in children.
   e. **True.** Compartment syndrome is suspected by the presence of intractable pain in the limb exacerbated by passive extension of the digits. There may be associated paraesthesia or numbness in a peripheral nerve distribution. If symptoms are not relieved by releasing all constricting dressings, fasciotomy should be undertaken sooner rather than later.

EMI answers

1. Theme: Diagnosis

1. D. Slipped upper femoral epiphysis presents in this way and may be a gradual, chronic slip due to obesity in adolescence.
2. H. The upper tibia is a common site for primary bone tumour in this age group.
3. C. This moderate-velocity injury to the exposed thigh could cause a femoral shaft fracture.

2. Theme: Complications

1. F. As the fracture heals with some overriding of the bone ends there will be *shortening* of leg length but this will correct as the limb grows. If the fracture were anatomically reduced there is a risk of *increased* leg length in response to the hyperaemia of fracture healing.
2. E. Premature physeal growth arrest on the lateral side of the elbow allows the development of valgus angulation as the medial side grows.
3. I. The blood supply to the capital epiphysis may be disrupted causing chondromalacia and ultimately avascular necrosis of the femoral head.

CRQ answers

CRQ 1

a. Bruising, swelling, deformity around the elbow.
b. Compromised blood supply to the forearm and hand. Absent radial pulse.
c. Straighten the arm and observe the return of the radial pulse.
d. AP and true lateral (See Fig. 35A)
e. Volkman's ischaemic contracture.

CRQ 2

a. The leg is held in external rotation, partial flexion and appears shorter. It is painful.
b. Frog-leg lateral shows the degree of displacement of the capital epiphysis most accurately.
   Pinning the displaced femoral head in situ. If severely displaced an osteotomy of the femoral neck can be planned later.

c. Chondrolysis and avascular necrosis of femoral epiphysis.
d. There may be an early slip in the opposite, unaffected hip.

OSCE answers

OSCE 1

a. Fracture of the lateral mass of the elbow.
b. Open reduction and internal fixation to secure anatomical position. K wires used to secure the fragment across the growth plate (see Fig. 41).
c. Premature closure of the lateral condylar physis and development of cubitus valgus.
d. Tardy ulnar palsy.

OSCE 2

a. Slipped lower radial epiphysis.
b. Dorsal.
c. Salter–Harris classification.
d. Manipulation under anaesthesia and moulded plaster cast with the wrist in flexion.

Viva answers

1. The presence of periosteal elevation suggests the presence of pus, blood or tumour between the bone cortex and periosteum. Investigation should focus on looking for an occult fracture in the cortex and a subperiosteal haematoma. The presence of infection should be eliminated by white cell count and plasma viscosity. A CT scan or MRI scan may be helpful in diagnosing a tumour.

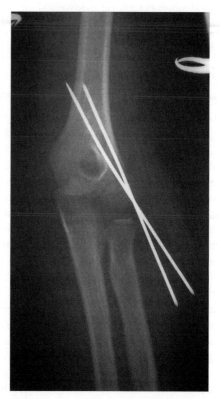

Fig. 41 Kirschner-wire fixation of the displaced fracture of the medial epicondyle.

2. A child in whom you suspect non-accidental injury should be admitted to hospital for observation. A skeletal survey is carried out to detect the presence of fractures at various stages of healing. A thorough clinical examination is required to detect the presence of soft tissue injuries. Help from the paediatrician and the social work department are required before the discharge of the child to a place of safety or back home.

4 Orthopaedic disorders of children

Chapter overview

A number of minor orthopaedic conditions occur in childhood which are usually transient or developmental. The important task for the doctor is to be able to distinguish these, provide appropriate reassurance and to recognise the serious debilitating conditions with which they may be confused.

Means of distinguishing these minor orthopaedic disorders are described together with the management of the more serious conditions.

4.1 Clinical examination

Learning objectives

You should:

- be able to develop a friendly, non-threatening approach to the examination of a child
- know how to perform the specific manoeuvres in the examination for CDH gently and accurately.

Before examining children it is important to have gained their confidence by friendly conversation or play and to avoid any sudden or potentially painful actions. It is important that the examination is carried out in a warm environment and that the doctor has warm hands. The examination is almost impossible if the child becomes unsettled or distressed because of your initial approach.

Examine the patient walking, standing and lying.

Walking. Observe for an antalgic gait or a Trendelenburg gait.

Standing. Observe the contour of the lumbar spine, the posture of the pelvis and whether the feet are flat on the floor. The presence of calcaneovalgus and associated flat foot should be observed. Flexion of the spine by asking the patient to touch the toes will unmask and exaggerate any scoliosis.

Lying. Put the hips through a full range of movement; internal rotation particularly is limited if there is a synovial effusion in the hip joint, and any movement of the hip will be impossible in the presence of acute septic arthritis. When examining a neonate for congenital dislocation of the hip (CDH) remember that Ortolani's and Barlow's tests must be carried out gently to avoid causing vascular damage to the capital epiphysis. With the patient sitting on the couch, carefully examine the foot and ankle. Three movements should be elicited: ankle movement, which is pure flexion and extension, subtalar movement, which involves moving the os calcis into inversion and eversion, and mid-tarsal joint movement, which includes internal and external rotation.

4.2 Minor disorders

Learning objectives

You should:

- remember that many apparent abnormalities in the lower limbs in children are developmental, transient and cause no long-term disorder.

Children with minor or transient conditions are frequently referred to paediatric orthopaedic clinics because parents are worried that a serious abnormality may be developing.

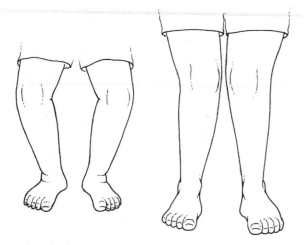

Fig. 42 During the first years of life, a child's knees change from a genu varus position through normal alignment to a genu valgus position by the age of 4 years.

In-toeing. Parents complain that their toddler is always tripping over his feet. Examination should exclude three common abnormalities which cause the leg or foot to rotate inwards: femoral neck anteversion, tibial torsion and metatarsus adductus. Usually each of these causes is self-limiting and is unlikely to require intervention.

Knock-knee. Normal physiological development of the lower limbs shows a progression from genu varus in the first 2 years of life through normal alignment at the age of 3 to genu valgus with a characteristic gap between the malleoli at the age of 4 (Fig. 42).

Flat feet. Postural or mobile flat feet are common in children and are caused by physiological ligamentous laxity, which disappears with age. The medial fat pad in the sole of the foot exaggerates the appearance. Calcaneovalgus is seen when the feet are viewed from behind but the heel corrects to normal alignment and the medial arch reappears when the child stands on tip toe. Rigid or spastic flat foot is much rarer and is caused by an underlying abnormality of the tarsal bones and associated muscle spasm.

4.3 Irritable hip

Learning objectives

You should:

- know how to make a diagnosis of transient synovitis and differentiate this from more serious hip disorders
- know how to manage the child through an acute episode.

Unwillingness to weight-bear or limping in a child is commonly the result of transient synovitis of the hip. This condition, as its name suggests, is a self-limiting inflammation of the joint lining resulting from synovial irritation. As such it is quite benign. However, several other diagnoses should be excluded:

- acute septic arthritis
- Perthes' disease.

Irritable hip can be due to:

- idiopathic causes
- recent upper respiratory tract infection
- minor trauma.

Clinical features
- **Listen** — history of recent intercurrent illness
- **Look** — the leg lies in mild external rotation
- **Feel** — typically there is tenderness
- **Move** — there is limited movement of the joint. Internal rotation is especially limited because this movement has the effect of tightening the joint capsule and so constricting the effusion even further and increasing the pain.

Diagnosis
Investigations are directed to eliminating the other possible causes of hip pain. An X-ray of the hip is taken to look for features of Perthes' disease.

A white cell count and plasma viscosity are used to exclude a diagnosis of septic arthritis.

A throat swab and ASO (antistreptolysin O) titre may help to confirm a recent upper respiratory tract infection.

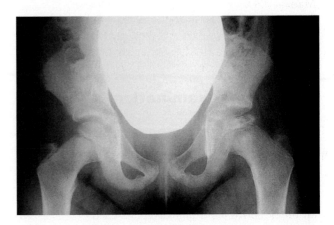

Fig. 43 Perthes' disease of the right hip compared with the opposite normal side. The capital epiphysis is flattened, sclerotic and fragmented.

Management

After a short period of bed rest, the child's symptoms usually settle. There are no long-term complications but the child may have another episode in the future.

4.4 Osteochondritis

Learning objectives

You should:

● be able to list the common sites of osteochondritis and recognise their common features

● know the principles of management for Perthes' disease.

Osteochondritis occurs in several locations and is usually caused by a transient interruption of the blood supply to an area of growing bone; the mechanism by which this occurs is unknown.

Perthes' disease

Boys between the ages of 5 and 10 years are usually affected. There is a recurring history of episodic pain in the hip, which causes a limp and limitation of movement. Internal rotation and extension are particularly affected.

Diagnosis

Radiographs show sclerosis and irregularity of the capital epiphysis (Fig. 43). Sequestration may be apparent and the head may be flatter than normal and appear to be extruding from the acetabulum.

Management

Treatment is aimed at *containing* the hip while maintaining movement. An abduction splint may be required but in milder cases limitation of activities during exacerbation of symptoms is sufficient. In severe cases, where the femoral head has extruded from the acetabulum, a femoral neck osteotomy is required to relocate the head in the acetabulum.

Other sites of osteochondritis

Osteochondritis dissecans. In the knee the lateral side of the medial femoral condyle is the usual site for an area of avascularity to develop. An island of bone demarcates and eventually may separate and become a loose body in the joint causing intermittent locking and pain.

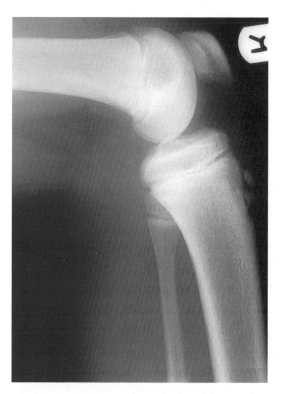

Fig. 44 Osgood–Schlatter's disease. The tibial tuberosity is elevated, sclerotic and fragmented.

Traction apopyhysitis. Osgood–Schlatter's disease is a common example of a traction apophysitis. Idiopathic aseptic necrosis of the tibial tuberosity causes knee pain in adolescence, which is usually exacerbated by vigorous activity. The tibial tuberosity is elevated and tender. Radiographs show elevation, sclerosis and fragmentation of the tuberosity and, in older patients, a fragment of bone is sometimes seen in the patellar tendon. Management consists of avoiding sports when symptoms are severe. Sometimes a splint or plaster cylinder is used to enforce this (Fig. 44).

Kienbock's disease. This condition presents in young adults with pain and stiffness of the wrist caused by avascular fragmentation and collapse of the lunate. Radiographs show increased density.

4.5 Congenital hip dysplasia

Learning objectives

You should

● recognise the predisposing factors and clinical features of CDH

● describe the different types of management required for presentation at different ages.

Opportunities to examine babies for possible congenital dislocation of the hip (CDH) are available in postnatal wards, paediatric clinics, the paediatric orthopaedic service and general practice. Although the quoted incidence of CDH is only between one and two per 1000 live births, the consequences of missing a case are severe and distressing for the child and the parents.

Predisposing factors are:

- family history
- developmental factors — intrauterine malposition, breech presentation
- environmental factors — swaddling.

Clinical features

- **Listen** — positive family history, difficult birth
- **Look** — asymmetrical buttock creases. Short leg or Trendelenburg gait when standing. If bilateral there is a characteristic waddling gait
- **Feel** — the hip may be felt to relocate during manipulation
- **Move** — there is loss of full abduction of the hips in flexion, a 'click' or 'clunk' noise may be heard from the hip while changing a nappy.

If the diagnosis is not made until adult life, the presentation is of hip pain, resulting from secondary osteoarthritis, and the presence of a positive Trendelenburg sign.

Diagnosis

Although lack of hip abduction in flexion is the more common presenting feature, Ortolani's and Barlow's tests are usually carried out in the neonatal period (Fig. 45). In Ortolani's test a 'clunk' sound and the sensation of the hip relocating can be elicited while the flexed hip is gently manipulated into abduction. The sensation and sound are quite different from the physiological soft tissue 'click' often heard from the hip in the neonatal period.

Radiographs do not show the capital epiphysis in the first months of life but it can be visualised by ultrasound or arthrography. Radiographs at the age of 6 months, however, can be used to predict the position of the capital epiphysis and to measure the acetabular angle. Von Rosen views, ultrasound or arthrography are used to predict whether the joint is dislocated and to confirm reduction (Fig. 46).

Management

If the diagnosis is made in the first 2 months of life, then effective treatment can be instituted early. This involves holding the hips in abduction and flexion in a von Rosen splint (Fig. 47) or Pavlik harness.

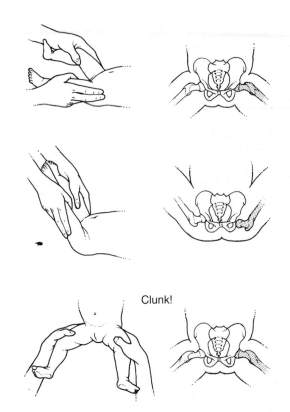

Clunk!

Fig. 45 Ortolani's test (see text for description).

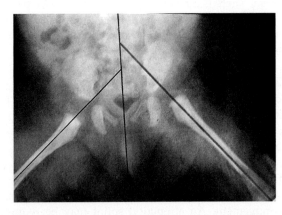

Fig. 46 A von Rosen view radiograph of the hips taken with the legs internally rotated. The long axis of the femur should point through the triradiate epiphysis if the hip is in joint, as on the right, but not if the hip is dislocated, as on the left.

After the age of 2 months, a period of traction and plaster immobilisation will be required.

By the age of 12 to 18 months, open reduction is necessary to remove limbus and capsule which may be blocking anatomical reduction. A subsequent derotation osteotomy is often required as the hip is only stable in the reduced position if fully internally rotated. A pelvic osteotomy to deepen the acetabulum (Salter's osteotomy) may also be necessary.

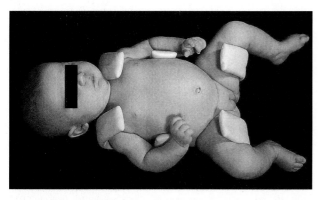

Fig. 47 A von Rosen splint used to keep the dislocated hip in the reduced position.

Complications

Complications arising from failure to make an early diagnosis include:

- persisting limp
- hip pain
- later osteoarthritis.

Complications that can occur as a result of treatment include:

- avascular necrosis of the femoral head
- recurrent dislocation.

4.6 Infection

Learning objectives

You should:

- be able to recognise the clinical features of infection in a bone or joint
- know how to begin appropriate urgent treatment.

Bone and joint infection in childhood, once a serious and common illness is now only rarely seen in westernised countries. Vigilance, however, is still important to ensure that a case is not missed, and the possibility of infection must always be considered in the differential diagnosis of any patient with joint pain or limp.

Acute osteitis

The metaphyseal area of a long bone is the usual site of acute osteitis and often the proximal tibia is the location. There may be a history of minor trauma to the area which causes a small haematoma. Bacteraemia from a remote infective source colonise this and produce an abscess, which may discharge onto the skin or, if the epi-

physis is within the joint capsule, into the joint itself, causing septic arthritis.

Clinical features

- **Listen** — there is intense pain at the site involved
- **Look** — the child is unwell with a pyrexia and sweating
- **Feel** — the infected area is tender, hot, swollen and red. A subperiosteal abscess may be palpable
- **Move** — any movement of the joint is resisted.

Diagnosis

Blood tests show positive blood cultures, elevated ESR (erythrocyte sedimentation rate) or plasma viscosity, and a polymorphonuclear leucocytosis. In later stages, radiographs will show periosteal elevation.

Management

Conservative treatment begins with elevation of the limb to reduce pain. When all investigations are under way, the 'best-guess' antibiotic can be commenced. This is usually a combination of fucidic acid and flucloxacillin, as the organism usually responsible is *Staphylococcus aureus*. Occasionally *Haemophilus influenzae* is isolated, in which case amoxycillin or cotrimoxazole are indicated. If the symptoms fail to settle, surgical exploration and drainage of the area is required.

Complications

- Brodie's abscess — an interosseus collection of pus which repeatedly becomes symptomatic
- chronic osteitis — characterised by sinus, sequestrum, involucrum and growth arrest.

Septic arthritis

A joint may become infected from adjacent osteitis, bacteraemia or a penetrating wound into the joint. Left untreated progressive bacterial destruction of the articular cartilage will occur.

Clinical features

The child is unwell and pyrexial. The joint is swollen, tender to touch and inflamed. Movement is resisted.

Diagnosis

White cell count, blood culture and plasma viscosity measurements are all required. Radiological examination is unlikely to be helpful.

Management

Early commencement of 'best-guess' antibiotics is necessary. Although *Staphylococcus aureus* is the most likely organism, gonococcal infection should not be forgotten. It is imperative that the joint is thoroughly washed out either by open operation or arthroscopically. Either way, joint fluid must be sent for bacteriological examination. Accessible joints can be treated by arthroscopy (see p. 119).

Complications

- secondary osteoarthritis
- spontaneous ankylosis
- chronic osteitis.

4.7 Talipes equinovarus

Learning objectives

You should:

- be able to distinguish postural TEV from fixed TEV
- know how to start conservative, corrective treatment for postural TEV.

Congenital (fixed) talipes equinovarus (TEV) in its severest form is an uncommon condition. There may be a positive family history. The condition is characterised by failure of development of the postero-medial muscles of the calf and also of the os calcis and forefoot.

A milder, more commonly seen, condition is postural TEV, which results from the position of the fetus in utero.

Clinical features

The affected foot is held in equinus and varus. In severe cases (structural TEV) the deformity cannot be corrected passively by manipulation (Fig. 48). There may be inter-

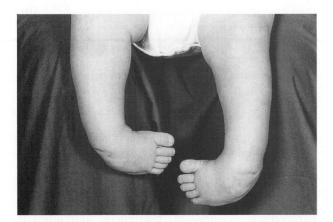

Fig. 48 Bilateral talipes equinovarus.

nal tibial torsion and forefoot adductus. The calf muscles seem small and the os calcis is underdeveloped.

Diagnosis

The diagnosis is easily made on clinical examination, but failure to start treatment promptly may compromise a satisfactory result.

Management

Within the first 6 weeks of life, daily manipulation of the foot can stretch out the deformity and this will be entirely effective in patients with pure postural TEV. More severe cases may require subsequent elastoplast strapping or plaster of Paris splinting.

If correction has not been achieved by the age of 6 months, a postero-medial release of the restraining ligaments and tendons should be considered. After the age of 5 years, bony abnormalities are established and a wedge of tarsal bones must be removed from the lateral side to enable the foot to be put in a plantigrade position on the ground.

Complications

- incomplete correction
- rocker-bottom foot — due to failure to correct the equinus hindfoot aspect of the deformity
- small foot — even when corrected there will still be loss of normal development of the foot.

4.8 Scoliosis

Learning objectives

You should:

- be able to describe the different types of scoliosis
- know the principles of radiological monitoring of a spinal curve.

Although uncommon, it is necessary to be able to recognise the presence of scoliosis, as missed cases may progress to produce severe cosmetic deformity. Scoliosis is excessive spinal curvature in a coronal plane. It can be classified as postural or structural. Structural scoliosis may have varying causes:

- idiopathic
- congenital
- neuromuscular
- miscellaneous.

Idiopathic scoliosis is the most common variety and it is more common in girls than in boys.

Clinical features

The cosmetic deformity of a thoracic curve, usually convex to the right, is reported as an incidental finding by the family. The degree of deformity becomes progressively severe during adolescence until growth ceases. Forward flexion exacerbates the deformity. In later stages, secondary osteoarthritic degeneration in the spine may cause pain and stiffness.

Diagnosis

Radiology confirms the diagnosis by showing the presence of rotated vertebrae. The degree of curve is classically measured as the angle between the end plates of the normal vertebrae above and below the abnormal section (Cobb's angle) (Fig. 49).

Management

Because cases only present rarely, it is best if management of all but the mildest curves is carried out in regional specialist spinal centres. Plaster of Paris immobilisation has been recommended for infantile idiopathic scoliosis but this condition may resolve spontaneously with time. The role of corrective orthoses has probably been overstated in the past and is now less popular.

Extensive corrective spinal surgery is carried out in progressive, severe disease with dramatic results but at the risk of the considerable complications of implant failure or even spinal cord damage.

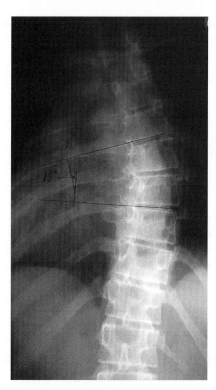

Fig. 49 A mild thoracic scoliosis with a Cobb's angle of 15°.

Complications

- progression of the curve and development of a rib hump
- secondary osteoarthritis
- cardiopulmonary embarrassment in progressive cases starting in infancy.

Self-assessment: questions

Multiple choice questions

1. The following are possible sequelae of acute osteitis:
   a. Looser's zones found on radiograph
   b. sequestrum formation
   c. septic arthritis
   d. fracture of the affected bone
   e. myositis ossificans

2. Talipes equinovarus:
   a. is associated with CDH
   b. necessitates tendon transfer in its management
   c. necessitates repeated and frequent reviews
   d. is associated with dislocating patellae
   e. certain types respond to simple manipulation and splinting

Extended matching items questions (EMIs)

1. Theme: Diagnosis

A Osgood–Schlatter's disease
B osteochondritis dissecans
C congenital hip dysplasia
D transient synovitis
E Perthes' disease
F bow legs
G flat feet
H knock-knee (genu valgum)
I in-toeing
J infective arthritis

Which diagnosis from the list above is most likely indicated by the clinical findings below:

1. Intermalleoli distance of 20 cm in a 4 year old.
2. Upper respiratory infection followed by pain and resistance to internal rotation of the hip.
3. Pain around the knee in an adolescent made worse by football.

2. Theme: Diagnosis

A Osgood–Schlatter's disease
B osteochondritis dissecans
C congenital hip dysplasia
D transient synovitis
E Perthes' disease
F bow legs
G flat feet
H knock-knee (genu valgum)
I in-toeing
J infective arthritis

Which diagnosis from the list above is most likely indicated by the clinical findings below:

1. Recurrent episode of pain on weight–bearing with evidence of progressive bone fragmentation on X-ray.
2. Intermittent pain and locking of the joint during normal movement in an adolescent.
3. Asymmetrical buttock creases and a block to full hip abduction in a 6-month-old baby.

Constructed response questions (CRQs)

CRQ 1

A teenage sportsman complains of pain in his left knee which has been getting worse since training. He had a similar episode last year but this has been getting worse now for three weeks and is causing limping. He has localised tenderness at the tibial tuberosity but no swelling or hotness.

a. What is the most likely diagnosis?
b. Of what group of conditions is this an example?
c. What radiological findings are associated with this condition?
d. What is the initial treatment?
e. How can this be enforced?

CRQ 2

You have been asked to examine a baby who has been born with a clicking hip.

a. What questions would you ask the parents about predisposing factors?
b. What clinical examination would you carry out?
c. The results of your clinical examination confirm a dislocatable hip on the left. How would you manage the baby at this stage?
d. Despite this treatment, you are not certain that the hip has remained reduced. When the infant is 9 months old you request an X-ray. What view would you ask for?
e. What other investigation would be helpful?

f. The hip is obviously still out of joint. Closed manipulation fails and surgery is indicated. What abnormalities might you expect to find during the operation?

Objective structured clinical examination questions (OSCEs)

OSCE 1

Study the clinical photograph of a 2-year-old child (see Fig. 50)

a. What abnormality of posture can you see?
b. What manoeuvre would you ask the child to carry out while you observe the feet and what would you expect to find in the majority of cases?
c. What is contributing to the appearance of the foot?
d. The parents are concerned that the child's shoes are wearing down quickly on the medial side. What could you suggest to help?

OSCE 2

Study the laboratory data presented below.

White cell count: elevated
CRP: elevated
ASO titre: normal

You have been asked to see a child admitted as an emergency with a painful hip on weight bearing. The results of previous investigations are available.

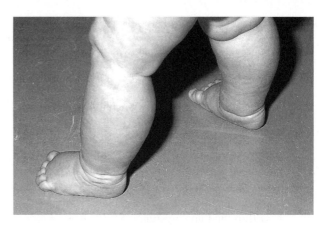

Fig. 50 Feet of a 2-year-old child.

a. The child is pyrexial with a temperature of 39.5°. What do you think is the most likely diagnosis at this stage?
b. What emergency procedure is indicated?
c. What is the most likely causative agent?
d. What would be the best-guess treatment to use?
e. What are the sequelae if this condition remains untreated?

Viva questions

1. Describe the investigations used to diagnose CDH.

2. Describe how you would examine and investigate a teenage girl presenting with scoliosis.

Self-assessment: answers

Multiple choice answers

1. a. **False.** Looser's zones are associated with osteomalacia.
   b. **True.** A portion of cortex may lose its blood supply as a result of the surrounding infection and become sequestrated as an island of dead bone.
   c. **True.** Osteitis in the metaphysis may spread to involve the adjacent joint, if the area of infection is within the joint capsule.
   d. **True.** The architecture of the infected bone is less strong than normal bone.
   e. **False.** Myositis ossificans is associated with calcification of an intramuscular haematoma and is, therefore, associated with fractures particularly around the elbow.

2. a. **True.**
   b. **False.** Initial management depends on manipulation and splintage. Later lengthening of the Achilles tendon and medial tendons is required.
   c. **True.**
   d. **False.**
   e. **True.** Postural talipes equinovarus responds well to simple manipulation and splinting while the more severe types associated with underdevelopment of the calf and os calcis usually require early surgery.

EMI answers

1. Theme: Diagnoses

1. H. Knock-knee (genu valgum) is common in children around the age of 4 years until it gradually corrects with growth.
2. D. Transient synovitis (irritable hip) may occur following an intercurrent infection. It causes a reactive joint effusion in the hip. The capacity of the hip joint is greatest in external rotation. Internal rotation tightens the joint capsule, compresses the joint fluid and increases pain.
3. A. Osgood–Schlatter's disease is a traction apophysitis of the tibial tuberosity. The bone in this growing area is partially avulsed by the patellar tendon so is more painful during resisted knee extension movements.

2. Theme: Diagnosis

1. E. Perthes' disease causes hip pain but can be differentiated from transient synovitis by X-ray changes showing patchy areas of avascular necrosis and eventually fragmentation and flattening in the femoral head.
2. B. Osteochondritis dissecans is characterised by separation of a portion of the intra-articular surface of the knee. The loose body formed causes mechanical locking of the knee by intermittently jamming between the joint surfaces during movement.
3. C. A dislocated hip in a baby causes a block to full abduction in flexion. It may subsequently reduce with a 'clunk' and then permit full abduction (positive Ortolani test).

CRQ answers

CRQ 1

a. Osgood–Schlatter's disease.
b. Osteochondritis.
c. Lateral radiograph will sometimes show elevation of a small portion of the tongue of the tibial apophysis or occasionally a separate ossicle.
d. Rest and lighter sports.
e. By a splint to maintain the leg in extension and prevent flexion.

CRQ 2

a. Family history
   Evidence of intrauterine malposition e.g. breech presentation
   Oligohydramnios.
b. Ortolani's test
   Barlow's test.
c. Abduction splint
   Pavlik harness.
d. A von Rosen view.
e. Ultrasound scan.
f. In-turned limbus
   Long ligamentum teres
   Underdeveloped acetabulum and a small femoral head
   Hourglass capsule from psoas tendon pressure.

OSCE answers

OSCE 1

a. Flat feet.
b. Ask the child to stand on tiptoes

The medial plantar arch should reform and the calcaneo-valgus deformity correct so that the heel lines up with the Achilles tendon.

c. A large medial fat pad in the plantar arch
    Ligamentous laxity around the ankle.
d. Wedged insoles
    Shoes with firm uppers
    A heel seat insert.

OSCE 2

a. Septic arthritis of the hip.
b. Open irrigation of the joint.
c. *Staphylococcus aureus.*
d. Flucloxacillin and Fucidin.
e. The septic arthritis may proceed to osteoitis of the hip with subsequent destruction of articular cartilage and the development of premature osteoarthritis.

Viva answers

1. The following investigations may be used to diagnose CDH. Before the age of 9 months, the capital epiphysis is not visible radiologically but the cartilaginous head can be outlined by the intra-articular injection of contrast medium. This will show the configuration of the joint and whether the head is subluxated or not. A less invasive investigation is an ultrasound scan, but the findings are difficult to interpret.

    In a child over the age of 9 months, a plain X-ray of the pelvis may indicate whether the head of the femur is in joint or not. The acetabular angle may indicate whether the acetabulum is likely to be dysplastic or normal, and von Rosen views are used to predict whether the joint is dislocated.

2. The patient's spine must be observed from behind and any scoliosis or rib hump noted. Asking the patient to touch the toes will exacerbate the deformity. Postural scoliosis resulting from leg length inequality is neutralised when the patient's back is observed when sitting down. Radiographs of the spine are used to visualise the deformity and calculate the angle of the curve (Cobb's angle).

5 Backache and neckache

Chapter overview

This chapter describes both cervical spine and lumbar spine problems and shows how the methods of differentiation of mechanical pain from radicular pain due to nerve root compression are similar for both locations. The important diagnoses of prolapsed intervertebral disc and compression of the cervical lower spinal cord and cauda equina are described. There is a brief description of spondylolisthesis, ankylosing spondylitis and spinal column problems caused by tumour or infection.

5.1 Clinical examination

Learning objectives

You should:

- be able to carry out a local examination of the cervical and lumbar spine looking for abnormalities and limited range of movement
- be able to carry out a neurological examination of the arms and legs to determine symptoms caused by dysfunction of any particular nerve root
- know the pattern of dermatome distribution in the limbs and which myotomes are associated with different movements.

Examination includes both a local examination of the axial skeleton and a neurological examination of the limbs.

Local examination

Cervical spine. Observe any abnormal posture of the neck and the presence of muscle spasm. Localised tenderness can be elicited with one-finger palpation of the vertebral spines. Full range of flexion, extension, lateral flexion and rotation should be attempted.

Lumbar spine. The patient should be examined standing. The lumbar spine is observed from behind and from the sides for loss of the normal lumbar lordosis and the presence of paravertebral muscle spasm. Full range of spinal extension, flexion and lateral flexion and rotation should be elicited. Pain associated with spinal extension classically suggests facet joint or posterior column pathology, while pain associated with forward flexion suggests intervertebral disc or anterior column pathology. A patient with sciatica often shows a scoliosis to one side in an attempt to relieve traction on the compressed nerve root.

Neurological examination

In cervical spondylosis and brachalgia, observation of the arms may show muscle wasting. Areas of altered sensation should be sought by careful examination in each dermatome. Muscle weakness and diminished reflexes may be present.

Patients with sciatica should be examined lying supine. The legs are observed for muscle wasting. Sensation is examined in a dermatome pattern and weakness or diminished reflexes looked for. Exacerbation of pain by straight leg raising should be sought in both legs.

With the patient prone, sensation in the sacral dermatome can be tested by examining perianal sensation. In all cases of disc prolapses, a rectal examination should be carried out to detect any loss of normal anal tone suggestive of a central disc prolapse. The femoral nerve stretch test, which involves extension of the hip, can also be attempted in this position.

In some cases, additional examination for inappropriate signs associated with functional overlay may be appropriate.

5.2 Mechanical back pain

Learning objectives

You should:

- know which features of the history and clinical examination indicate that symptoms are mechanical (arising in joints, muscles and ligaments) rather than neurogenic (due to nerve root involvement)

Backache is the cause of many lost hours from work and many visits to orthopaedic clinics. The vast majority will be due to mechanical backache and only a small minority will result from prolapse of an intervertebral disc or other specific abnormality.

Clinical features
Patients complain of acute onset of back pain, which may radiate to the buttock and knee on the affected side but not any further. There is a history of some heavy lifting or of a long period of sitting with the spine in a flexed position as when driving a car. There are no neurological deficits on examination of the legs.

Diagnosis
Radiological examination is unremarkable but an incidental finding of some disc space narrowing and an occasional osteophyte may be seen. However, the radiographs must be carefully scrutinised for the presence of an occult tumour, usually a metastasis from a primary bronchial, breast or renal tumour. Any questionable areas must be further investigated by CT scan.

Management
Management of mechanical back pain involves:

- rest from heavy work (but not from normal daily activities) until the initial symptoms settle
- analgesics
- heat and gradual spinal extension exercises
- lumbosacral support (this sometimes helps)
- learning correct posture and lifting techniques.

Surgery for back pain is usually inappropriate.

Complications
Patients' interpretation of their symptoms may be complicated by:

- functional overlay
- an outstanding claim for compensation.

5.3 Nerve root entrapment

Learning objectives

You should:

- be able to obtain an accurate history of nerve root compression and be able to deduce from this and subsequent examination which nerve root is affected
- describe the investigations used to detect a prolapsed intervertebral disc
- know how to differentiate this from bony nerve root entrapment and spondylolisthesis.

Prolapsed intervertebral disc

The lumbar disc is composed of the annulus fibrosus, which surrounds the nucleus pulposus. As the disc loses its water content as part of the degenerating process, the annulus fibrosus softens, allowing the nucleus pulposus to bulge posteriorly towards the spinal canal. Compression of a nerve root may result. Extruded fragments of degenerate disc may become lodged in a nerve root canal (Fig. 51).

Clinical features
Patients complain of the local effects of pain in the back and of lower motor neurone symptoms in the legs.

- **Listen** — pain is more severe in the leg than the back and radiates to below the knee. In classical sciatica, pain is felt on the dorsum of the foot in the dermatome distribution of L5 or S1
- **Look** — examination of the spine shows spasm in the paravertebral muscles, loss of lumbar lordosis and possibly scoliosis at the involved level
- **Feel** — sensation may be diminished in the dermatomes supplied by the involved spinal nerves (Fig. 52)
- **Move** — straight leg raising is diminished, tendon reflexes may be absent or depressed and power is weakened in the appropriate myotomes.

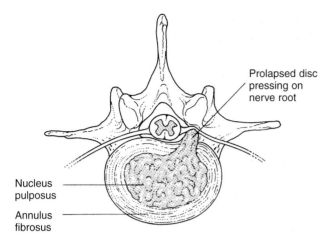

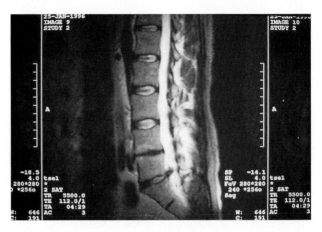

Fig. 53 MRI scan showing posterior prolapse of the disc at L5/S1.

Fig. 51 Pressure on a lumbar nerve root due to herniation of the nucleus pulposus through the annulus fibrosus of the intervertebral disc.

Management

Cauda equina lesions need emergency decompression if permanent bowel and bladder dysfunction are to be avoided.

The majority of the remaining cases, however, will settle as the disc shrinks again with a period of reduced activity. A caudal epidural injection of steroid and local anaesthetic may be used for temporary relief. Disc excision by fenestration of the lamina is required for patients for whom conservative treatment fails or who are in severe pain. Microdiscectomy under operating microscope control may be used to minimise the morbidity associated with more extensive surgery.

Complications

- persisting back pain
- interfacet joint degeneration
- arachnoiditis
- missed diagnosis of spinal tumour.

Other causes of nerve root entrapment

Two conditions must be considered:

- bony nerve root entrapment
- spinal stenosis.

Bony nerve root entrapment

In bony nerve root entrapment there is impingement of osteophytes on a spinal nerve root in the root canal (Fig. 54).

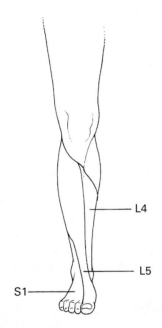

Fig. 52 Dermatome distribution in the leg.

Patients with a central disc prolapse may develop urinary retention and a neurogenic bladder from compression of the sacral nerve roots of the cauda equina. Physical examination shows loss of anal tone and perianal anaesthesia.

Diagnosis

An MRI scan will show the nerve roots and the site of compression. L4/5 and L5/S1 are the most frequently affected levels for disc prolapse (Fig. 53). A CT or radiculogram using an intrathecal injection of radioopaque contrast material may also visualise the site of root compression.

Clinical features

Usually the patient is older than those with prolapsed intervertebral disc. There is pain in a dermatome distribution but, in addition, there is an ill-defined pain from osteoarthritic degeneration of the facet joints. Pain is

61

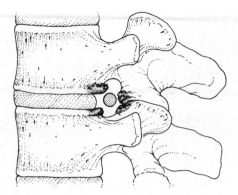

Fig. 54 In bony nerve root entrapment the spinal nerve is compressed by osteophytosis from the adjacent joints.

usually less severe than with prolapsed intervertebral discs.

Diagnosis
An MRI is the most useful investigation for identifying the site of nerve root compression.

Management
Simple methods of local pain relief are used initially. In selected patients decompression of the nerve root canal may help.

Spinal stenosis

Even a mild degree of osteophytosis will cause impingement in the spinal canal if this is already narrow. In such patients, a minor degree of congestion in the spinal canal produces symptoms.

Clinical features
Exercise-induced pain in the buttocks and legs, especially when walking, gives rise to the description of symptoms as 'spinal claudication'. Symptoms are exacerbated by standing and extending the spine and relieved by sitting and flexing.

Diagnosis
A narrow spinal canal can be diagnosed from the MRI scan.

Management
Weight reduction and limitation of activities that involve extension of the spine may help. A multilevel decompression is required in some patients to decompress the spinal cord.

Complications

- arachnoiditis
- missed diagnosis of spinal tumour
- spinal instability after laminectomy.

5.4 Spondylolisthesis

Learning objectives

You should:

- be able to list different types of spondylolisthesis
- recognise diagnostic features in the history
- understand the principles of management.

There are several causes of spondylolisthesis, but the underlying abnormality in them all is a forward slip of one vertebra on another, usually of L5 on S1, caused by a defect in the pars interarticularis, the part of the vertebrae between the superior and inferior articular facets.

Different types of spondylolisthesis include:

- dysplastic
- isthmic
- degenerative
- traumatic
- pathological.

The isthmic type is the most common.

Clinical features
The patient is classically a young active person who complains of low back pain radiating to the buttocks. On examination, a step may be felt in the tender area at the base of the lumbar spine.

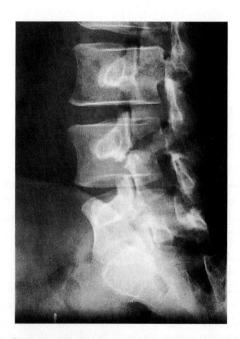

Fig. 55 Oblique radiograph of a 20 year old showing a spondylolysis at L4 but without any forward slip of the vertebrae.

Diagnosis

Oblique radiographs are required and show either a lucent area in the pars interarticularis or a slip of one vertebrae on the other at this point (Fig. 55).

Management

Rest during acute episodes, a spinal support and extension exercises may all help. A lumbo-sacral fusion is indicated for progressive slips.

Complications

- persisting back pain.

5.5 Ankylosing spondylitis

Learning objectives

You should:

- be able to recognise the radiological features of ankylosing spondylitis.

This uncommon inflammatory disease affecting young males between the ages of 15 and 30 years is part of a complex multijoint disease.

Clinical features

There is stiffness in the lumbar spine and low back pain. There is often a positive family history. In severe cases, gross flexion and fusion of the entire spinal column is seen and chest wall expansion becomes limited. Other joints may also be involved.

Diagnosis

Radiological examination in patients presenting early shows fusion of the sacro-iliac joints. Eventually the characteristic 'bamboo spine' develops (Fig. 56).

Management

Rest and non-steroidal anti-inflammatory analgesics followed by mobilisation are aimed to keep the patient's spine as mobile and comfortable as possible.

Complications

In addition to the natural progression of the conditions, other systems can be involved:

- colitis
- uveitis.

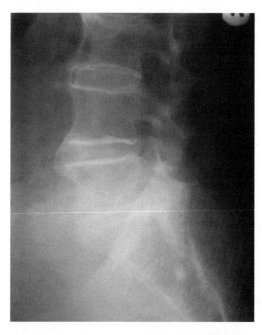

Fig. 56 Calcification of the soft tissues in ankylosing spondylosis producing the characteristic 'bamboo spine'.

5.6 Tumours and infection

Learning objectives

You should:

- be able to list the common sites of primary tumours which metastasise to bone

- list the spinal canal tumours which may cause spinal cord or nerve root compression

- indicate the principles of management of infection in the spinal column.

Tumours

Secondary metastatic tumour must always be considered in cases of undiagnosed pain in the back. The usual sites for the primary tumour are:

- prostate
- breast
- kidney
- bronchus.

Osteoblastoma, giant cell tumour and multiple myeloma are examples of primary bone tumours that may be seen; primary spinal canal tumours such as neurofibroma and meningioma are also occasionally encountered.

Clinical features

There is localised back pain, possibly of long duration, that is severe and unrelenting. Root signs may be absent.

Diagnosis

Metastatic deposits are seen as lytic lesions on plain radiographs and are usually sited in the pedicles of the vertebrae. Unlike the other metastases, prostatic metastases can also be sclerotic. A myelogram or MRI scan will demonstrate a spinal canal tumour (Fig. 57).

Management

Management involves decompression and radiotherapy.

Complications

● vertebral collapse
● nerve root invasion
● spinal cord compression resulting in paraplegia.

Infection

Patients with acute infective discitis are usually adolescents or immunosuppressed. Blood-borne infection may involve the disc and an adjacent vertebra. Tuberculous discitis is rare in westernised countries.

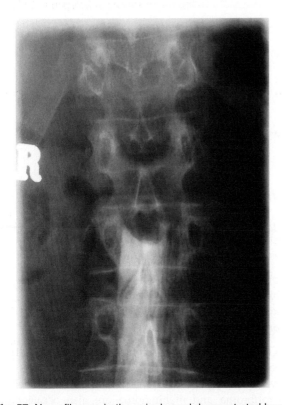

Fig. 57 Neurofibroma in the spinal canal demonstrated by a lumbar myelogram.

Clinical features

Severe back pain is present but pyrexia may be absent. Plasma viscosity and ESR are elevated, but the expected leucocytosis is absent.

Diagnosis

A needle biopsy will retrieve pus for bacteriological examination but sometimes an open biopsy is required.

Management

High doses of 'best-guess' antibiotics are required while laboratory results are awaited. Spontaneous intervertebral fusion tends to occur when the infection is cured.

Complications

● kyphosis
● spinal cord compression.

5.7 Cervical spondylosis

Learning objectives

You should:

● be able to describe the pathophysiology of cervical spondylosis

● understand how this may cause mechanical neck pain, radiculopathy or myelopathy

● be able to examine the upper limb to determine the site of nerve root compression

● know the principles of investigation and management of cervical spondylosis.

Cervical spondylosis is the name given to chronic degeneration of the cervical spine involving the intervertebral discs and the ligamentous and osseous structures associated with them. It can be responsible for a spectrum of problems ranging from mechanical neck pain to cervical cord compression.

Figure 58 shows the normal anatomical relationship between the intervertebral foramen and the two adjacent vertebral bodies. The intervertebral disc lies anteriorly and the facet joint posteriorly. The emerging nerve root is shown end-on.

Figure 59 shows how degeneration of the cervical disc and the associated osteophyte formation around the vertebral end-plates can press on the nerve roots and on the spinal cord itself. With increasing age, the intervertebral disc loses its water content and shrinks. In doing so, its height decreases and movement at the interfacet joints is altered. Osteoarthritic degeneration of these joints can then occur (Fig. 60).

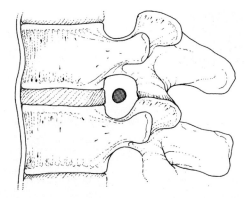

Fig. 58 Normal anatomical relationship between the intervertebral foramen and the two adjacent vertebral bodies. The nerve root exits through the intervertebral foramen.

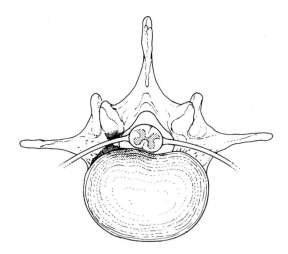

Fig. 59 Compression of the spinal nerve root and the cord itself following cervical disc degeneration and associated osteophytosis of the adjacent joints.

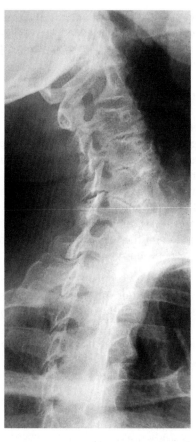

Fig. 60 Oblique view of the cervical spine showing osteophytes narrowing the intervertebral foramen at C5/6 especially.

Radiological evidence of degeneration of the cervical discs is seen in 50% of the population over the age of 50 and 75% of the population over the age of 65. However, this may be an incidental finding and the patient may have no symptoms. However, if the spinal canal measures less than 13 mm on CT scan, its contents are more at risk from compression and symptoms will ensue.

Acute cervical disc prolapse is uncommon (unlike lumbar disc prolapse). Severe trauma to the cervical spine is necessary to produce this injury. When it occurs, it is usually in young patients. More commonly, cervical disc herniation is an acute-on-chronic phenomenon seen in older patients.

The following syndromes are associated with cervical spondylosis:

- mechanical neck pain
- radiculopathy
- myelopathy.

Mechanical neck pain

This is the most common presentation of cervical spondylosis.

Clinical features

- **Listen** — neck pain and associated muscle spasm originating from facet joint degeneration radiates to the occiput and shoulders but there is no pain radiating down the arms. Symptoms are worse with activity and in the morning.
- **Look** — the neck may be held to one side
- **Feel** — localised tenderness in the paravertebral muscles
- **Move** — there is only slightly decreased range of movement in the cervical spine because 50% of rotation takes place at the atlanto-axial joint, which is not usually affected.

Management

The majority of patients respond to simple treatment. A cervical collar may provide a comfortable support but little more. Heat treatment, cervical traction and non-steroidal anti-inflammatory analgesics may all be tried. In the majority of patients, however, the symptoms will settle with time.

Radiculopathy

Clinical features
Radiculopathy is the name given to the symptoms produced when a nerve root is compressed by or stretched around an osteophyte or prolapsed intervertebral disc. The settling down of one facet joint on another following shrinking of the intervertebral disc causes narrowing of the intervertebral foramen, which also contributes to compression on the nerve root. Patients complain of lower motor neurone symptoms in the arms.

- **Listen** — patients complain of pain in a dermatome distribution in the arm (brachalgia) (Fig. 61)
- **Look** — wasting of the muscles in the myotome involved
- **Feel** — there may also be decreased sensation in the appropriate dermatome
- **Move** — Muscle weakness and depressed tendon reflexes.

Diagnosis
An oblique radiograph will show encroachment of osteophytes at the intervertebral foramen. More detail will be gained by an MRI scan (Fig. 62).

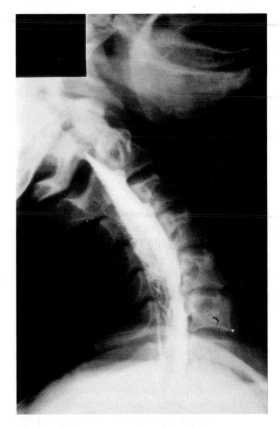

Fig. 62 Cervical myelogram showing indentation of the contrast medium by osteophytes at C5/6.

Management

Conservative
- cervical traction
- analgesics.

Surgical. When conservative measures fail, decompression of the compressed nerve root by excising the adjacent osteophytes (see below) can be carried out electively.

Myelopathy

Clinical features
Pressure from a protruding cervical disc or the associated osteophytes may cause pressure on the spinal cord itself. This is present when patients exhibit upper motor neurone signs in the legs and lower motor neurone signs in the arms. Patients complain of the insidious onset of weakness, clumsiness and dysaesthesia in the hand and may develop difficulty in walking because of spasticity and weakness of the lower limbs and retention of urine due to a neurogenic bladder.

Diagnosis
MRI.

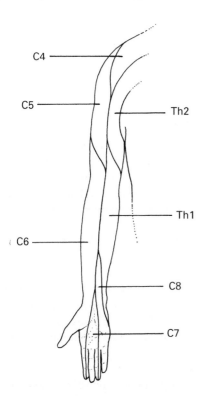

Fig. 61 Pattern of dermatomes in the upper limb.

Management

Surgical decompression is urgently required for patients who develop symptoms of cervical cord compression. In the classic operation of anterior cervical decompression, a core of vertebral body and intervertebral disc is drilled out and prolapsed material removed. Osteophytes can be trimmed through the same approach to decompress the spinal cord and the nerve root canal.

Self-assessment: questions

Multiple choice questions

1. In a 40-year-old patient with a prolapsed intervertebral disc affecting S1 root, the following signs and symptoms are classically found:
   a. Limited straight leg raising in the affected leg
   b. Absent knee jerk
   c. Absent ankle jerk
   d. Weakness of extensor hallucis longus
   e. Weakness of plantar flexion of the ankle

2. In cervical spondylosis:
   a. The majority of patients respond to conservative treatment
   b. Pressure on a cervical nerve root causes upper motor neurone signs to be present in the arms
   c. Assessment of the lower motor neurone deficits helps to identify the level of the cervical lesion
   d. Wasting of the interossei muscles in the hand suggests a C5/6 disc prolapse
   e. Unlike a prolapsed lumbar intervertebral disc, a prolapsed cervical disc does not merit surgical intervention

Extended matching items questions (EMIs)

1. Theme: Pathology

A   S1 nerve root entrapment
B   spondylolisthesis
C   central cord compression
D   T1 root entrapment
E   C 5/6 root entrapment
F   L3 root compression on the left
G   infection in body of L5
H   spinal tumour
I   cauda equina lesion
J   L3 root compression on the right side

Match the clinical presentations below to the most appropriate pathology listed above:

1. Neck pain and wasting of the interossei muscles in the hand.
2. Depressed right knee-jerk reflex and weakness of knee extension.
3. Pain shooting from the back down the side of the leg to the lateral side of the foot.

2. Theme: Pathology
A   S1 nerve root entrapment
B   spondylolisthesis
C   central cord compression
D   T1 root entrapment
E   C 5/6 root entrapment
F   L3 root compression on the left
G   infection in an intervertebral disc
H   spinal tumour
I   cauda equina lesion
J   L3 root compression on the right side

Match the clinical presentations below to the most appropriate pathology listed above:

1. Back pain in a 60-year-old without radiation associated with pyrexia, high white cell count and 'hot spot' on bone scan.
2. Bilateral leg pain with back pain and urinary retention.
3. Loss of ankle jerk on examination.

Constructed response questions (CRQs)

CRQ 1

A 58-year-old man consults you complaining of a 4-week history of pain in the back of his neck experienced down the outside of the same arm into the hand, thumb and index fingers.

a. What dermatome distribution is being described?
b. What physical finding would you expect to find on examining this area?
c. You continue your examination of myotomes. Which movement would you expect to be weak?
d. You proceed to examination of the reflexes. Which reflex would you expect to be diminished?
e. You decide to X-ray the patient's neck. What views would you ask for and why?

CRQ 2

A 40-year-old offshore worker injures his back while lifting heavy weights. He is seen by the medic on the oil rig and a diagnosis of mechanical back pain is made. There are no neurological symptoms.

a. What would be the appropriate management at this stage?
b. He subsequently arrives home and attends your surgery. What would you expect to find when you examine his back?

c. In addition he tells you that there is now pain radiating down the legs to the heel and lateral sides of both feet. Which dermatome is he describing?
d. What is the significance of this bilateral symptom?
e. What else must you examine or ask at this stage?
f. What is the emergency management of this?

Objective structured clinical examination questions (OSCEs)

OSCE 1

Study the diagram of a prolapsed invertebral disc (Fig. 63).

a. Name the portions indicated by the lines.
b. What investigation could be used to show the lesion like this?
c. What is the route of approach for decompression and excision of the prolapsed disc?

OSCE 2

> A 70-year-old patient complains of low back pain which has been going on for some time but has been more intense for the last two weeks. Plain X-rays show minor degenerative changes only (Fig. 64).

a. What is the main finding on the bone scan?
b. What three possible conditions could cause this finding?
c. The patient also complains of urinary outflow obstruction. Blood tests reveal an elevate prostatic specific antigen. What is the most likely diagnosis now?
d. How would you confirm this?

Viva questions

1. Differentiate the radiological features of spondylolysis from spondylolisthesis.

2. In a patient complaining of backache and sciatica describe the features that are usually thought to be inappropriate clinical findings and indicative of functional overlay.

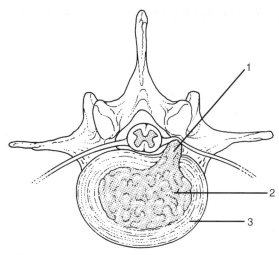

Fig. 63

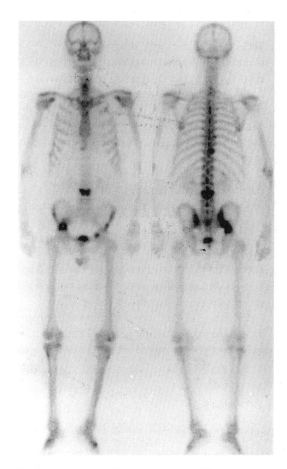

Fig. 64 Bone scan of a 70-year-old man with lower back pain. (Courtesy of Dr N. Kennedy, Nuclear Medicine Unit, Ninewells Hospital and Medical School, Dundee.)

Self-assessment: answers

Multiple choice answers

1. a. **True.** Symptoms from S1 nerve root compression are exacerbated by traction on the nerve to which this root contributes. Stretching the sciatic nerve by flexing the hip with the knee fully extended, therefore, exacerbates the symptoms.
   b. **False.** The knee jerk is supplied by nerve roots L3 and 4. The ankle jerk is supplied by S1.
   c. **True.** The ankle jerk is absent as it is supplied by S1.
   d. **False.** Extensor hallucis longus is supplied by L5 and is, therefore, functioning.
   e. **True.** Plantar flexion of the ankle is controlled by S1 and is, therefore, weak.

2. a. **True.** In most patients, simple analgesics, heat, rest and sometimes longitudinal traction will relieve symptoms of cervical spondylosis.
   b. **False.** Pressure on a nerve root produces lower motor neurone signs, but if the cervical cord is compressed in the spondylitic process then upper motor neurone signs may be present in the lower limbs.
   c. **True.** The pain and paraesthesia in a particular dermatome will help to elicit the level of the cervical nerve root compression. The neurological level can be confirmed by looking for weakness or loss of tendon reflexes in the appropriate myotome.
   d. **False.** The interossei muscles are supplied by the T1 root and are, therefore, weak or wasted when the compression is at this level.
   e. **False.** Surgical decompression at the appropriate level is required in the presence of unremitting pain, progressive motor weakness or evidence of cord compression.

EMI answers

1. Theme: Pathology

1. D. The first thoracic nerve root controls the interossei. Wasting of these muscles is eventually seen in T1 root entrapment.
2. J. The knee jerk reflex and knee extension are both usually innovated by the third lumbar spinal nerve root.
3. A. The first sacral nerve root dermatome extends in this distribution.

2. Theme: Pathology

1. G. A septic discitis will produce reactive hyperaemia in the adjacent vertebral body, which will show as an area of increased isotope uptake on the bone scan.
2. I. A central disc prolapse at the L5/S1 level may cause cauda equina compression and a neurogenic bladder. Bilateral S1 dermatome signs are a warning feature.
3. A. The ankle jerk reflex is controlled by the first sacral nerve root.

CRQ answers

CRQ 1

a. C6.
b. Diminished touch sensation.
c. Wrist dorsi flexion and elbow flexion.
d. Supinator reflex.
e. An oblique view of the cervical spine gives the clearest view of the intervertebral (neural) foramena. Osteophyte formation here will show as a 'figure of 8' deformity indicating that there is nerve root compression.

CRQ 2

a. Early return to normal activities. Rest from heavy work, and analgesia until symptoms subside.
b. Muscle spasm
   Scolosis
   Paravertebral tenderness
   Restriction of lumbar spine movement.
c. S1.
d. It suggests central disc prolapse causing cauda equina compression.
e. The patient may have altered perineal sensation and urinary retention.
f. Urinary catheterisation
   Emergency MRI scan
   Neurosurgery to decompress the nerve roots and cauda equina.

OSCE answers

OSCE 1

a. 1. Prolapsing disc
   2. Nucleus pulposus
   3. Annulus fibrosus

b. MRI scan.
c. Fenestration of the lamina to gain access for excision of the prolapsed disc.

OSCE 2

a. Increased uptake of radioactive technitium in the third lumbar vertebra.
b. Vertebral body crush fracture
   Vertebral body or disc infection
   Secondary deposit in a vertebral body.
c. Secondary deposit from prostatic carcinoma.
d. Core biopsy from the lesion under X-ray control to get a histological diagnosis.

Viva answers

1. An oblique radiograph of the lumbar spine in spondylolysis will show a radiolucent defect across the pars interarticularis. When present, this finding appears like a collar on a bony shape resembling a 'Scottie dog'. In patients where a slip has occurred (spondylolisthesis) at this area, there will be a step in the vertebral alignment between two adjacent vertebral bodies as one has slipped forward on the other.

2. Inappropriate clinical findings indicative of functional overlay include exacerbation of pain by axial loading of the skeleton, pain experienced by hip flexion but without the knee in extension and the ability to sit forwards on the examination couch while the legs are still fully extended.

6 Shoulder and elbow disorders

Chapter overview

Both the elbow and shoulder joint are relatively subcutaneous, so that during palpation it is possible to acquire quite a detailed picture of any pathology and relate it to a knowledge of the underlying anatomy. Shoulder pain is usually associated with loss of full range of movement but it is necessary to determine whether this is the result of inflammation, degeneration or tears in the rotator cuff or because of inflammation or degenerative changes in the joint. Rheumatoid arthritis (RA) is commonly seen in the upper limb and may eventually require surgery. A variety of operative procedures are available and the indications and limitations of each should be known.

Anterior dislocations of the shoulder are common presentations to the Accident and Emergency department but it is important not to miss the less common posterior dislocation. Patients who have had multiple dislocations are a special group and often need surgical management. Soft tissue problems around the elbow are a common presentation in General Practice where they can often be reliably diagnosed and treated.

6.1 Clinical examination

Learning objectives

You should:

- be able to relate your clinical examination to your knowledge of the underlying anatomy
- practice the 'listen, look, feel and move' approach to examination.

Examination of the shoulder and elbow provides plenty of opportunity to exercise the routine of 'listen, look, feel and move'.

Shoulder

Listen. Is there a history of trauma or gradual onset of symptoms? Which movements aggravate the symptoms or are impossible? Can the patient reach to the back of the head and the buttock?

Look. With the patient suitably undressed, the shoulders can be observed from all sides and compared. It is helpful to sit the patient down and observe the shoulders from above as well as from the front and sides. Loss of normal lateral contour is indicative of a dislocation of the shoulder or wasting of the deltoid. Scars, swelling and inflammation can also be looked for.

Feel. Bony outlines of the pectoral girdle can be felt, beginning at the sternoclavicular joint, continuing along the clavicle to the acromioclavicular joint and tracing around the point of the acromion along the spine of the scapula. Finally the angle of the scapula can be palpated. The upper humerus and tuberosities may be felt in thin people. Tenderness over the joints can be noted.

Move. The full extent of flexion and extension is observed. When assessing abduction, the angle of the scapula should be palpated to determine how much abduction is true glenohumeral movement and how much is scapulothoracic rotation. With the elbows tucked into the sides, external rotation and internal rotation can be noted. Because the abdomen gets in the way of internal rotation, this movement can be further assessed by observing how far the patient can reach up their back with each hand.

Elbow

Listen. Did the onset follow a particular activity or injury? Are other joints similarly painful? Can the elbow stretch out and the hand be brought to the mouth?

Look. An effusion in the elbow and swelling of the olecranon bursa are easily seen at the elbow. Rheumatoid nodules over the olecranon are a common finding.

Feel. The bony prominences of the medial and lateral epicondyles and of the olecranon are readily palpable and form the points of an equilateral triangle. The radial head can be palpated and during pronation and supination of the forearm, crepitus may be felt here by the examining thumb.

Move. Any loss of full extension of the elbow can be measured and the range of flexion noted. Supination and pronation must be examined with the elbows stabilised against the chest wall to eliminate any contributory movements from the shoulder. Varus or valgus laxity of the elbow should be sought.

6.2 Shoulder disorders

Learning objectives

You should:

- be able to recognise and treat acute symptoms of supraspinatus tendinitis
- be able to differentiate subacromial impingement from rotator cuff tear
- be able to recognise the features of shoulder instability
- know a procedure to reduce an anterior dislocation of the shoulder.

Shoulder pain

Pain in the shoulder is a common complaint. It may be referred pain from the cervical vertebrae, radicular pain from cervical nerve root entrapment or intrinsic pain caused by specific pathology in the shoulder joint itself.

Acute supraspinatus tendinitis

This condition is seen in early middle age and occurs commonly. Inflammation of the supraspinatus muscle in the rotator cuff produces a swollen area on the rotator cuff which becomes squashed beneath the acromion during abduction.

Clinical features

- **Listen** — there is sometimes a history of unaccustomed heavy use of the shoulder prior to the onset of symptoms
- **Look** — patients prefer to keep the shoulder still
- **Feel** — there is tenderness over the anterior rotator cuff
- **Move** — initially abduction is comfortable, but between 30 and 60° it becomes painful; beyond 60, however, when the inflamed portion of the rotator cuff advances beyond the tight area beneath the acromion, pain is relieved.

Diagnosis

Radiological examination occasionally may show the presence of calcification in the supraspinatus tendon. The diagnosis is then 'acute calcific tendinitis', which is excruciatingly painful, unresponsive to analgesia, but relieved by 'needling' the deposit while injecting a steroid.

Management

Rest and non-steroidal analgesics are the first line of management. If symptoms are very severe or persistent, local infiltration of hydrocortisone and local anaesthetic into the subacromial bursa produces dramatic relief (Fig. 65).

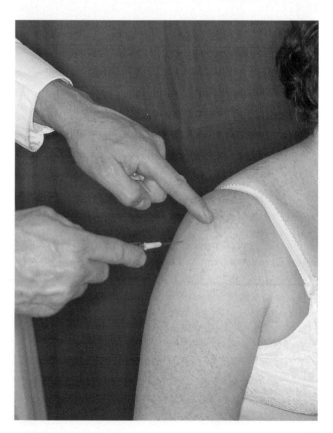

Fig. 65 The subacromial bursa can be injected from the lateral side as shown or anteriorly. The needle is passed under the acromion into the bursa and not into the rotator cuff itself.

Complications

- intratendonous injection with steroids may cause a tear in the rotator cuff.

Subacromial impingement

In older patients (40–60 years) there is chronic thickening of the rotator cuff from repeated 'wear and tear'. Associated with this may be arthritic degeneration of the acromioclavicular joint with osteophytes causing further impingement on the rotator cuff.

Clinical features

Patients present with similar symptoms and signs to those with supraspinatus tendinitis, but:

- **Listen** — there is a long history of repeated episodes of shoulder pain. Reaching upwards with the arm exacerbates the pain
- **Look** — patients tend to shrug the shoulder rather than abduct it
- **Feel** — there is tenderness over the rotator cuff
- **Move** — painful abduction can be demonstrated.

Management

This chronic impingement of a thickened rotator cuff in a narrowed subacromial space will not respond to anti-inflammatory agents and requires more space to be made by subacromial decompression of the rotator cuff by arthroscopic acromioplasty or open procedure may be required including acromioclavicular joint excision.

Complications

- rotator cuff tear.

Rotator cuff tear

Rotator cuff tears may be acute or degenerative, full thickness or partial thickness. Severe injuries to the shoulder in a young person produce an acute tear, but in an elderly person a trivial injury may be sufficient to produce an acute tear in a degenerative rotator cuff.

Clinical features

There is pain on attempting to move the shoulder. In full thickness tears, active movement is impossible. Initiation of abduction, particularly, is absent, but further abduction is possible by the action of the deltoid. In partial thickness tears, movement is possible but there is pain and weakness.

Diagnosis

An arthrogram (Fig. 66) or MRI scan will show the defect on the rotator cuff.

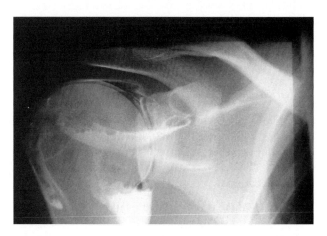

Fig. 66 Arthrogram of the shoulder showing a partial thickness tear of the rotator cuff.

Management

In the young person, an acute rotator cuff tear can be treated by surgical repair. In the elderly, degenerative changes make repair unsuccessful, but a course of heat treatment until symptoms settle followed by strengthening exercises over a full range of movement will produce an acceptable result.

Complications

- shoulder stiffness — disuse of the shoulder for whatever reason results in shrinking of the capsule and loss of movement in all directions.

Frozen shoulder

Idiopathic adhesive capsulitis (frozen shoulder) may follow any minor trauma but may be caused by an autoimmune reaction in the rotator cuff.

Clinical features

Initially a painful restriction of movement in all directions followed by marked stiffness (frozen) lasting up to 12 months. Some movement gradually returns

Management

Analgesics, physiotherapy and manipulation under anaesthesia are each used in the various stages of this condition.

Sporting shoulder injuries

Dislocations and fractures of the shoulder can occur particularly in those involved in sports.

Dislocations can be:

- anterior
- posterior

- inferior (luxatio erecta — very rare)
- associated with a fracture
- recurrent.

Anterior dislocation

This injury occurs with an abduction and extension force on the shoulder (Fig. 67). It is associated with falls and with sports.

Clinical features

- **Listen** — there is a history of a fall or a twisting injury of the shoulder
- **Look** — the affected shoulder appears flatter than normal on the lateral aspect. The tip of the acromion is prominent and is in line with the lateral epicondyle of the elbow giving a 'squared off' appearance to the shoulder on the affected side
- **Feel** — the humeral head may be palpable anteriorly. Loss of sensation on the 'badge-patch' area must be sought, as if present it denotes damage to the axillary nerve at the humeral neck.
- **Move** — normal shoulder movements are impossible.

Diagnosis

The diagnosis is usually obvious clinically but a radiograph should be taken to exclude an associated fracture. Radiographs can sometimes be difficult to interpret. Posterior dislocations are notorious for being overlooked as the humerus appears to be in joint. Close inspection, however, shows the characteristic 'light bulb' shape of the humeral head as the tuberosities are not seen in their usual position.

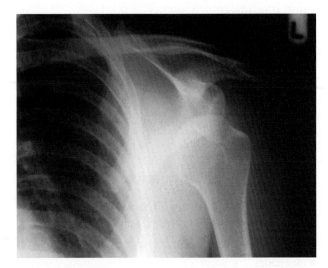

Fig. 67 Anterior dislocation of the shoulder.

Management

Occasionally, the shoulder may reduce spontaneously or by the 'hanging arm' technique in which the patient lies prone allowing the affected arm to hang vertically over the side of the couch. More usually, however, reduction under anaesthesia is required. Kochner's manoeuvre is commonly used, in which the arm is externally rotated and abducted; the arm is then swung into internal rotation and adducted across the patient's chest to be nursed there in a broad arm sling for 3–4 weeks while the anterior capsule heals. Alternatively, traction on the arm against counter-traction from a colleague's hand in the axillary can be used.

Complications

- axillary nerve damage: this may occur during the injury or during the manipulation; the integrity of the nerve must always be checked prior to attempting reduction. Absence of sensation over the point of the acromion suggests the nerve is damaged and, if it is, there will be resulting paralysis in the deltoid
- associated humeral fracture
- arterial damage: the axillary artery may be damaged
- shoulder stiffness
- irreducible dislocation: this is present if the humeral head button-holes through the rotator cuff. This happens only rarely but requires open reduction
- recurrent dislocation occurs if postoperative splintage is inadequate allowing resultant laxity of the soft tissues to develop.
- iatrogenic humeral fracture (especially a risk in osteoporotic patients).

Posterior dislocation

This condition is unusual but easily missed. Ligamentous laxity gives some patients the ability to voluntarily dislocate the shoulder posteriorly.

Diagnosis

The radiograph shows the characteristic 'light bulb' shape of the humeral head.

Management

Manipulation under anaesthesia followed by 3 weeks' immobilisation and subsequent physiotherapy.

Recurrent dislocation

Recurrent anterior dislocation occurs with extension and external rotation movements usually without any further trauma. Some patients report their shoulder dislocating while simply turning over in bed.

Diagnosis

Radiological examination shows flattening of part of the humeral head; the Hill–Sach's lesion. Elevation of the anterior glenoid rim and subscapularis muscle (the Bankart lesion) may be demonstrated by arthrography or MRI.

Management

Recurrent dislocation requires stabilisation of the shoulder by securing the soft tissues back to their anatomical positions. Reefing the subscapular tendon or providing a dynamic anterior support by the transfer of the conjoint tendon through the subscapularis are more extensive procedures with their own complications.

Fractured clavicle

This common injury is often associated with sports but can occur with any fall on the outstretched hand.

Clinical features

Pain and tenderness. The patient characteristically supports the weight of the arm with the opposite hand.

Diagnosis

The majority of injuries are in the middle third and occasionally there is overriding of the bone ends.

Management

The arm should be rested in a broad arm sling; sometimes a figure-of-8 bandage provides a comfortable brace for the shoulders.

Complications

- malunion
- damage to the subclavicular vessels
- non-union; this may be asymptomatic but, occasionally, requires open reduction, internal fixation and bone grafting
- deformity
- brachial plexus damage.

Acromioclavicular joint disruption

A fall on the point of the shoulder, classically during a rugby game, produces this injury (Fig. 68).

Clinical features

The injury may be a sprain, a subluxation or a dislocation. The clavicle springs upward at the acromioclavicular joint producing a characteristic step on the shoulder.

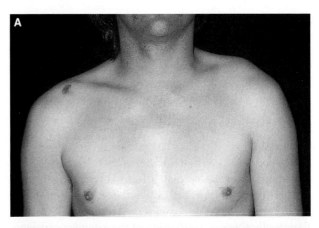
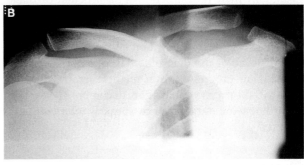

Fig. 68 A. 30-year-old man with acromioclavicular dislocation of his left shoulder. **B.** X-ray appearance of both acromioclavicular joints.

Diagnosis

Radiographs comparing both shoulders while the patient carries weights in the hands are used to confirm a diagnosis and to differentiate between subluxations and dislocations.

Management

Conservative treatment is often all that is required, but occasionally fixation of the clavicle to the coracoid (Weaver–Dunn procedure) is carried out for those patients who require their shoulder for heavy work.

Complications

- pain
- weakness.

6.3 Rheumatoid arthritis

Learning objectives

You should:

- be able to list the radiological features of rheumatoid arthritis

- be able to describe the different contributions of medical (non-operative) management
- be able to describe various operative procedures which may be used and list the possible complications associated with each.

Rheumatoid arthritis (RA) is an inflammatory systemic disease of unknown aetiology, characterised by relapses and remissions, which may affect many joints simultaneously. An autoimmune inflammatory reaction in the synovium produces synovial hypertrophy and effusion. Eventually there is destruction of the articular cartilage, ligamentous laxity and erosion of the subchondral bone. These combine to result in mechanical derangement of the joint leading to subluxation and eventually permanent dislocation and deformity. The care of the rheumatoid patient progresses from medical treatment, often supervised by a rheumatologist, to combined care with an orthopaedic surgeon once surgical intervention is required.

Shoulder

Clinical features
- **Listen** — morning stiffness is characteristic. The shoulder is painful and limits function. It is difficult to comb the hair and reach to the perineum comfortably. Patients complain that they are unable to lie on the affected side
- **Look** — muscle wasting around the shoulder girdle
- **Feel** — joint swelling is not easy to detect. There may be tenderness at the acromioclavicular joint.
- **Move** — movements of the joint are painful and restricted, especially abduction and external rotation.

Diagnosis
Features of systemic disease may be present, such as a raised ESR and plasma viscosity. A positive RA latex may also be apparent but in approximately 30% of patients, this test is negative. Classically, radiographs of the wrists are used to look for early signs of rheumatoid arthritis. Radiological examination of the affected joint shows:

- joint space narrowing
- marginal erosions
- osteopenia
- irregular joint surface
- eventually features of secondary osteoarthritis develop (Fig. 69).

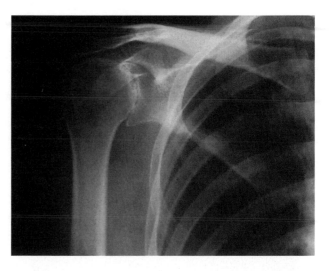

Fig. 69 Secondary osteoarthritis in the glenohumeral joint.

Management
Medical management includes:

- drugs: therapy progresses from simple analgesics and NSAIDs to disease-modifying drugs such as Sulfasalazine, Methotrexate, Penicillamine and gold; intra-articular injection of steroid, radioactive Yttrium and Systemic steroids
- physiotherapy: preserves useful joint movement
- appliances to aid in the activities of daily living.

Surgical management includes:

- arthroscopic synovectomy
- hemiarthroplasty of the humeral head is usually sufficient (Fig. 70)
- total shoulder replacement is required if the glenoid is severely eroded.

Complications
Complications of the disease:

- joint destruction
- dislocation
- rotator cuff degeneration.

Complications of prosthetic replacement:

- infection
- loosening.

Elbow

Clinical features

Patients with rheumatoid arthritis involving the elbow may have involvement of the humero-ulnar, humero-radial, proximal radio-ulnar joint or a combination of

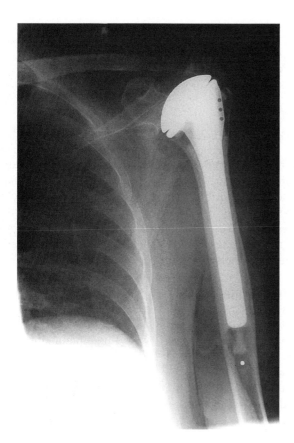

Fig. 70 Hemiarthroplasty of the shoulder for rheumatoid arthritis.

any of them. In addition, there may be disease at the distal radio-ulnar joint.

- **Listen** — patients complain of pain and loss of function in the elbow. There may be difficulty with eating and washing, and patients may complain of neck pain secondary to stretching forwards in an attempt to bring the mouth to the hand
- **Look** — swollen joint from synovial effusion; deformity of the bony contours due to subluxation
- **Feel** — crepitus and swelling
- **Move** — when the humero-ulnar joint is involved, the patient loses full flexion and extension and is unable to get the hand to the face. If the humero-radial or distal radio-ulnar joints are involved, there is loss of supination and pronation.

Diagnosis
Radiological examination shows features of RA (see Fig. 71, p. 82), but in addition excess bone resorption may be seen, which allows the olecranon to migrate proximally between the supracondylar ridges of the distal humerus.

Management
Conservative treatment includes drug therapy (p. 78) and splinting. Surgical management includes synovectomy, usually combined with radial head excision in cases of humero-radial joint involvement. Destruction of the humero-ulnar joint requires a total elbow replacement.

Complications
Complications of the disease include:

- progressive loss of function
- instability
- weakness.

Complications of surgery include:

- infection
- dislocation
- ulnar neuritis
- loosening of the prosthesis.

6.4 Elbow disorders

Learning objectives

You should:

- be able to recognise and treat enthesopathies around the elbow

- be able to differentiate and treat infective and inflammatory olecranon bursitis.

Elbow injuries associated with sport

Enthesopathy is the name given to discomfort at the site of origin of a muscle. It is caused by a tear in the muscle origin near the bone following repetitive activities involving lifting or stretching.

Tennis elbow/golfer's elbow

Clinical features
In tennis elbow there is pain over the lateral epicondyle of the elbow, which limits normal use. Local tenderness is found at the common extensor origin and symptoms can be exacerbated by stressing these muscles by forced palmar flexion of the wrist.

In golfer's elbow similar symptoms and signs are found on the medial side of the elbow at the common flexor origin. In this case, forced dorsiflexion of the wrist or resisted palmar flexion is painful.

Diagnosis
Radiological examination is unremarkable.

Management

Resting the elbow and avoiding particular activities may be all that is required. An above-elbow splint can be used to enforce this. Infiltration of the common extensor or flexor origin with local anaesthetic and steroid may produce some relief and can be repeated up to three times. Occasionally, surgical release is indicated, but the results are unpredictable.

Complications

Complications can arise from steroid injection:

- subcutaneous fat necrosis
- loss of skin pigmentation
- persisting symptoms.

Osteoarthritis

Arthritis in the elbow may be the result of heavy manual work or sports such as cricket.

Clinical features

There is pain, crepitus and loss of the full range of motion in the elbow.

Diagnosis

Radiological examination shows the features of osteoarthritis: joint space narrowing, osteophytes and subchondral sclerosis.

Management

Symptoms may be relieved by changing occupation and avoiding the use of the arm for strenuous activities. Occasionally, surgical debridement of osteophytes and release of joint capsule contractures can improve the range of movement but the results are often not maintained. In severe cases, total elbow replacement may be carried out, but the arm cannot be used for heavy activities after this procedure.

Complications

- continuing pain
- loss of full range of movement.

Bursitis

Olecranon bursitis

This is either inflammatory or infective. Inflammatory bursitis is associated with rheumatoid arthritis, gout, other crystal arthropathies or direct trauma to the olecranon. Classically, this was described as resulting from pressure or friction on the olecranon, hence the original name of 'student's elbow'. Infective bursitis is usually due to staphylococcal infection.

Clinical features

There is a large fluctuant swelling at the olecranon associated with pain and redness. In infective bursitis, there is oedema, tenderness and spreading inflammation.

Diagnosis

Aspiration will help to identify the infecting organism and also to relieve the acute symptoms of inflammatory bursitis.

Management

A course of non-steroidal anti-inflammatory analgesics is sufficient for mild inflammatory disease. An appropriate antibiotic is necessary in addition for infected cases. Surgical excision of the bursa prevents recurrence.

Complications of surgery

- poor wound healing.
- sinus formation.

Self-assessment: questions

Multiple choice questions

1. In the 'painful arc syndrome':
   a. Calcification in the region of the supraspinatus tendon may be seen on plain radiographs
   b. The cause is a tear of the supraspinatus tendon
   c. Typically there is severe pain on initiating abduction
   d. Tenderness is generalised
   e. If untreated shoulder stiffness often results

2. In rheumatoid arthritis:
   a. Radiographic features of osteoarthritis may be superimposed on those of rheumatoid arthritis
   b. Crepitus and pain may be produced by palpating the radial head while pronating/supinating the forearm
   c. Joint laxity allows a full range of shoulder movement to be retained in most patients
   d. Ulnar nerve dysfunction is rarely seen
   e. Synovectomy and radial head excision may relieve symptoms in the early stages of disease

Extended matching items questions (EMIs)

1. Theme: Diagnoses

A   medial epicondylitis
B   osteoarthritis
C   rotator cuff tear
D   subacromial impingement
E   acute supraspinatus tendinitis
F   bursitis
G   rheumatoid arthritis
H   posterior dislocation of the shoulder
I   recurrent shoulder dislocation
J   fractured clavicle

Match the most appropriate diagnosis from the list above to each of the clinical histories below:

1. Pain in the mid-range of shoulder abduction.
2. Elevation of the anterior glenoid labrum and subscapularis seen on arthrogram or MRI scan.
3. Inability to initiate shoulder abduction.

2. Theme: Diagnoses

A   medial epicondylitis
B   rheumatoid arthritis
C   dislocation
D   painful arc syndrome

E   synovitis
F   tennis elbow
G   bursitis
H   golfer's elbow
I   ulnar neuritis
J   osteoarthritis

Match the most appropriate diagnosis from the list above to each of the clinical histories below:

1. Localised pain, swelling and redness at the point of the elbow.
2. Gradual onset of pain, crepitus and loss of full range of elbow movement in an otherwise fit 58-year-old manual worker.
3. Lateral side elbow pain worse with stressing the extensor muscles in the forearm.

Constructed response questions (CRQs)

CRQ 1

A 70-year-old woman trips and falls onto her right shoulder. She complains of pain and inability to move the joint. She has localised tenderness around the humeral head. There is some swelling and bruising and localised tenderness around the greater tuberosity.

a. What might you expect to see on plain AP X-ray?
b. The X-ray is reported as normal. What is a possible diagnosis now?
c. How could you visualise this lesion?
d. In a younger person how might this be treated?
e. Why might this treatment not be suitable in an older person and what would you suggest instead?

CRQ 2

A 50-year-old accountant complains of pain in his dominant right shoulder after a weekend spent painting his house. Physical examination reveals well-localised acute tenderness, just lateral and superior to the coracoid process.

a. What diagnosis does this suggest?
b. What initial treatment would you suggest?
c. He attends two weeks later feeling no better. What would you expect to find on physical examination?

d. How would you treat him now?

e. Your treatment is satisfactory on this occasion. The patient presents some years later following several further episodes but now with a longer history of continued pain exacerbated by abduction. What would you expect to find on examination?

f. Your previous treatment does not help on this occasion. X-ray of the shoulder shows no evidence of arthritis. How would you manage this patient now?

Objective structured clinical examination questions (OSCEs)

OSCE 1

Study the photograph of an X-ray of the elbow (Fig. 71).

a. Label features marked A and B. What important structure passes near the eroded area of bone marked C?

b. What is abnormal about the radial head?

c. Looking at the elbow as a whole, what do you think is the likely diagnosis?

d. What are the classical features of this condition?

e. If you were to recommend a total elbow replacement for this patient, list two advantages and two complications to warn the patient about.

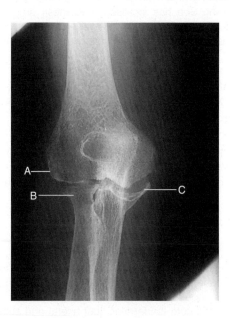

Fig. 71

OSCE 2

Study the photograph of an X-ray of the left shoulder of a man who has suffered an injury in a fall at football (Fig. 72).

a. What sensory examination should you carry out on a patient with this condition?

b. Describe the procedure used in the management of this condition.

c. What two contrasting complications are associated with this injury?

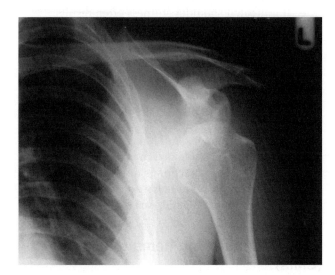

Fig. 72

Viva questions

1. Discuss the presentation and clinical findings in tennis elbow.

2. Demonstrate how the elbow can be examined to determine the range of movement.

Self-assessment: answers

Multiple choice answers

1. a. **True.** 'Painful arc syndrome' is caused by inflammation in the supraspinatus area of the rotator cuff, and calcification may occasionally be seen here on radiological examination.
   b. **False.** A tear of the supraspinatus part of the rotator cuff causes loss of ability to initiate abduction; although there may be pain in the shoulder, the painful arc is not present.
   c. **False.** The severe pain of painful arc syndrome is during the range from 30° to 60° as the inflamed, swollen area of the rotator cuff passes beneath the acromion. There is no pain during the initiation of abduction.
   d. **False.** There is acute localised tenderness over the rotator cuff.
   e. **True.** If the patient is inhibited in the use of the shoulder because of pain then the capsule contracts and a frozen shoulder results.

2. a. **True.** Once the joint is destroyed by rheumatoid arthritis, secondary osteoarthritis may develop.
   b. **True.** Crepitus from motion between the two joint surfaces and pain on movement are readily found at the radial head during supination and pronation.
   c. **False.** Usually the destruction of the joint and the long period of immobility resulting from the pain have resulted in a loss of full shoulder joint movement.
   d. **False.** Ulnar neuritis is often associated with rheumatoid disease involving the elbow or wrist.
   e. **True.** Excision arthroplasty of the radial head and synovectomy reduce the disease process and painful movement of the elbow. Dramatic relief can be achieved.

EMI answers

1. Theme: Diagnoses

1. E. Pain in the mid-range of shoulder abduction is the classical painful arc of discomfort associated with acute supraspinatus tendinitits.
2. I. Elevation of the anterior glenoid labrum with a potential space extending beneath subscapularis is a classical finding on an arthrogram or MRI scan and is associated with a history of recurrent dislocation of the shoulder.
3. C. A significant tear in the rotator cuff will make it impossible to initiate abduction as this action is carried out supraspinatus.

2. Theme: Diagnoses

1. G. Bursitis affecting the olecranon, either infective or inflammatory, causes localised pain and swelling at the point of the elbow.
2. J. Osteoarthritis associated with heavy work would be characterised by pain crepitus and loss of full range of movement.
3. F. Tennis elbow is an enthesopathy of the common extensor origin at the lateral epicondyle.

CRQ answers

CRQ 1

a. Fractured tuberosity or complex intra-articular fracture.
b. Rotator cuff tear.
c. MRI scan or arthrogram.
d. Operatively by formal rotator cuff repair.
e. Surgical treatment is often not possible in an older person because the tear may be large and the rotator cuff muscles friable. This makes it impossible to reoppose the edges of the tear and suture them together. Instead conservative management is usually carried out with physiotherapy and ultrasound.

CRQ 2

a. Acute supraspinatus tendinitis.
b. Rest
   Anti-inflammatory analgesics
   Ultrasound treatment from the physiotherapist.
c. Painful arc of abduction.
d. If he is not getting any relief, it may be appropriate to consider long-acting steroid and anaesthetic injection into the subacromial bursa.
e. Painful abduction in an older patient suggests a diagnosis of subacromiol impingement as the rotator cuff is swollen and frayed beneath the arch of the acromiom.
f. Subacromial impingement is best managed by an acromioplasty or acromioclavicular joint excision if associated with arthritis of this joint.

OSCE answers

OSCE 1

a. A–Lateral epicondyle
   B–Radial head
   C–Ulnar nerve.

b. It is flattened and eroded.
c. Rheumatoid arthritis.
d. Joint space narrowing
   Irregular joints surface
   Margin erosions
   Osteopenia.
e. **Advantages:**   **Complications:**
   Pain-free joint   Persistent ulnar neuritis
   Increased functional use   Infection, dislocation or
   Possible increased range   loosening of the
   of movement.   prosthesis.

OSCE 2

a. Examination for numbness over the 'badge-patch' area checking for damage to the axillary nerve.
b. General anaesthesia or muscular relaxation is required. Kocher's manoeuvre involves external rotation and abduction of the shoulder followed by adduction while internally rotating. Counter-traction with the help of a colleague's hand in the axilla may be required.
c. Shoulder stiffness
   Recurrent dislocation.

Viva answers

1. Tennis elbow presents with a history of pain over the lateral epicondyle of the elbow, which limits normal use. There may be a history of repetitive activities such as lifting or stretching. Physical examination shows well-localised tenderness in the common extensor origin exacerbated by resisted dorsiflexion of the wrist or by full palmar flexion.

2. Movements that take place at the elbow are flexion, extension, supination and pronation. With the patient's arms fully stretched forwards, the elbows are in full extension. The affected side can be compared with the normal side. The range of movement from full extension to full flexion can be measured and compared with the opposite side. Usually full extension is recorded as 0° and full flexion as 130°. To determine pronation and supination, it is important that the patient's elbows are tucked into the waist to prevent any auxiliary movement from the shoulder. With the hand in a fist and the palm upwards, the range of movement from full supination to full pronation can be observed and compared with the opposite side. Full supination is usually recorded as 90°, neutral (with the fist vertical) 0° and full pronation as approximately 80°.

7 Hand and wrist disorders

Chapter overview

Hand problems compose a significant percentage of the number of referrals to the orthopaedic department, both from general practice and from the Accident and Emergency department. Fractures and dislocations of the phalanges and metacarpals are common and the majority can be treated conservatively. Unstable or multiple fractures, however, require internal fixation or specific splintage. Penetrating injuries in the palm should always be explored as there is a significant risk that underlying tendons, nerves or ligaments will have been damaged.

The risk of infection in the hand should always be anticipated and the presence of any infection diagnosed and treated promptly. This may require surgical decompression and lavage. Although fractures in general are usually easily recognised, fractures of the carpal bones may be more difficult to identify and it is important to be familiar with the normal radiological pattern of the carpus to avoid missing these. Anterior dislocation of the lunate is often overlooked. Even if nothing appears abnormal on X-ray, the presence of intercarpal ligament disruption should always be considered if the patient fails to improve.

Rheumatoid and osteoarthritis in the hand may appear more deforming than disabling so surgery should only be considered to control pain or improve hand function rather than for cosmetic reasons alone.

7.1 Clinical examination

Learning objectives

You should:

- know how to take an appropriate history from a patient with a hand injury
- ask for details of the patient's injury, occupation, hobbies and whether the patient is right- or left-handed
- be able to examine the injured hand and consider which underlying structures may have been damaged
- understand the importance of splintage and therapy for rehabilitation of the injured hand.

Because of their exposed position in the body and their busy prehensile activity, the hand and wrist are vulnerable to injury in a variety of ways:

- cuts and bites
- fractures/dislocations
- burns
- crushing
- infection
- high pressure injection.

Almost any combination of structures within the hand may be damaged in these ways so for any injured hand a checklist should be made of all the structures that could possibly be injured:

- skin
- tendons
- nerves

- vessels
- bone
- joints
- ligaments.

Much information can be gained from the careful examination of the hands not only for local pathology but also because the hands often manifest signs associated with remote or systemic diseases. Patients who have suffered a hand injury are very anxious and distressed about the effect this will have on normal hand function. Patients with infection in the hand will be in acute pain and resist the slightest attempts at examination. With so much information to be found from the hands, it is important to carefully follow the pattern of 'listen, look, feel, move'.

Listen. Several important questions must be asked, concerning:

- details of the injury
  — position the hand was in at the time
  — mechanism of injury
  — duration of contact of the hand with the injury force, e.g. crush from industrial rollers
- right- or left-handed
- occupation
- hobbies
- other activities involving precision use of the hand.

Look. Systematically look at each joint in the hand and wrist and remember to look at both palmar and dorsal surfaces. Do not forget to inspect the nails closely. In an exam, always describe what you are looking for and what you find to the examiner. Note any abnormal posture in the hand such as that associated with loss of function of a flexor or extensor tendon.

Feel. Palpate the surface of any swelling and determine whether it is in the skin or beneath the skin. See if the lesion moves in relation to the flexor tendon. Try to locate areas of tenderness very precisely with single digit palpation. Areas of altered sensation should be assessed by light touch and especially the moving two point discrimination test. Patients should be able to discriminate between the points of a pair of dividers or the ends of a paper clip two millimetres apart when they are being moved on the skin surface.

Move. Observe the passive and active range of movement of the joint. Remember that at the wrist ulnar and radial deviation can be measured and compared with the opposite side. Examine the fingers for integrity of the flexor digitorum superficialis (FDS) and flexor digitorum profundus (FDP) tendons.

A careful history and examination should make it possible for you to predict exactly which structures have been injured.

Therapy

The worst complication of any injury to the hand is stiffness and contracture due to failure to prevent swelling or to encourage mobilisation. Sometimes, however, mobilisation is not possible and the hand must, therefore, be correctly splinted to avoid the development of joint contractures.

The correct position for splinting the hand is with the metacarpophalangeal joints in flexion and the proximal interphalangeal (PIP) joints in extension. In this position, the collateral ligaments of the joint are at their longest and, therefore, cannot contract. To aid this position, some dorsiflexion of the wrist is also used and can be maintained by a plaster back slab. A bulky dressing on the palm of the hand is made with layers of fluffed gauze. If only the wrist is to be immobilised, it is important that the dressing does not impede full flexion of the metacarpophalangeal joints.

7.2 Fractures and dislocations

Learning objectives

You should:

- recognise what fracture patterns in the phalanges and metacarpals are likely to be unstable and require internal fixation or splintage rather than early mobilisation

- be able to recognise disruption of the ulnar collateral ligament of the thumb MCP joint clinically and radiologically

- be able to recognise a scaphoid fracture or dislocation of the lunate but equally to be aware that the absence of a bony injury does not exclude the absence of a ligamentous injury to the wrist, especially at the scapholunate junction.

Phalanges

Clinical features

Fractures are caused by either twisting or angulating forces, may be stable or unstable and may be displaced or undisplaced (Fig. 73). The pull of the interossei on the proximal fragment causes it to flex, resulting in dorsal angulation at the fracture site as the extensors pull on the middle phalanx.

Management

Stable, undisplaced fractures can be splinted by the adjacent finger or a short metal splint, but interosseous wiring, crossed Kirschner wires or the AO minifragment technique may be necessary to stabilise an unstable fracture.

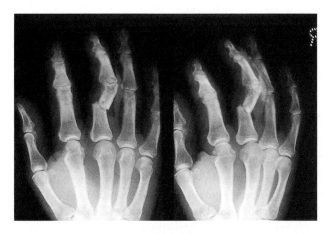

Fig. 73 Unstable transverse fracture of the proximal phalanx of the middle finger with posterior angulation and displacement.

Dislocation of the interphalangeal joint

This common injury is usually easily reduced but is associated with either disruption of the collateral ligaments or volar plate. There may be an associated avulsion fracture from the base of the adjacent phalanx.

Management
Reduction and splinting to the adjacent finger are usually sufficient but a large intra-articular fragment will require accurate internal fixation.

Complications

- stiffness caused by adhesion of extensor tendon at the fracture site
- malunion responsible for the rotated position of the finger, which becomes apparent with flexion
- flexion contraction due to scarring of the volar plate.

Metacarpals

Fifth metacarpal

The most commonly encountered fracture in the hand is a fracture of the neck of the fifth metacarpal (boxer's fracture). The metacarpal head is usually rotated and angled towards the palm.

Management
Unless this angulation is more than 40° from the long axis of the metacarpal shaft, it can be ignored so long as rotation is controlled by strapping the small and ring fingers together. Angulation of more than 45° often requires reduction and stabilisation of the fracture by percutaneous Kirschner wires.

Complications

- extension lag
- stiff finger
- painful lump in the palm.

First metacarpal

Fractures of the first metacarpal may be:

- extra-articular: the fracture is usually transverse and above the level of the carpal joint
- intra-articular: the fracture is oblique, unstable, often displaced and involves part of the articular surface (Bennet's fracture; Fig. 74).

Clinical features
There is usually a history of a staving or punching injury. The base of the first metacarpal is prominent.

Management
Undisplaced fractures can be held in a plaster cast that is well moulded to the base of the metacarpal and extended to the tip of the thumb. Displaced fractures require reduction and fixation either by an interfragmentary screw or by stabilising the position of the first metacarpal relative to the second by transverse Kirschner wires from one to the other.

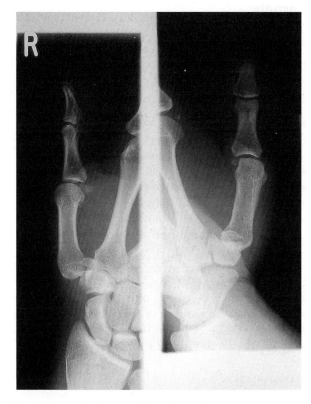

Fig. 74 Bennet's fracture of the first metacarpal.

Complications

- malunion
- osteoarthritis.

Multiple metacarpal fractures

These fractures are usually unstable and if displaced will require internal fixation with minifragment plates or Kirschner wires.

Ulnar collateral ligament disruption at the MCP joint of the thumb

Acute abduction of the metacarpophalangeal joint of the thumb tears the ulnar collateral ligament and may avulse its origin on the base of the proximal phalanx. This injury commonly occurs in skiing or bike accidents. Chronic laxity, 'gamekeeper's thumb', is due to repeated ligamentous injury.

Management
A Bennet's-type plaster is appropriate for partial tears but open reduction and intraosseous fixation are required if the bony fragment is widely displaced or if the joint is very lax. In these cases the adductor aponeurosis will be interposed between the avulsed ligament and its insertion on the proximal phalanx.

Carpals

Scaphoid

Clinical features
Falls on the outstretched hand in young people, usually at sports, may result in a fracture to the scaphoid.

- **Listen** — today the injury is often associated with sports, although at one time it was due to the kickback from a motor-car starting handle.
- **Look** — swelling in the anatomical snuffbox
- **Feel** — there is localised tenderness in the anatomical snuffbox
- **Move** — pain is exacerbated by radial deviation of the wrist and on axial compression of the thumb.

Diagnosis
Radiographs of the wrist in ulnar deviation show the scaphoid best and the type of fracture (stable, oblique, displaced) can be observed. Occult fractures may be more apparent if re-X-rayed a week later.

Management
Most scaphoid fractures can be treated conservatively in a plaster cast to immobilise the wrist while healing

occurs. Unstable or displaced fractures are probably best treated by early open reduction and internal fixation with a screw or K wires.

Non-union is a risk with these types and if present should be treated with bone graft either in isolation (Russe bone graft) or with an internal fixation device (Herbert screw).

Complications

- non-union
- avascular necrosis of the proximal fragment due to the retrograde blood supply to the scaphoid
- osteoarthritis and carpal collapse (SLAC wrist — scapholunate advanced collapse)
- persisting pain
- weak grip.

Dislocation of the lunate

A hyperextension injury of the wrist may dislocate the lunate anteriorly (Fig. 75) and produce acute symptoms of median nerve compression. Other more complex dislocations are associated with fractures of the scaphoid or capitate.

Management
Closed reduction may be possible followed by percutaneous wire stabilisation of the lunate, but often it is best to carry out an open reduction, repair the tear in the wrist capsule and decompress the carpal tunnel at the same time.

7.3 Soft tissue injuries

Learning objectives

You should:

- be able to describe the five zones of the hand and relate them to flexor tendon injuries
- be able to describe the principles of flexor tendon surgery and rehabilitation
- be able to list the clinical features of other types of hand injury.

Sharp injuries

Cuts to the hand frequently occur from falls onto broken glass or from cuts on a knife or metal edge. The skin wound often looks trivial so the depth of the wound and hence the damage to the underlying structures are frequently missed when patients attend the casualty department.

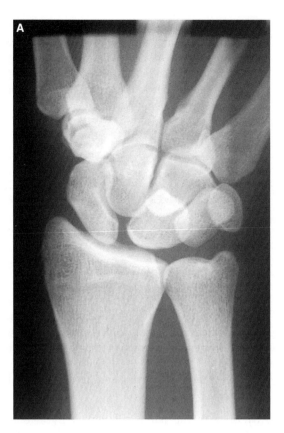

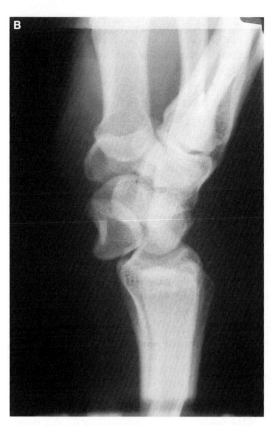

Fig. 75 Anterior–posterior (**A**) and lateral (**B**) radiographs of the wrist showing anterior dislocation of the lunate.

Clinical features

- **Listen** — An exact description of the mechanism of the injury should be elicited. The position of the hand at the time of the accident is important. For example, if the fingers were cut gripping the blade while trying to resist a knife attack then, when straightened, the position of the flexor tendon injury will be distal to the cut in the skin.

- **Look** — If a flexor or extensor tendon is divided, the affected finger will be out of cadence with the other fingers, which normally fall into a resting position of partial flexion that increases from the index to the small finger. The site of the skin wound should be noted. Injuries on the palmar aspect of the proximal phalanx may have divided both flexor tendons as they pass through the fibro-osseous tunnel in zone II (Fig. 76).

- **Feel** — Sensation on each side of the finger should be checked, although absence of touch sensation is not registered immediately by patients despite division of a digital nerve. Eventually the denervated side of the finger feels very dry due to loss of sudomotor innervation.

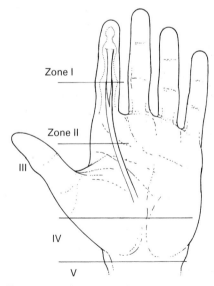

Fig. 76 Five zones of the hand showing the site of the fibro-osseous tunnel in zone II containing both flexor digitorum superficialis and flexor digitorum profundus in the fibrous flexor sheath.

- **Move** — Complete division of flexor digitorum superficialis (FDS) causes loss of proximal interphalangeal joint flexion. If the adjacent fingers are held straight, the injured finger is unable to flex at the proximal interphalangeal joint as this manoeuvre disables the mass action muscle, flexor digitorum profundus (FDP) from flexing both joints of all fingers. FDS in contrast controls each finger independently. Complete division of flexor digitorum profundus causes loss of distal interphalangeal joint flexion when the finger is held straight at the proximal interphalangeal joint. Partial division is associated with painful weakness of these movements. If an extensor tendon is divided, the finger hangs lower than its neighbours and cannot extend actively.

Diagnosis

The extent of injury to the underlying structures can be made clinically in most cases. If the injury was caused by a radio-opaque material, a radiograph is useful to exclude any particles remaining in the wound.

Management

Tendons, nerves and vessels can all be repaired. The principles of surgery on the hand include the use of a bloodless field (produced by a tourniquet on the limb), magnification and appropriately fine instruments and suture material. The patient's hand should be rested on a table that is wide enough to allow the surgeon to rest his elbows on it while operating. In this way hand tremor is reduced. If digital vessels and nerves are to be repaired, the operating microscope should be used, but operating loupes magnifying between two and three times are sufficient for most procedures. Postoperative splinting to protect the repair together with exercises supervised by a hand therapist are required if a good result is to be achieved after these injuries.

Complications

- stiffness
- tendon adhesions
- cold intolerance
- numbness
- neuroma formation
- scar contracture.

Bites

Human or animal bites are usually seen at the knuckles or fingertips. The skin wound is ragged and the extensor tendon may be partially or completely divided. Occasionally the underlying joint capsule is open and in very severe injuries a digit may be partially or completely amputated.

Management

Infection is the main problem. Copious lavage, surgical debridement and best-guest antibiotics, usually benzylpenicillin, are needed.

Wounds should be left open initially and reinspected at 24 hours before being closed.

Thermal injuries

Burns

Hands are also at risk from thermal injuries. As well as hot objects, other agents such as steam, liquids, flames, electricity and chemicals can cause burns, as can cold objects and liquids.

Clinical features

Burns are classified (see Fig. 77) as:

- superficial (epidermal damage only) — epithelial cells remain in the hair follicles and sweat glands
- deep dermal (epidermis and some of the dermis are lost)
- full thickness (epidermis and dermis are totally destroyed).

Any burn of the hand is followed by swelling. This swelling interferes with movement of the hand and may

A

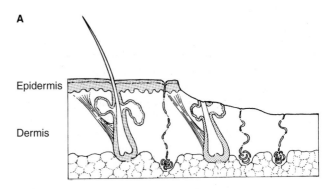

B

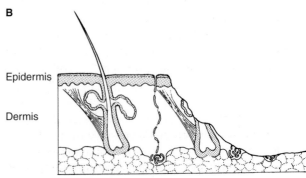

Fig. 77 **A.** In a superficial burn portions of the hair follicles and sweat glands with their associated epithelial linings remain to be the focus of epithelial regeneration. **B.** In a full thickness burn the epidermis and dermis are destroyed leaving no ability for epithelial regrowth to occur except from the wound edges.

cause permanent stiffness. It also interferes with healing of the skin. Larger and more severe burns are associated with more severe swelling.

Management

Minor burns are treated with small dressings that do not interfere with movement. More extensive burns are usually treated by occlusion by placing the hand in a plastic bag with an antibacterial cream and instructing the patient on elevation and mobilisation. Fingers must be put through a full range of movement to prevent stiffness and reduce the oedema, and thus promote healing. Deep dermal and full thickness burns will require excision and covering with a split thickness skin graft, which limits the risk of infection and the extent of scar contracture.

Cold injuries

Exposure of the fingers to extreme cold may lead to frostbite.

Clinical features

There is discoloration, blistering and, ultimately, necrosis of the fingertips.

Management

The principles of treatment are the same as for burns. The hand should be elevated to prevent swelling and the patient encouraged to exercise the digits. Eventually the areas of necrosis will demarcate with dry gangrene of peripheral ischaemic areas. These will ultimately separate spontaneously, but amputation of necrotic areas will hasten the healing process.

Crush injuries

With crush injuries, it is important to know the nature of the crushing object. Often the injury involves industrial machinery. The size, weight, temperature or velocity of the equipment responsible may be of relevance. The length of time the hand was crushed may also be relevant.

Clinical features

A hand crushed between blunt objects or rollers may be swollen and bruised without definite injury to any of the internal structures. However, the skin may have been sheared (degloving injury) from the underlying structures and become devascularised. Loss of capillary return helps to confirm this diagnosis. The defatted skin however, may be reapplied to the underlying raw tissue as a skin graft.

High pressure injection injuries

Paint, lubricants or other solvents may be injected under pressure into the hand or digits.

Clinical features

The entry wound is small and the severity of the injury is easily underestimated initially. After a few hours, there is increasing pain and swelling.

Management

Surgical opening of the area reveals the extent of spread of the injected substance. Mechanical lavage and surgical debridement are necessary. Closure should be delayed until swelling subsides.

7.4 Infection

Learning objectives

You should:

- be able to recognise infection in the hand and know how this should be managed as an emergency.

Clinical features

Staphylococcal infection in the hand presents as a web-space infection, paronychia (nail-fold infection) or a tendon-sheath infection. There is a collection of yellow pus, inability to move the affected finger and inflammation. Streptococcal infection is associated with a more insidious spreading infection, cellulitis, and ascending lymphangitis without the presence of pus at the original site.

Management

Pus under pressure must be released and the area washed out. Specimens are sent for bacteriological examination and intravenous antibiotics commenced. Flucloxacillin and Fucidin are the 'best guess' for staphylococcal infections, but penicillin must be used if streptococcal infection is suspected.

Complications

- swelling
- contracture
- stiffness
- skin necrosis is seen in some cases of streptococcal infection
- a digit may be lost if its vessels become thrombosed following infection.

7.5 Entrapment neuropathy

Learning objectives

You should:

- be able to describe the clinical features of carpal tunnel syndrome and differentiate these from ulnar nerve compression at the elbow.

Pressure on a peripheral nerve in its fibro-osseous tunnel causes pressure on a localised section of the nerve, which results in neuronal dysfunction causing characteristic features.

Carpal tunnel syndrome

Clinical features
Patients are usually female.

- **Listen** — The classical history is of pain at night in the radial three and a half digits (the distribution of the median nerve). There may be numbness, tingling, dysaesthesia and clumsiness.
- **Look** — There may be wasting of the muscles of the thenar eminence, especially abductor pollicis brevis, which is always innervated by the median nerve.
- **Feel** — There is altered or diminished sensation in the palmar aspect of the radial three and a half digits but not in the palm of the hand as the superficial branch of the median nerve supplying this area does not pass through the carpal tunnel.
- **Move** — There is weakness of abductor pollicis brevis. Tinel's sign, percussion over the median nerve at the carpal tunnel, exacerbates the symptoms, as does palmar flexion of the wrist (Phalen's sign).

Diagnosis
The diagnosis is usually made clinically but in equivocal cases nerve conduction studies are helpful, showing characteristic decreases in nerve conduction velocities at the wrist if the median nerve is significantly compressed.

Management
Conservative. A dorsiflexion splint to wear at night prevents wrist flexion during sleep and relieves symptoms. Local infiltration of a steroid into the carpal tunnel may be effective.

Surgical. Division of the flexor retinaculum achieves a dramatic improvement in symptoms. In cases of advanced thenar muscle wasting, an opponensplasty to restore thumb opposition to the other digits can be achieved using palmaris longus, if present, or flexor digitorum superficialis from the ring finger.

Cubital tunnel syndrome

Clinical features

- **Listen** — Pressure or traction on the ulnar nerve at the elbow causes pain and tingling in the distribution of the ulnar nerve.
- **Look** — There may be wasting of the hypothenar eminence and of the interossei. This is best seen in the first web space where the first dorsal interosseus is easy to see.
- **Feel** — There is altered sensation or numbness in both palmar and dorsal aspects of the ulnar one and a half digits.
- **Move** — There is weakness of abductor digiti minimi and of abduction and adduction of all the fingers. Adductor pollicis is also weak resulting in a positive Froment's sign in which interphalangeal joint flexion of the thumb occurs to increase pinch grip.

Diagnosis
Nerve conduction studies will confirm the diagnosis and localise the constricting lesion — usually a fibrous band between the two heads of flexor carpi ulnaris at the elbow.

Management
The ulnar nerve can be decompressed in the cubital tunnel by dividing the fibrous band. Traction on the nerve can be relieved by an anterior transposition, which relocates the nerve on the anterior side of the medial epicondyle.

7.6 Ganglia

Learning objectives

You should:

- be able to describe the common sites of appearance of a ganglia and describe the usual clinical features.

The presence of a lump on the wrist or hand is a frequent presentation at the hand clinic. Ganglia are seen at the following sites:

- wrist: palm or dorsal aspects
- flexor tendon sheath
- distal interphalangeal joints.

The pathology causing a ganglion to develop is somewhat uncertain. Although ganglia communicate with a synovial-lined cavity, such as a joint or the flexor tendon sheath, the fluid they contain is more gelatinous than pure synovial fluid. Although a pedicle can often be found connecting them to a joint (at the wrist this is usually the scapholunate joint), abnormal areas of joint capsule are found near the base where mucoid degeneration is taking place. Intraosseous and intratendinous ganglia are occasionally found.

Clinical features

Patients complain of a lump on the dorsum of the wrist or on the line of the flexor tendon sheath or on the dorsum of the distal interphalangeal joints. The lumps characteristically come and go but when present can be quite large and painful. Grip strength is impaired and the wrist may ache after prolonged use. Flexor tendon sheath ganglia are small and hard. They remain static during finger movement and cause pain when gripping objects tightly. Ganglia at the distal interphalangeal (DIP) joints (usually referred to as mucous cysts) are unsightly. There is underlying osteoarthritis of the joint and the associated osteophytes are readily palpable.

Wrist ganglia are fixed to the underlying structures but not to the overlying skin. Their surface is smooth and they are often large and fluctuant but may be small and tense. On the palmar side, they are frequently in close conjunction to the radial artery.

Ganglia compressing the ulnar nerve as it passes through Guyon's canal, between the pisiform and the hook of the hamate may present with weakness of the muscles innervated by the ulnar nerve or altered sensation on the palmar aspect of the ulnar one and a half digits or with both motor and sensory abnormalities.

Diagnosis

Clinical examination is usually sufficient to make the diagnosis. A radiograph of the fingers will show the underlying changes of osteoarthritis associated with a mucous cyst.

Management

Wrist ganglia were classically treated by dispersion as they were ruptured by being hit with a heavy object. Recurrence, however, is frequent after this procedure. Small ganglia can be managed by aspiration and injection of hydrocortisone, and this method is sometimes effective in flexor tendon sheath ganglia. The most reliable method is surgical excision. At the wrist, ganglia

must be carefully dissected from the radial artery and the stalk dissected back to the joint. Any abnormal areas of joint capsule must be removed at the same time. Flexor tendon sheath ganglia must be removed with a similar surrounding area of abnormal flexor tendon sheath. Careful dissection to ensure that the excision is complete will avoid recurrence. Mucous cysts require to be carefully dissected from the overlying skin. Osteophytes can be trimmed and the skin repaired. Sometimes a small rotation flap is necessary to close the defect.

Complications

- recurrence.

7.7 Dupuytren's contracture

Learning objectives

You should:

- be able to recognise the predisposing features associated with the development of Dupuytren's contracture

- know when a patient should be referred for surgery.

Dupuytren's disease is a progressive contracture of the palmar fascia of the hand or foot of uncertain aetiology but it is more commonly seen in Celtic and Scandinavian races than others. Factors associated with the development of Dupuytren's contracture are:

- positive family history
- alcohol abuse
- diabetes
- anticonvulsant medication.

Clinical features

The disease usually affects the hands symmetrically and the ring and small fingers are usually the most severely involved. The condition may begin as a pit or a nodule in the palm before spreading distally as a cord to the digit and proximally to the base of the palm. Contracture of the cord produces flexion of the metacarpophalangeal and proximal interphalangeal joints. The presence of knuckle pads, involvement of the plantar fascia and a positive family history are associated with a poor prognosis and an increased recurrence rate after surgery.

Management

Surgical excision of the contracted cord is indicated if the metacarpophalangeal joint is flexed more than 40° or if there is any flexion of the proximal interphalangeal joint.

Great care must be taken to protect the neurovascular bundles during the excision of the Dupuytren's tissue, which often winds round the neurovascular bundle to produce a spiral cord. Postoperative extension exercise and splintage are required to keep the finger straight.

Patients with recurrence often require multiple operations. Full thickness skin grafts are sometimes helpful to achieve healthy skin cover, but after several operations, amputation of the affected digit may be necessary.

Complications

- recurrence in the same area after surgery
- extension to other parts of the hand
- maceration if left untreated
- cold intolerance } if the neurovascular bundles
- numbness } have been damaged.

7.8 Arthritis

Learning objectives

You should:

- recognise the presenting features of arthritis in the hand

- know when surgery should be recommended and what surgical options are available

- recognise the classic sites of osteoarthritis in the hand and know the surgical procedures available.

Rheumatoid arthritis

The wrist and hand are common sites to be affected by rheumatoid arthritis.

Clinical features

Movements are restricted and painful.

- **Listen** — Painful joints cause difficulty with tasks of everyday life.
- **Look** — Swollen joints due to synovial hypertrophy and effusion are present. Muscle wasting may be seen in later stages. Characteristic deformities in the hand occur when the joints have become lax. They include radical deviation of the carpus and metacarpals, ulnar deviation of the phalanges, Z-shaped thumb, and Boutonnière and swan neck deformities of the fingers (Fig. 78).
- **Feel** — Synovial effusion and hypertrophy may be felt over the metacarpophalangeal joints.

- **Move** — Joints may be immobile or very lax, allowing movement in any direction. If tendon ruptures have occurred then individual fingers will be floppy.

Diagnosis

Radiological features of rheumatoid arthritis are:

- osteopenia
- joint space narrowing
- marginal erosions
- joint subluxation and dislocation

and in later stages

- confluent, spontaneous arthrodesis of the carpus.

Management

Conservative

- splints
- analgesics, non-steroidals and disease-modifying agents
- intra-articular steroids.

Surgical

- arthroplasty — replacement of the metacarpophalangeal joints and wrist
- arthrodesis — for any severely destroyed joints and for stabilisation of the interphalangeal joints
- excision arthroplasty — excision of the distal ulna allows pain-free supination and pronation, and prevents further extensor tendon ruptures.

Complications

- progressive deformity
- loss of function
- loss of independence.

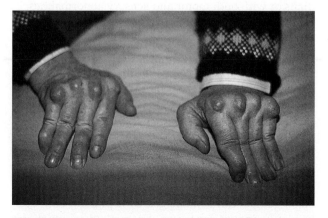

Fig. 78 Rheumatoid hand showing dislocation of the metacarpophalangeal joints and swan neck deformity of the fingers.

Osteoarthritis

In the hand, primary osteoarthritis is often seen in females over the age of 60 years. The sites affected are:

- distal interphalangeal joints
- carpometacarpal joint of the thumb
- triscaphie joint (between the scaphoid, trapezium and trapezoid)
- the proximal interphalangeal joint is rarely affected.

Secondary osteoarthritis may develop due to:

- intra-articular fractures
- septic arthritis
- carpal collapse — seen following scaphoid non-union
- Keinbock's disease (avascular necrosis of the lunate)
- rheumatoid arthritis.

Clinical features

- **Listen** — patients complain of pain, weak grip and loss of function.
- **Look** — the affected joints are swollen and stiff. There is deformity caused by osteophyte formation and eventually loss of function. At the dorsal interphalangeal joint, mucous cyst formation is seen as an eccentric dorsal swelling.
- **Feel** — tenderness and swelling.
- **Move** — movements are limited and painful. Crepitus may be present.

Diagnosis

Radiological examination shows features of osteoarthritis:

- joint space narrowing
- subchondral sclerosis
- cysts
- osteophyte formation
- collapse.

Management

Conservative

- analgesics, splints

Surgical

The following surgical options should be considered:

- arthrodesis for the distal interphalangeal joint and triscaphie joint
- interposition arthroplasty for the carpometacarpal joint of the thumb
- excision arthroplasty for the carpometacarpal joint of the thumb
- joint replacement for the interphalangeal joint of the middle or ring fingers.

Complications

- adduction deformity of first metacarpal following subluxation of arthritic first carpometacarpal joint
- first web space contracture
- weak pinch grip
- chronic pain.

Self-assessment: questions

Multiple choice questions

1. The radial nerve supplies:
   a. The extensors of the wrist
   b. The radial flexors of the wrist
   c. Abductor pollicis brevis
   d. Extensor pollicis longus
   e. Sensation to the tip of the thumb

2. In the hand:
   a. Boutonnière deformity results from rupture of the flexor digitorum tendon
   b. 'Trigger finger' may be caused by tightness of the flexor tendon sheath
   c. 'Mallet finger' is a flexion deformity of the proximal interphalangeal joint associated with trauma
   d. A functioning first dorsal interosseous muscle indicates intact motor function of the ulnar nerve
   e. Stenosing tenosynovitis (de Quervain's) affects the extensor pollicis longus tendon

Extended matching items questions (EMIs)

1. Theme: Diagnoses

A carpal tunnel syndrome
B rheumatoid arthritis
C tendon sheath infection
D rheumatoid nodule
E Dupuytren's contracture
F cubital tunnel syndrome
G osteoarthritis
H ganglion
I phalangeal fracture
J trigger finger

Which of the diagnoses listed above is the most likely cause of the symptoms described below:

1. Pea-sized firm spherical mass in the line of the flexor tendon at the proximal interphalangeal joint.
2. Painless inability to fully extend the proximal interphalangeal joint of the index finger.
3. Paraesthesia on both dorsal and palmar surfaces of the ring and small fingers.

2. Theme: Diagnoses

A carpal tunnel syndrome
B rheumatoid arthritis
C tendon sheath infection
D rheumatoid nodule
E Dupuytren's contracture
F cubital tunnel syndrome
G osteoarthritis
H ganglion
I phalangeal fracture
J trigger finger

Which of the diagnoses listed above is the most likely cause of the symptoms described below:

1. Pain and dorsal angulation in relation to the proximal phalanx.
2. Fixed flexion of the proximal interphalangeal joint and hyperextension of the distal interphalangeal joint in the ring finger.
3. Painful inability to flex or extend a red, swollen index finger.

Constructed response questions (CRQs)

CRQ 1

A 30-year-old female keyboard operator complains of pain in her right hand and fingers by the end of the week. Symptoms are becoming worse and the discomfort and altered sensation becoming permanent. Further questioning reveals that it is the radial three digits which are involved.

a. What other questions might you ask about her symptoms?
b. Physical examination reveals wasting of abductor pollicis brevis in the thenar eminence. Why should this be present?
c. What special clinical tests can be carried out?
d. These tests are all positive. What is your diagnosis?
e. Is it possible that her symptoms could be related to her occupation?

CRQ 2

A 60-year-old woman complains of pain in the radial side of her wrist and base of her thumb when knitting. On examination the first metacarpal is adducted and there is prominence at the carpometacarpal joint suggesting subluxation. Her thumb is developing a 'Z-shaped' deformity, her other hand is satisfactory.

a. What diagnosis does this suggest?
b. On manipulating the joint and attempting to reduce the subluxation of the carpometacarpal joint, what symptoms would you expect to produce?

c. What conservative management could be tried initially?

d. Her symptoms fail to settle over the following few months, and you arrange an X-ray. What do you expect this to show?

e. Is a repeat of the management you suggested in 'c' likely to help at this stage?

f. What would be your next line of management?

Objective structured clinical examination questions (OSCEs)

OSCE 1

Study the clinical photograph below (Fig. 79).

a. What action is this patient unable to do with his finger?

b. What structure do you think has been damaged?

c. The cut in the patient's hand is on the palmar aspect of the middle phalanx. Why is he still able to flex the proximal interphalangeal joint?

d. What other structures may be damaged?

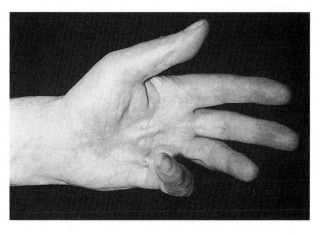

Fig. 80

OSCE 2

Look at the clinical photograph above (Fig. 80).

a. What condition of the hand does it show?

b. List three predisposing factors for this condition.

c. What are the indications for recommending surgery?

d. What structures are in jeopardy during the operation and what postoperative complications should the patient be aware of?

Viva questions

1. Discuss the cause of the sudden loss of ability to extend the ring and small fingers in a rheumatoid hand. How can this disability be managed?

2. Demonstrate the examination of the hand required to assess the integrity of the flexor digitorum superficialis (FDS) and profundus (FDP).

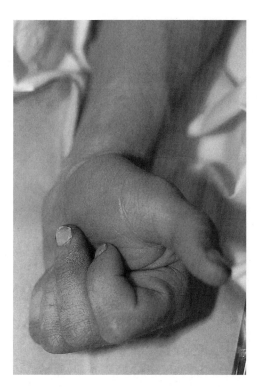

Fig. 79 Injury to the palmar aspect of the middle finger.

Self-assessment: answers

Multiple choice answers

1. a. **True.**
   b. **False.** Flexor carpi radialis is supplied by the median nerve.
   c. **False.** Abductor pollicis brevis is supplied by the median nerve.
   d. **True.**
   e. **False.** Sensation at the tip of the thumb is supplied by the median nerve.

2. a. **False.** The Boutonnière deformity is caused by rupture of the central slip of the extensor tendon over the proximal interphalangeal joint.
   b. **True.** Constriction at the mouth of the flexor tendon sheath at the level of the first annular pulley produces local swelling of the tendon, which prohibits its gliding into the mouth of the tendon sheath, producing a snapping movement called triggering.
   c. **False.** 'Mallet finger' is used to describe the inability to extend the distal interphalangeal joint following traumatic rupture of the extensor tendon or avulsion of a bony fragment from the base of the terminal phalanx.
   d. **True.** The first dorsal interosseous muscle is supplied by the ulnar nerve and its muscle belly can be readily seen in the first web space.
   e. **False.** De Quervain's tenosynovitis refers to symptoms related to the first dorsal compartment containing the tendons of abductor pollicis longus and extensor pollicis brevis.

EMI answers

1. Theme: Diagnoses

1. H. This is a classic description of a tendon sheath ganglion. The lesion is fixed to the tendon sheath and does not move with the tendon as the finger flexes and extends. They are always painful when squashed. Patients complain of discomfort when gripping objects.
2. E. Flexion and contraction of the proximal interphalangeal joint caused by Dupuytren's contracture causes a painless block on full extension.
3. F. Paraesthesia and numbness localised to the ulnar one and a half digits is the classical distribution of altered sensation seen in compression of the ulnar nerve at the cubital tunnel. Compression occurring more distally

(i.e. in Guyon's canal) would not cause numbness on the dorsal surface of the fingers as the dorsal cutaneous branch leaves the main nerve more proximally.

2. Theme: Diagnoses

1. I. A transverse fracture of the proximal phalanx is dorsally angulated by the pull of the extensor tendon on the middle phalanx and flexion of the proximal fragment by the interosseii. A fracture is painful.
2. B. The deformity described is a Boutonnière deformity characteristic of rheumatoid arthritis.
3. C. The finger is red and swollen and movements are painful and resisted. This is characteristic of a tendon sheath infection; prompt decompression is required.

CRQ answers

CRQ 1

a. Does the patient wake up at night with an exacerbation of altered sensation, pins and needles or tingling with numbness in these digits? Is she aware of clumsiness or inability to distinguish articles by touch?
b. The recurrent motor branch of the median nerve comes off the main nerve distal to the carpal ligament so compression of the nerve causes muscle atrophy.
c. Phalen's test
   Tinel's test.
d. Carpal tunnel syndrome.
e. Possibly.

CRQ 2

a. Osteoarthritis of the carpometacarpal joint.
b. Pain and crepitus.
c. Splintage
   Intra-articular steroid injection
   Non-steroidal anti-inflammatory analgesics.
d. Joint space narrowing at the joint between the first metacarpal and the trapezium
   There may be osteophytes and sclerosis
   The joints between the trapezium, the scaphoid and the trapezoid may also be affected (pan-trapezoidal arthritis).
e. No.

f. Trapezectomy or prosthetic replacement of the trapezium.

OSCE answers

OSCE 1

a. Flexion at the distal interphalangeal joint of the left middle finger.
b. Flexor digitorum profundus to the middle finger.
c. Flexor digitorum superficialis has not been damaged at this level.
d. The digital nerve and vessel to the finger.

OSCE 2

a. Dupuytren's contracture.
b. Family history
   Alcohol abuse
   Diabetes or antiepileptic medication.
c. Metacarpophalangeal joint contracture more than 40°
   Any proximal interphalangeal joint contracture.
d. Neurovascular bundles may wind around Dupuytren's cords and are at risk of injury during surgery
   Numbness and cold intolerance may be problems if they are damaged
   Recurrence and inability to regain full extension despite the surgery.

Viva answers

1. In rheumatoid arthritis, the extensor tendons may rupture spontaneously at the wrist, especially under the extensor retinaculum where they are invaded by rheumatoid synovium. Attrition rupture can also occur at this site if the tendons rub on the exposed head of the ulna.

   Treatment for rupture of extensor tendons in rheumatoid arthritis consists of suturing the ruptured tendon to an intact neighbour. Tendons that have been cut can be sutured together directly, but tendons that have spontaneously ruptured or worn through cannot, because their ends are frayed and thin.

2. The integrity of flexor digitorum superficialis is assessed by examining the hand with the fingers fully extended. Allowing the affected finger to flex at the proximal interphalangeal joint demonstrates its action. With all the fingers held in full extension, the terminal phalanges are allowed to flex together. This action indicates the integrity of the flexor digitorum profundus.

8 Hip disorders

Chapter overview

Many clinical signs can be elicited by careful examination of a patient with either osteoarthritis or rheumatoid arthritis of the hip, but it is a detailed history of the extent and degree of their pain and the limitation of ability which will help you decide whether or not surgery is indicated. Hip injuries in young people are usually associated with high velocity injuries and polytrauma, and as a result, require a different approach to management than femoral neck fractures in elderly people. Additional investigations may be required especially if a fracture through the femoral head is suspected.

Dislocation of the hip requires prompt assessment and treatment to prevent prolonged damage to the sciatic nerve and the development of avascular necrosis of the femoral head. Fractures of the pelvis are a potentially life-threatening injury as a result of circulatory collapse and both experience and additional imaging will be required to assess the stability of the pelvic ring. However, prompt reduction of an 'open' pelvis in the Accident and Emergency department using an external fixator may be life saving. Open reduction and internal fixation of an acetabular fracture is a complex and specialist procedure for the orthopaedic traumatologist.

8.1 Clinical examination

Learning objectives

You should:

- in addition to listen, look, feel and move, remember to observe the patient lying, standing and walking, which may reflect an underlying disorder
- observe the patient standing to look for short leg length or a positive Trendelenberg sign
- observe the patient lying to measure true and apparent leg lengths.

In addition to the usual 'listen, look, feel, move', examination of the hip includes observation of the patient walking, standing and lying.

Walking. Observe for short leg gait, antalgic gait or Trendelenburg gait.

Standing. Observe the pelvic tilt while standing on each leg in turn. A positive Trendelenburg sign is present when the patient's pelvis dips to the opposite side while weight-bearing on the affected leg (Fig. 81).

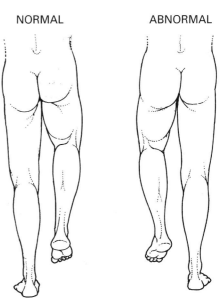

NORMAL   ABNORMAL

Fig. 81 Normal test standing on the *unaffected* left hip. Positive Trendelenburg test when standing on the *affected* right hip.

Lying. With the patient lying supine, movements of the hip joint can be measured. These include flexion and extension, abduction and adduction, and internal and external rotation. Care must be taken to ensure that the pelvis does not move during these manoeuvres, and this can best be achieved by stabilising the pelvis with one hand while manipulating the leg with the other. Thomas's test, which unmasks a fixed flexion deformity of the hip, should be performed by flexing the un-affected hip up to the chest wall and observing whether the leg on the affected side rises off the couch during this manoeuvre. The test should be carried out with the examiner's hand under the lumbar spine to check that the secondary lumbar lordosis has been abolished by this manoeuvre. Finally, true and apparent leg lengths should be measured. True leg length is measured with the hips in the identical degree of adduction, measuring from the anterior superior iliac spine to the medial malleolus. Apparent leg length is measured with the legs parallel to each other measuring from the umbilicus to the medial malleolus.

8.2 Arthritis

Learning objectives

You should:

- be able to carry out Thomas's test for fixed flexion deformity

- recognise the radiological features of osteoarthritis in the hip

- know the rare occasions when osteotomy, arthrodesis or excision arthroplasty of the hip may be indicated

- outline the technique for total hip replacement

- be able to list the general complications, the specific early complications and the specific late complications of this operation.

Osteoarthritis of the hip is a common condition, affecting patients usually in their sixties and seventies. Primary osteoarthritis occurs idiopathically but is sometimes associated with a positive family history.

Secondary osteoarthritis can develop following previous insults to the joint from:

- trauma
- infection
- avascular necrosis
- Perthes' disease.

The sequence of pathological changes in the articular cartilage begins with fibrillation and cleft formation of the articular surface secondary to breaks in the normal arcades of collagen fibres. Clefts develop in the articular cartilage and the intracellular enzymes released cause synovial irritation. The resulting inflammation leads to contracture of the capsule. Eventually, articular cartilage is destroyed and subchondral bone becomes exposed. Cysts may develop in the subchondral bone and contribute to the femoral head collapse.

Clinical features

The main clinical features are:

- pain
- stiffness
- loss of function.

Listen. The severity of pain should be graded to assess the severity of the condition. A useful scale is one ranging from pain that is present with vigorous activity, through pain that is present with weight-bearing, to pain that is present at rest and, ultimately, pain that prevents sleep. Pain is often referred to the groin and thigh and sometimes the misleading symptom of isolated pain at the knee is the presenting feature of hip disease. Does the patient need regular analgesics and use a walking stick?

Look. Examination of the patient walking may show an antalgic gait, a Trendelenburg gait or a short-leg gait (see Fig. 81).

Feel. Because the hip joint is deeply situated, little can be felt by palpation, but tenderness may be elicited by percussion over the greater trochanter.

Move. There is limited range of movement and in particular there are flexion and abduction contractures with loss of internal rotation. Flexion contractures can be unmasked by Thomas's test, which corrects the secondary hyperlordosis of the lumbar spine.

Diagnosis

Radiological examination shows joint space narrowing, subchondral sclerosis, osteophyte formation and subchondral cysts (Fig. 82).

Management

General. Some simple advice may be helpful. The patient may be able to live within the limits of their discomfort without further treatment. Weight reduction may help. The use of a walking stick in the opposite hand decreases the load crossing the painful hip. If there is leg length inequality, a shoe raise is used to correct the

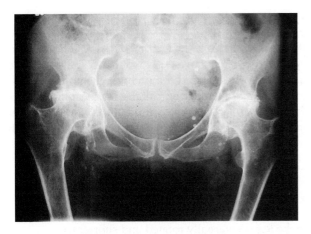

Fig. 82 Bilateral osteoarthritis of the hips with loss of the joint space, subchondral sclerosis, osteophytes and subchondral cysts. Very extensive femoral head collapse.

gait and so relieve secondary back pain. Physiotherapy has a role in keeping other joints mobile.

Medical management. Analgesics and non-steroidal anti-inflammatory drugs are useful, although there is a risk of gastrointestinal haemorrhage with these.

Surgical management. The mainstay of surgical management has become a total joint replacement, but this is not always the most appropriate option. Other procedures to be considered include:

- osteotomy
- arthrodesis
- excision arthroplasty.

Osteotomy

Cutting the femur in the area of the trochanters and displacing the fragments can be used to rotate the head and realign the joint (Fig. 83). This has the effect of altering the weight-bearing surface, reducing the load across the hip joint and achieving vascular decompression of the bone. Symptoms may be relieved and joint function improved. Osteotomy is appropriate for a young patient with only an isolated point of arthritis in the joint.

Arthrodesis

Fusion of the hip joint with a bone graft achieves pain relief but at the expense of loss of movement. The knee, back and contralateral hip must have free painless movement to compensate for the arthrodesed joint. This debilitating operation may be considered in severe arthritis in a young patient.

Excision arthroplasty

If the affected joint is excised, the 'gap' fills with fibrous tissue. The leg is several centimetres shorter after this procedure but painless movement is possible. This is

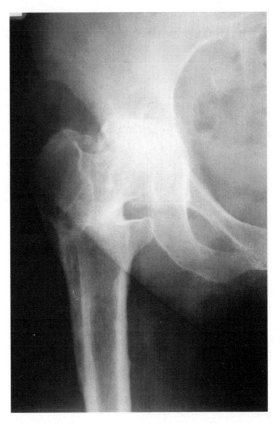

Fig. 83 Osteoarthritis of the hip which has previously been treated by an intertrochanteric displacement osteotomy.

usually reserved as a revision operation following removal of an infected joint replacement.

Total joint replacement

A total joint replacement involves replacement of both the acetabular and femoral parts of the joint. An acetabular cup made of high-density polyethylene and a metal femoral component are used (Fig. 84). These are cemented into the bone with acrylic cement. Prophylactic antibiotics and precautions against deep venous thrombosis and pulmonary embolism are usually required. Reliably good results can be achieved but there is a long-term risk of recurrence of hip pain if the implant becomes loose or infected. Revision surgery is then required. Patients should be prepared to limit their activities in an attempt to avoid the development of loosening and further surgery.

Complications of surgery

- chest infection
- urinary tract infection
- pressure sores
- deep vein thrombosis and pulmonary embolus.

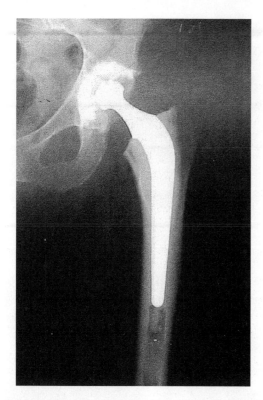

Fig. 84 Arthritis of the hip treated by a Charnley total hip replacement.

Specific complications

- early
  — haematoma formation
  — wound dehiscence
  — wound infection
  — dislocation
- late
  — aseptic loosening
  — deep infection.

8.3 Hip injuries

Learning objectives

You should:

- know that hip injuries in young people are different from those in the elderly population

- recognise the clinical appearance of a dislocated hip. Understand why this is a surgical emergency

- be able to identify a fractured pelvis radiologically

- differentiate stable from unstable pelvic fractures. Remember that the complications of hypovolaemic shock and uretheral damage may be present.

Hip injuries in young people

Whereas fractures of the femoral neck are commonplace low-energy injuries in elderly women, a similar fracture in a young adult is uncommon but, when present, indicates the involvement of a high-energy injuring force. Fractures are, therefore, commonly comminuted and may extend into the upper third of the femur (sub-trochanteric fractures) or involve the femoral head.

Clinical features

- pain
- excessive swelling of the hip and thigh
- the leg is externally rotated and shortened
- injuries to adjacent soft tissues
- injuries elsewhere.

Diagnosis
Plain radiographs will show the fracture fragments.

Management
High fractures of the femoral neck are stabilised by screw fixation, but subtrochanteric fractures can be more difficult. Operative stabilisation with an intramedullary device such as the 'reconstruction nail' is used and allows early active movement and weight-bearing (Fig. 85).

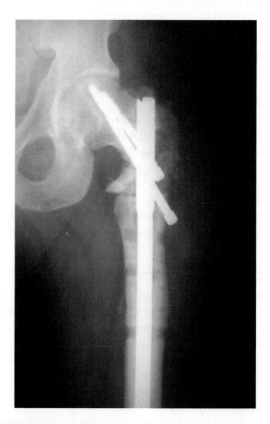

Fig. 85 Reconstruction nail used in the treatment of a subtrochanteric fracture previously treated unsuccessfully with a sliding nail plate.

Complications

- of the injury
  - shock
  - damage to adjacent soft tissues
- of surgery
  - wound infection
  - delayed union
  - non-union.

Dislocation

A high-energy injury is required to dislocate the hip. Involvement in a road traffic accident is a common history. Dislocations can be classified as:

- posterior dislocation
- anterior dislocation
- central dislocation.

Posterior dislocation

As the hip has dislocated posteriorly, there may be an associated fracture of the posterior lip of the acetabulum or of the head of the femur itself.

Clinical features

- **Listen** — There is a history of a direct blow to the knee while seated, often from the car dashboard in a road traffic accident.
- **Look** — The leg lies in a characteristic position of adduction and internal rotation and appears short. There is often flexion of the hip and knee. There may be a telltale injury over the knee.
- **Feel** — Sciatic nerve compression from the displaced femoral head causes altered sensation in the leg.
- **Move** — Hip movements are resisted, and with sciatic nerve compression there may be weakness of ankle movement.

Diagnosis
Plain radiographs show the dislocation and any major fractures of the acetabular margin, but small fractures, especially displaced fragments of a femoral head fracture, will be best seen by CT scan (Fig. 86).

Management
Urgent reduction of the dislocation is required as avascular necrosis of the femoral head will occur if stretching of the capsular vessels to the femoral head is prolonged. Open reduction may be required, especially if exploration of the sciatic nerve is thought to be necessary or if there is a posterior acetabular lip fragment requiring

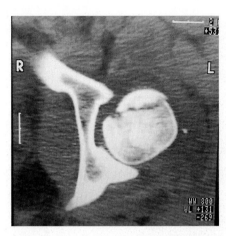

Fig. 86 CT scan of a reduced dislocation of the hip showing an associated fracture of the femoral head.

internal fixation. Small bone fragments within the joint must be removed, but a large fragment from the femoral head should be secured back in place with screws.

Complications

- sciatic nerve damage
- avascular necrosis
- secondary osteoarthritis.

Anterior dislocation

This injury is rare. The leg lies in external rotation, abduction and flexion. The dislocation can be reduced by manipulation under anaesthesia. Again, avascular necrosis is a complication.

Central dislocation

High-energy injury is required to produce this dislocation, which is really a fracture of the floor of the acetabulum.

Diagnosis
A plain radiograph shows a comminuted fracture with central displacement of the femoral head into the pelvis (Fig. 87A). There are various degrees of displacement of the femoral head and multiple fragments of bone may be present, which can best be identified by a CT scan (Fig. 87B). This will assist in planning the stabilisation of the fracture by internal fixation.

Management
The hip can be reduced by manipulation under anaesthesia, although internal fixation of the fragments of the acetabular floor by contoured plates and screws is a preferable but more difficult approach requiring considerable expertise.

A

B

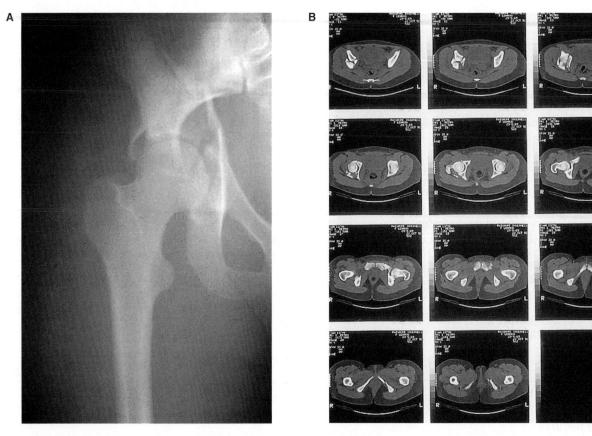

Fig. 87 A. Central dislocation of the hip with a comminuted fracture of the acetabulum. **B.** CT scan showing the position of the multiple fragments of an acetabular fracture.

Complications

- secondary arthritis.

Fractured pelvis

Fractures of the pelvis can range from trivial to life threatening.

Fractured pubic rami

A minor fall in an elderly patient is often the cause of a fracture of one or two pubic rami.

Clinical features

After a minor fall, the patient complains of discomfort around the hip and groin. Clinical examination reveals no evidence of fracture of the femoral neck or greater trochanter (which are other likely sites of injury) but there is localised tenderness at the pubic rami and maybe bruising and swelling here later.

Diagnosis

Plain radiographs will confirm the diagnosis. Both pubic rami on the same side are usually injured.

Management

The patient rests until the discomfort has settled and then gradual mobilisation begins over the following few days.

Complications

- none except those related to bed rest.

Fractures of the pelvic ring

Depending on the mechanism of injury, fractures may be classified as due to:

- AP compression — 'open book' and 'floating segment' fractures
- lateral compression — the acetabulum is involved
- shear type injuries — both anterior and posterior elements are fractured

All types of pelvic ring fracture carry a risk of massive haemorrhage, DIC and urethral or bladder damage.

'Open book' fracture

The pelvic rim is disrupted both anteriorly and posteriorly and has 'hinged' open like a book. An external fixator between the anterior iliac crests should be used in the emergency room to 'fold' the pelvis together and so control bleeding.

'Floating segment' fracture

Clinical features. A direct blow from the front may fracture all four pubic rami, creating a floating segment incorporating the fragments attached to the pubic symphysis, the bladder and the urethra (Fig. 88). There is a boggy swelling and bruising in the perineum. There may be extraperitoneal extravasation of urine, haematuria or blood at the urinary meatus.

Diagnosis. Plain radiographs show the fracture but the presence of urinary tract rupture must be sought by retrograde urethrograms.

Management. Initially, circulating volume must be restored as internal bleeding may be extensive. A single attempt is usually made to pass a urethral catheter, but if this fails, suprapubic drainage must be commenced, usually by a urologist. Bladder and urethral repair may be required. Definitive open reduction and internal fixation can be attempted later.

Acetabular fractures

Major trauma to the pelvis, directed via the greater trochanter or along the axis of the femur, fractures either the anterior or posterior columns of the acetabulum. These columns represent the strong bony margins of the pelvis that enclose the acetabulum.

Clinical features. There is localised tenderness and bruising around the pelvis with pain on stressing the pelvic ring. The patient may be profoundly shocked from extensive bleeding from the pelvic veins.

Diagnosis. X-rays at 45° will show the anterior and posterior columns more effectively than antero-posterior films. CT scan will show the details of the injury more precisely.

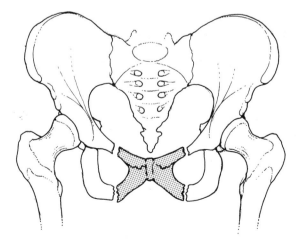

Fig. 88 Fracture of all four pubic rami creating a floating segment.

Management. Initial management involves the restoration of acute blood loss by intravenous fluids. In the younger patient, open reduction and internal fixation with malleable plates is required. A preoperative arteriogram may be necessary if damage to a major vessel at the fracture site is suspected. Alternative treatment in an elderly or debilitated patient is traction until the fracture stabilises.

Complications

- acute blood loss
- other injuries to the axial skeleton
- damage to the bladder or ureter.

Shear type injuries

Clinical features. Disruption of the pelvic ring with anterior and posterior injuries creates an ipsilateral segment of one half of the pelvis. There may be fractures of two ipsilateral pubic rami, together with a posterior fracture of the ilium or a separation of the sacroiliac joint. Stressing the pelvis produces pain. One half of the pelvis is obviously higher than the other creating a difference in leg length.

Diagnosis. X-rays show the extent of the disruption.

Management. Again early stabilisation with an external fixator restores haemodynamic stability but definitive internal fixation will be necessary later.

Complications

- circulatory collapse
- sacral nerve root disruption.

8.4 Avascular necrosis

Learning objectives

You should:

- list the predisposing causes of avascular necrosis of the hip.

Avascular necrosis of the femoral head may be idiopathic but is also associated with alcohol abuse and deep-sea diving. Sometimes it is secondary to infection or to intracapsular fractures or dislocations of the hip. The avascular bone becomes sclerotic, collapses and dies.

Clinical features

The hip joint is stiff and painful and the patient walks with a limp.

Diagnosis

MRI or plain radiographs will show collapse and sclerosis of the avascular femoral head with osteoporosis of the surrounding bone.

Management

Treatment of the early painful phase of avascular necrosis is difficult. Osteotomy and core excision of the femoral neck and head have been used in an attempt to stimulate revascularisation. An operation to insert a vascularised iliac crest bone graft has also been used in an attempt to bring a new external blood supply to the femoral head. Once osteoarthritic changes have developed total joint replacement is necessary.

Complications

- secondary osteoarthritis.

Self-assessment: questions

Multiple choice questions

1. Emergency management of the patient with a high-velocity pelvic ring fracture includes:
   a. Longitudinal traction to the affected limb
   b. Passing a urethral catheter
   c. Institution of intravenous infusion with large volumes of crystalloids
   d. Exclusion of other life-threatening injuries
   e. External fixation of the pelvic fractures

2. Which of the following radiographic features are commonly seen in osteoarthritis:
   a. Subchondral cysts
   b. Marginal erosions at the joint
   c. Osteophytes
   d. Looser's zones
   e. Heterotopic calcification

Extended matching items questions (EMIs)

1. Theme: Clinical presentation

A external rotation and shortening of the leg
B fixed flexion
C adduction contracture
D increase in true leg length
E apparent lengthening
F bruising down the iliotibial tract
G bruising over the trochanteric bursa
H perineal swelling and bruising with blood at the urinary meatus
I abduction deformity
J internal rotation and shortening of the leg

Identify the clinical presentation from the list above which is mostly commonly associated with the conditions described below:

1. A front seat car passenger involved in a head-on collision injures her knee on the dashboard. Her hip is painful.
2. Subtrochanteric fracture.
3. High-energy fracture of multiple pubic rami.

2. Theme: Clinical presentation

A posterior dislocation
B subtrochantic fracture
C kyphosis
D apparent shortening
E normal Thomas's test
F Loss of external rotation
G positive Trendelenberg test

H true shortening
I secondary increase in lumbar lordosis
J fixed internal rotation

Which of the clinical findings above are most closely associated with the conditions below:

1. Adduction contracture of the hip.
2. Flexion contracture of the hip.
3. Loss of hip abduction.

Constructed response questions (CRQs)

CRQ 1

> A 50-year-old labourer presents with a 12-month history of increasing pain in his right hip. He is having annoying side effects from the analgesics he has been using. He has read about the benefits of total hip replacement and wishes to have surgery.

a. How would you define how severe his pain is?
b. You begin your examination with him standing up. He has a positive Trendelenberg test. Why should this be?
c. On examining him on the couch he has a fixed flexion deformity of the affected hip. What test would you do now?
d. You place his legs parallel to each other and measure from the midline to the medial malleolus on each side. You record a discrepancy of 4 cm in this measurement. What is the name of this type of shortening and why should it occur?
e. What other treatment option may be appropriate? Why may a total hip replacement be unsatisfactory for him?

CRQ 2

> An 84-year-old woman weighing 95 kg presents having fallen in her home. She is unable to weight-bear on the right leg. There is little to see on physical examination but moving the hip is painful. You suspect a fracture of the femoral neck and arrange an X-ray. This is reported as negative.

a. What other fracture may she have sustained?
b. You decide to manage her conservatively with bed rest. What are the risks of bed rest for this patient?

c. After a week she is reluctant to recommence weight-bearing but the nursing staff think she should be made ready for discharge. Who might help you with this patient at this stage?

Objective structured clinical examination questions (OSCEs)

OSCE 1

This is a photograph of an X-ray of the pelvis of a 45-year-old barmaid who complains of pain in the left hip (Fig. 89).

a. What underlying features can be seen?
b. She has a history of previous dislocation of this hip from a car accident some years ago. What is the significance of this and what other predisposing factors do you know?
c. How should the patient be managed initially?
d. Her condition deteriorates. What subsequent treatment may be necessary?

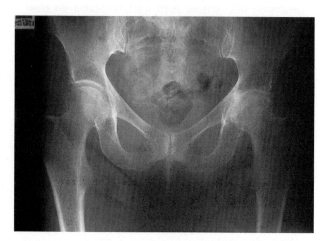

Fig. 89

OSCE 2

A young man has bilateral hip injuries from a motorbike accident. Study the photograph of an X-ray of the right hip (Fig. 90A and B).

a. What injury is shown?
b. What further information would you require about this fracture?
c. On the left side he has had a posterior dislocation of the hip, which has been reduced urgently in the casualty department. CT scan of this site shows an abnormality. How has this occurred?
d. How should both these injuries be treated?

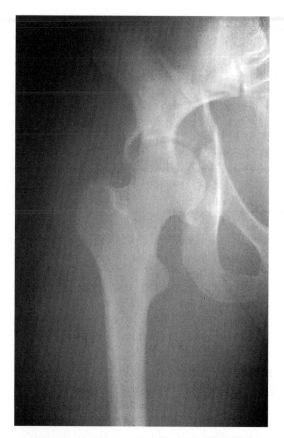

Fig. 90A

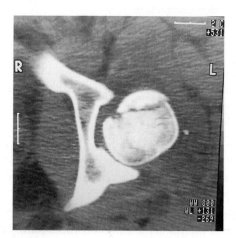

Fig. 90B

Viva questions

1. List the surgical methods of treating arthritis and illustrate each of them with reference to a particular joint.

2. What would be the duties of a preregistration house officer attending a patient the day after a total hip replacement?

Self-assessment: answers

Multiple choice answers

1. a. **False.** Disruption of the pelvic ring requires urgent reduction to compress the pelvis. Longitudinal traction on the leg would not achieve this.
   b. **True.** Urethral damage is suspected in the presence of perineal bruising, scrotal haematoma or blood at the urethral meatus. The integrity of the urethra can be verified by passing a catheter.
   c. **True.** Large volumes of blood are lost from pelvic fractures and rapid intravenous restoration of the circulating volume is mandatory.
   d. **True.** The presence of one high-velocity injury should alert you to the possibility of other severe injuries to the chest or abdomen.
   e. **True.** An external fixator placed between the iliac crests will reduce a displaced fracture of the pelvic ring and decrease haemorrhage.

2. a. **True.**
   b. **False.** These are associated with rheumatoid arthritis.
   c. **True.**
   d. **False.** These are associated with osteomalacia.
   e. **False.** This can be the sequelae of an intramuscular haematoma.

EMI answers

1. Theme: Clinical presentation

1. J. This is a classical story of a posterior dislocation of the hip. The characteristic clinical presentation for this is internal rotation and shortening.
2. A. In a subtrochanteric fracture the leg will lie in external rotation with shortening.
3. H. In a high-energy injury with multiple fractures of the pubic rami, there will be a perineal swelling and bruising, with possible damage to the urethra presenting with blood at the urinary meatus.

2. Theme: Clinical presentations

1. D. In the presence of an adduction contracture of the hip, there will be apparent shortening in that leg as a patient adapts to stand with legs parallel.
2. I. In order to compensate for a flexion contracture of the hip, a patient will develop a secondary lumbar lordosis.

3. G. If the hip cannot abduct because it is stiff, there will be a positive Trendelenberg test as the patient is unable to centralise their centre of gravity over the affected hip when weight-bearing, consequently they 'dip' to the opposite side with this manoeuvre (positive Trendelenberg test).

CRQ answers

CRQ 1

a. Severity of pain can be graded according to how much it interferes with activities and rest. How much is his ability to work and his walking distance limited?
b. He has limited or absent ability to abduct the right hip.
c. Thomas's test.
d. Apparent shortening because of an adduction contracture of the affected hip.
e. Hip arthrodesis only if his other hip and spine are satisfactory. Total hip replacement in a young working man has an increased chance of loosening thus requiring revision at an early date.

CRQ 2

a. Fracture of the greater trochanter or fracture of a pubic ramus.
b. Pressure sores
   DVT
   Urinary tract infection
   Chest infection.
c. Physiotherapist
   Walking aids
   Occupational therapist for home visit and assessment for any additional aids in the house.

OSCE answers

OSCE 1

a. Sclerosis of the femoral head and flattening of the normal shape
   No osteophytes.
b. A dislocated hip may cause loss of blood supply to the femoral head resulting in subsequent avascular necrosis. Alcohol abuse and deep-sea diving are associated with the spontaneous onset of avascular necrosis.
c. Medical treatment
   Analgesics
   Physiotherapy.

d. Osteotomy, core excision, ultimately a total hip replacement.

OSCE 2

a. Central dislocation of a comminuted fracture of the acetabulum.
b. CT scan to determine the anatomy of the fragments.
c. This is a displaced fracture of the femoral head, which has been sheared off during the dislocation of the head by the posterior acetabular lip.
d. Open reduction and internal fixation is required on the right side. The femoral head fragment on the left side may require internal fixation if large.

Viva answers

1. The following surgical methods of treating arthritis are available:

   Osteotomy. A lateral closing wedge osteotomy of the upper tibia is used to treat medial compartment arthritis in the knee (see Ch. 9).

   Arthrodesis. Hallux rigidus can be treated by arthrodesis of the first metatarsophalangeal joint in the appropriate degree of dorsiflexion (see Ch. 10).

   Excision arthroplasty. Arthritis around the radial head can be treated by excision arthroplasty of the radial head without the use of a prosthetic spacer (see Ch. 6).

   Interposition arthroplasty. Arthritis of the basal joint of the thumb can be treated by interposition arthroplasty with a silastic spacer or soft tissue 'anchovy' (see Ch. 7).

   Total joint replacement. This is the final method of treating arthritis and involves replacing both surfaces of the joint with components of metal and high-density polyethylene.

2. The house officer would be responsible for:

   - pain relief
   - prophylactic measures to prevent postoperative infection and deep venous thrombosis
   - fluid balance
   - assessing the need for blood transfusion
   - monitoring of temperature, blood pressure and heart rate
   - requesting a radiograph to check the position of both the acetabular and femoral components of the prosthesis.

9 Knee disorders

Chapter overview

The knee lends itself to physical examination as many of its anatomical landmarks are palpable and pathological features may readily be detected on physical examination. The presentation of a painful swollen knee is common in both elective orthopaedic practice, where it may be associated with rheumatoid or osteoarthritis, and in trauma surgery, where haemathrosis is commonly seen in sports players and signifies some internal derangement in the joint.

Arthroscopic surgery has revolutionised the approach to knee surgery for many patients and the duplications of this treatment should be understood. Both rheumatoid and osteoarthritis remain common problems in the knee and recent years have seen considerable development in the design of total knee replacements. The indications for surgery and postoperative management should be clearly understood. Intra-articular fractures, especially of the tibal plateau, remain a technical challenge for orthopaedic surgeons. Loose bodies and infection in the knee are less common but, as with many other knee problems, much can be gained by careful attention to history and physical examination.

9.1 Clinical examination

Learning objectives

You should:

- be able to examine the knee and relate your findings to the underlying anatomy
- know how to detect an effusion of the knee joint
- know how to carry out tests for ligamentous laxity.

The knee joint is very superficial, so much of its structure can be observed and palpated. Examination can be very precise, and if done carefully will help extensively in making a diagnosis. Being asked to examine the knee is a common question in undergraduate clinical examinations as patients with specific clinical findings are readily available. It is very important, therefore, to be proficient at the examination technique involved. This, as always, includes 'listen, look, feel and move'. Do not forget to observe the patient walking and standing as well as lying down.

- **Listen.** Key features in the history include:
  - mechanism of injury
  - pain
  - instability
  - swelling or locking.
- **Look:**
  - quadriceps muscle wasting
  - varus/valgus alignment
  - effusion in the suprapatellar pouch
  - scars from previous injury or surgery
  - do not forget to look behind the knee for a popliteal cyst.
- **Feel** — With the knee extended, feel for retropatellar tenderness or a small effusion. With the knee flexed to 90°, the medial and lateral joint lines are easily palpated. The origins and insertions of the medial and lateral collateral ligaments may be tender if they have been stretched or torn.
- **Move** — Carry out the anterior drawer sign to check for anterior cruciate laxity. Observe for the presence of a posterior sag suggestive of posterior cruciate ligament rupture. Apply varus and valgus stresses to

the partially flexed knee to check the integrity of the medial and lateral collateral ligaments. Observe the knee for evidence of locking (a block to full extension) and demonstrate that full flexion is possible.

9.2 The 'sportsman's knee'

Learning objectives

You should:

- be able to recognise a history suggestive of a meniscal lesion

- be able to differentiate the clinical findings of a torn miniscus from a collateral ligament injury

- know the emergency management of a haemarthrosis.

Knee injuries are often caused by sporting activities.

Meniscus

Meniscal tears are the most common injury to the knee. They are caused by twisting injuries while weight-bearing on the affected leg. Those associated with sports are usually vertically orientated (Fig. 91) and may form part of a triad of injuries which includes damage to the medial collateral and anterior cruciate ligaments. In an older patient the meniscus becomes degenerate and minor twisting forces may be enough to cause meniscal tears, which are usually orientated horizontally.

Clinical features

The key features of meniscal damage are:

- pain
- instability
- swelling
- locking.

Listen. Patients complain of pain in the knee and instability, especially on stairs. There is often a history of an injury while playing sports.

Look. A swelling may be seen in the para-patellar recesses or, if large, in the suprapatellar pouch. The effusion must be very large before the patella rises away from the femoral condyles and a patellar tap can be elicited by balloting it back down. A swelling occurring within hours of an injury is usually due to bleeding and is a haemarthrosis. A swelling which occurs slowly is usually due to synovial fluid from the inflamed or irritated synovial lining.

Feel. There is well-localised jointline tenderness usually on the medial side

Move. A block to full extension is called 'locking' and is due to trapping of an intra-articular structure, usually the displaced meniscus, within the joint. Twisting and compression manoeuvres may reproduce the pain and 'lock' or 'unlock' the joint (McMurray's test).

Diagnosis

MRI scan will show a torn meniscus but careful clinical examination will make the diagnosis in the majority of cases. Examination under anaesthesia followed by arthroscopy will make it possible to proceed to a therapeutic procedure on the same occasion. Other knee conditions with some of the same clinical features can also be seen arthroscopically. These include loose bodies (see p. 118), discoid meniscus and cystic meniscus.

Management

A large haemarthrosis should be drained urgently to relieve pain. When the diagnosis has been confirmed by arthroscopy, a small meniscal tear can be trimmed or a bucket handle tear removed (Fig. 92). A peripheral detachment of the meniscus can be sewn back if several operating portals into the knee are used to place the arthroscope and other necessary instruments accurately. This minimally invasive procedure ensures that rehabil-

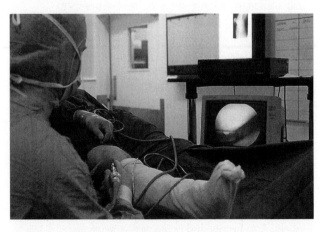

Fig. 92 Arthroscopic examination of the knee.

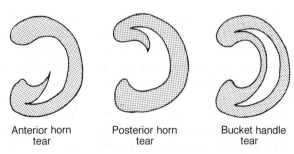

Anterior horn tear   Posterior horn tear   Bucket handle tear

Fig. 91 Three types of vertical tears seen in the meniscus.

itation can occur in the quickest possible time. An open procedure for total meniscectomy is therefore rarely indicated today.

Complications. The articular surface of the knee may be damaged by repeated trauma from long-standing fragments of displaced meniscus.

Cruciate ligaments

The anterior cruciate ligament (ACL) arises at the anterior tibial spine and passes backwards across the knee joint to be inserted on the medial side of the lateral femoral condyle. It prevents the tibia sliding off the front of the femur.

Clinical features

A tear of the ACL is a common sporting injury (Fig. 93). Rupture of the ACL accounts for 75% of haemarthrosis associated with sports.

Listen. There is a history of a twisting injury, a direct blow behind the upper tibia or a hyperflexion injury. The patient often describes a snapping sound and sensation from the knee.

Look/Feel. A haemarthrosis develops quickly.

Move. If the knee is examined before swelling and muscle spasm occur then a positive anterior drawer sign will be easily demonstrated. Lachmann's test can be done if the knee joint is too swollen and painful to allow full flexion for the anterior drawer test. It involves gliding the extended tibia forwards at the knee while holding the thigh steady with the other hand. The pivot shift test involves moving the knee into different positions of flexion while internally rotating the tibia and

applying a valgus stress. It is most usefully carried out under anaesthesia.

Diagnosis

A lateral radiograph may show an avulsion of the anterior tibial spine but usually the tear is in the mid-substance of the ligament and requires MRI to visualise it.

Management

Initial treatment involves aspiration of the knee and early physiotherapy to regain stability by hamstring function. As a rough guide, a third of patients become asymptomatic with this regime. A second third remain symptomatic but adjust their lifestyle to having a knee which is unstable when making sudden changes of direction at speed. Sports, such as squash, that involve cutting and turning movements are not possible but other types of physical exercise can comfortably be carried out.

The final third require a reconstruction to regain a knee which is more stable for sporting activities. The usual method is with a composite bone — patellar tendon — bone transfer or a hamstring autograft. In the rare cases of an avulsion of the anterior tibial spine, open reduction and internal fixation can be carried out.

Complications

● instability, especially on uneven ground. Loss of proprioception from the knee probably accounts for some of this problem.

Posterior cruciate ligament

The posterior cruciate ligament (PCL) arises on the posterior aspect of the tibia and passes anteriorly to be inserted on the lateral side of the medial femoral condyle. This ligament holds the tibia forward under the femur and prevents it dropping backwards. Injuries to the PCL are less frequently seen than ACL injuries.

Clinical features

There is a history of hyperextension or forced posterior displacement of the tibia on the femur. There is a haemarthrosis and an obvious posterior sag to the knee.

Diagnosis

MRI or arthroscopic examination confirms the diagnosis.

Management

Conservative management involves aspiration of the joint and physiotherapy to the quadriceps muscles to stabilise the knee.

Surgical management will involve open reduction and internal fixation of any avulsed bony fragment from the PCL insertion. Mid-substance PCL tears require autograft reconstruction.

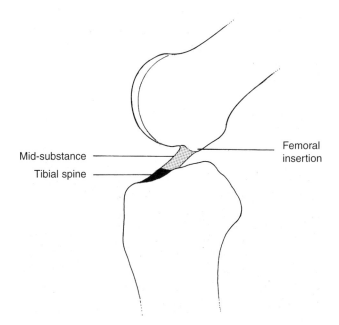

Mid-substance
Tibial spine
Femoral insertion

Fig. 93 Sites of disruption of the anterior cruciate ligament.

Complications

- Chronic instability.

Medial collateral ligament

Damage to the medial collateral ligament is usually associated with both a medial meniscus tear and damage to the anterior cruciate ligament. Injuries are usually the result of twisting forces on the knee. Isolated, pure valgus injury is unusual.

Clinical features

Clinical presentation will include:

- bruising
- swelling
- tenderness
- laxity.

Tears may be in the mid-substance of the ligament or at its origin or insertion on the femur or tibia.

Diagnosis

Radiological examination may show an avulsed bony fragment at either end of the ligament. Stress radiographs may be helpful.

Management

Conservative. Splinting in an orthosis protects the collateral ligament but allows flexion and extension.

Surgical. Reconstruction of an associated anterior cruciate ligament rupture may help to regain stability if a complex derangement of the knee is present.

Complications

- Pellegrini–Stieda syndrome (calcification and discomfort in the medial collateral ligament)
- chronic ligamentous laxity.

Lateral collateral ligament

Isolated injuries to the lateral collateral ligament are less important than medial collateral ligament injuries but may be associated with lateral capsule damage and are usually part of a complex internal derangement of the knee.

Management

A functional brace protects the ligament while allowing flexion and extension.

Complications

- Chronic ligamentous laxity.

9.3 Arthritis

Learning objectives

You should:

- be able to differentiate between osteoarthritis and rheumatoid arthritis of the knee on clinical examination
- list the radiographic features of osteoarthritis and rheumatoid arthritis
- know the principles of management for both these conditions and their indications.

Rheumatoid arthritis and osteoarthritis are both frequently seen in the knee.

Osteoarthritis

Primary osteoarthritis may develop in the knee spontaneously and is sometimes associated with a positive family history.

Secondary osteoarthritis may follow trauma, infection or intra-articular derangement of the knee, such as a ligamentous disruption or meniscectomy.

The medial side of the joint is more frequently involved than the lateral side.

Clinical features

Listen. There is knee pain ranging in severity from being associated only with walking, especially on stairs, to being present at rest.

Look. Classically, there is varus alignment of the joint with synovial thickening and effusion. In late cases there is a flexion contraction.

Feel. There is a swelling in the suprapatellar pouch due to effusion. Marginal osteophytes can be felt at the tibial plateau.

Move. There is loss of full extension due to flexion contracture. A valgus strain applied to the knee will correct the varus alignment and reveal laxity of the medial collateral ligament. Moving the knee produces crepitus.

Diagnosis

Radiographs show:

- joint space narrowing
- sclerosis
- subchondral cysts
- osteophytes
- varus alignment

Management

Conservative management includes:

- physiotherapy
- non-steroidal anti-inflammatory drugs
- walking stick
- weight reduction
- limitation of activities.
- intra-articular steroid injection

Operative management

Lavage and debridement. Arthroscopic lavage gives some relief. Marginal osteophytes can be trimmed and fragments of damaged articular surface and menisci washed out of the joint. At the same time, the exact state of the articular cartilage can be assessed (Fig. 94).

Upper tibial osteotomy. A laterally based wedge of bone at the upper tibia is removed (Fig. 95). This

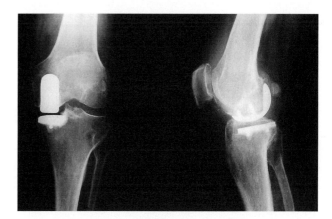

Fig. 96 Unicompartment arthroplasty.

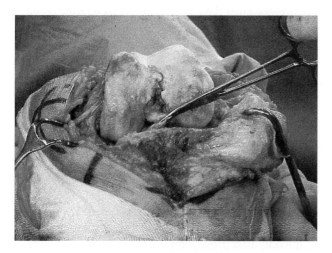

Fig. 94 The extent of osteoarthritic destruction of the articular surfaces can be seen. There is full-thickness loss of articular cartilage and osteophytosis at the intercondylar notch.

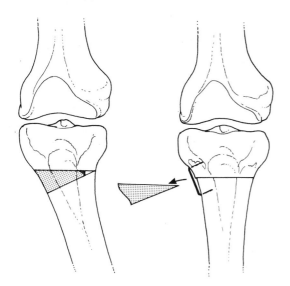

Fig. 95 Procedure of a tibial osteotomy.

realigns the tibia on the femur and redistributes load across the joint diverting high pressures from the damaged medial compartment to the undamaged lateral compartment. The osteotomy is secured with a staple. This operation is suitable for early disease in young patients.

Unicompartmental joint replacement. This replaces both the femoral and tibial sides of one half of the joint, usually the medial compartment (Fig. 96). The operation is only suitable for the early stages of the disease and has been shown to be of limited value.

Total knee replacement. A semi-constrained surface replacement by a metal convex femoral component and a metal-backed high-density polyethylene concave tibial component is used. The prosthesis can be cemented or uncemented to the bone. The stability of the joint depends on correct tensioning of the medial and lateral collateral ligaments and on the contour of the high-density polyethylene tibial component (Fig. 97 A and B).

Arthrodesis. Surgical fusion of the joint may be appropriate for a young patient with arthritis but may also be used to salvage a knee after infection.

Complications of total knee replacement

- wound dehiscence
- infection
- loosening of the components
- bone resorption
- instability
- revision surgery.

Rheumatoid arthritis (also see other sections on rheumatoid arthritis)

Rheumatoid arthritis begins as inflammation of the synovium as part of an autoimmune response. The inflammation ultimately spreads to the articular cartilage and destroys it. The presence of persisting synovial effusions stretches and damages the ligaments and capsule of the

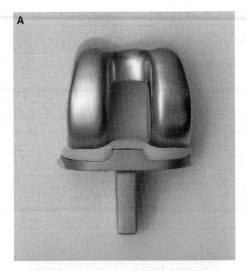

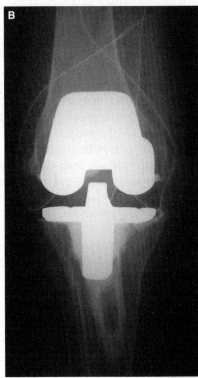

Fig. 97 A. Total knee prosthesis in flexion. **B.** Total knee prosthesis cemented in place with the knee extended.

joint. The joint surface becomes destroyed and the joint itself lax. This results in subluxation, deformity and painful movement.

Clinical features

- **Listen** — the joint is unstable; during exacerbation of the disease it becomes warmer and more painful
- **Look** — swelling
            — valgus alignment

- **Feel** — a joint effusion may be apparent
- **Move** — laxity of the lateral collateral ligament.

Diagnosis

Radiographic features of rheumatoid arthritis include:

- joint space narrowing
- irregular joint surface
- marginal erosions
- valgus alignment.

Management

Medical management includes the use of both analgesics and disease-modifying drugs. Synovectomy may prevent the progression of the disease. This can be done by injection of intra-articular radioactive Yttrium or as an arthroscopic or open procedure.

Operative management. All rheumatoid patients listed for surgery must have radiographs taken of the cervical spine in flexion and extension. This assesses the extent of subluxation of the odontoid process as there is a risk of cord compression with cervical spine manipulation during anaesthesia.

Arthroscopic synovectomy or total joint replacement may be indicated.

Complications

- as listed for knee surgery in osteoarthritis but in rheumatoid arthritis the bone is softer and the skin thinner and more easily damaged
- systemic manifestations: ligamentous laxity of the cervical spine may cause spinal cord compression by the odontoid process during intubation.

9.4 Loose bodies

Learning objectives

You should:

- be able to list the conditions which may give rise to loose bodies in the knee

- know how to examine the knee for 'locking'.

The following may cause loose bodies to be present in the knee:

- osteochondral fractures
- osteochondritis dissecans
- separation of articular cartilage
- synovial chondromatosis
- fragments of meniscus.

Clinical features

Osteochondral fractures occur in young adults, but separation of large portions of the articular cartilage are seen in older patients. Osteochondritis dissecans is more common in boys and usually occurs between the ages of 8 and 12. The lesion is initially on the medial femoral condyle.

The patient usually complains of:

- intermittent pain
- locking and unlocking of the knee which occurs in different degrees of knee flexion
- effusion.

Diagnosis

A plain radiograph will not always show a loose body in the joint as not all are radio-opaque. The fabella (a sesamoid bone in the medial head of gastrocnemius) can easily be mistaken on X-rays for a loose body in the joint. A lucent line around a small part of the medial femoral condyle may be seen in osteochondritis dissecans and if a portion has become loose then a crater will be seen at the same site.

MRI and arthroscopy will visualise a lesion more clearly.

Management

An unseparated fragment can be left alone if not loose. A loose fragment with sufficient bony component can be fixed back in place. Once separated, however, a fragment should be removed arthroscopically. Such fragments often make their way to the suprapatellar pouch. The base of the defect can be drilled to encourage fibrocartilage formation.

9.5 Infection

Learning objectives

You should:

- know how to identify infection in the knee by physical examination
- know the emergency management of an infected knee.

Infection may spread to the joint from osteitis in the adjacent bone. In children, the metaphysis of the proximal tibia is intra-articular. Bacteria from infection at a remote site may also be a cause. Direct intra-articular trauma is a rare cause of joint infection. However, patients with diabetes mellitus or rheumatoid arthritis are more at risk of joint infections. *Staphylococcus aureus* and gonococci are the traditional pathogens involved, but subacute infections in the elderly are probably more common. A more recent cause of knee infection is arthroscopic surgery.

Clinical features

Clinical features include:

- pain
- swelling
- heat
- tenderness
- resistance to active or passive movement.

Diagnosis

There is a raised temperature, white cell count and plasma viscosity. Radiographs may show hyperaemia of the bone in the early stages but are usually normal. The condition should be differentiated from gout, pseudogout or reactive arthritis.

Management

Left untreated, septic arthritis in the joint will ultimately discharge spontaneously through the skin and the joint will undergo a fibrous ankylosis.

When first suspected, the joint must be aspirated and specimens sent for bacteriological examination. Antibiotics must be commenced early. If pus is aspirated from the joint thorough irrigation via the arthroscope should be carried out. Sometimes continuous irrigation and drainage for several days is required. In later stages of infection, arthroscopic division of adhesions is indicated.

Complications

- chronic osteitis
- spontaneous fibrous or bony ankylosis.

9.6 Intra-articular fractures

Learning objectives

You should:

- be able to recognise different types of tibial plateau fracture from the radiological appearance
- know which of these require further imaging for assessment and which will require elevation of the tibial plateau and bone grafting.

Osteochondral fractures

In young adults, shearing forces or direct trauma will produce an osteochondral fracture that may separate entirely from its bed. Such a fragment may grow in the joint as it receives as nutrition from the synovial fluid.

Management

A small fragment should be removed arthroscopically, but a large fresh fragment should be reattached.

Tibial plateau fractures

Valgus forces directed to the knee will tear the medial collateral ligament and damage the lateral tibial plateau.

Clinical features

- **Listen** — history of an angulatory or twisting force to the knee
  - — pain on either side of the joint
- **Look** — medial bruising
  - — swelling
  - — haemarthrosis may be present
- **Move** — valgus laxity on stressing the joint

Diagnosis

Radiological examination may show:

- vertical split
- depression fracture (die punch)
- comminution of the whole lateral tibial plateau
- combination of split and depression fractures.

The different types of tibial plateau fracture are shown in Fig. 98.

Management

Cleavage fractures require screw fixation to restore the stability of the articular surface.

Depression fractures require elevation of the defect with a bone graft. A portion of the lateral meniscus may be found driven into the crater by the injury.

More complex fractures require elevation of the plateau and stabilisation by a buttress plate on the tibia. Bone graft is always necessary. Postoperatively, the knee is nursed in a functional brace, which allows the joint to mobilise but weight-bearing has to be avoided for 6 to 8 weeks.

Complications

- osteoarthritis requiring later total conversion to a total knee replacement
- valgus laxity
- stiff joint.

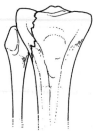
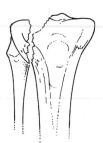

1. Cleavage   2. Cleavage and depression

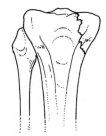
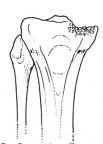

3. Depression

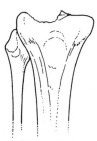

4A. Medial cleavage   4B. Comminution and depression

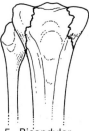
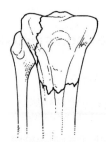

5. Bicondylar   6. Any fracture with discontinuity between diaphysis and metaphysis

Fig. 98 Classification of types of tibial plateau fracture.

Condylar fractures of the femur

Axial angulatory forces directed across the knee may fracture the distal femur.

Clinical features

Clinical features include:

- haemarthrosis
- joint laxity.

Diagnosis

Radiological examination shows a split fracture of a single condyle or a 'Y' shaped fracture of both condyles. There may be a comminuted fracture involving both condyles.

Management

The haemarthrosis is aspirated. Plaster immobilisation may be sufficient for an undisplaced unicondylar split fracture, but accurate anatomical reduction with screw fixation to prevent subsequent displacement is preferable for more complex fractures. Postoperatively, the knee is mobilised in a functional brace.

Complications

- valgus/varus angulation
- osteoarthritis.

9.7 Extensor mechanism injury

Learning objectives

You should:

- list the different types of extensor mechanism injury and relate these to different age groups
- know the principles of management of each injury.

Resisted extension of the knee damages different areas of the extensor mechanism at different ages (Fig. 99).

Adolescents

Avulsion of the tibial tuberosity

A traction injury to the tibial apophysis may elevate a portion causing localised pain, tenderness and a lump. Sometimes a similar condition (Osgood–Schlatter's disease) occurs in adolescence as a result of activity but with no specific injury. In both cases, the lesion is treated by rest and a back splint.

Young adults

Ruptured patellar tendon

Straight leg raising is inhibited and a palpable gap is present. Repair of the tendon is required.

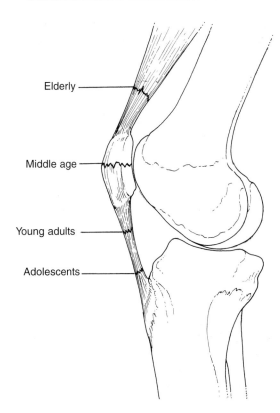

Fig. 99 Sites of rupture of the extensor mechanism at different ages.

Middle age

Transverse (avulsion) fractures of the patella

A palpable gap is present in the patella, sometimes accompanied by extensive lateral and medial bruising and swelling. This indicates a probable tear in the quadriceps expansion and, if present, straight leg raising will be impossible. Repair of the fracture with tension band wire and suture of the quadriceps tear are necessary. The articular surface must be carefully restored. Quadriceps-strengthening exercises and knee flexion can begin when comfortable.

Stellate fractures of the patella

These result from a direct blow on the patella so the quadriceps expansion is not usually torn. There is a haemarthrosis.

A radiograph shows the extent of comminution of the fracture.

Initially the joint is aspirated. A cylinder splint may be sufficient treatment, but with displaced fragments, cerclage wire or screw fixation is indicated.

The elderly

Rupture of quadriceps tendon or rectus femoris muscle

In degenerative tissues, the avulsion is at the osteo-tendinous junction.

Suture and bone anchors are used but the tissues are friable. Physiotherapy alone is usually sufficient to restore quadriceps function.

Complications of extensor mechanism injuries

Complications include:

- weak quadriceps and loss of straight leg raising
- a painful ossicle in the patellar tendon may follow tibial tuberosity avulsion.

Self-assessment: questions

Multiple choice questions

1. Knee pain:
   a. Related to the medial joint line in a 60-year-old patient with a normal knee X-ray is, in the majority of patients, caused by a cleavage lesion of the medial meniscus
   b. At the patellar femoral joint is often a finding in adolescent females
   c. Associated with painful intermittent locking suggests the presence of an intra-articular loose body
   d. In relation to the tibial tuberosity is most commonly found in active osteoporotic females
   e. Associated with intermittent effusions suggests an acute infective synovitis

2. In acute septic arthritis:
   a. *Staphylococcus aureus* is the usual infecting organism
   b. Movement of the infected joint is restricted by adhesions
   c. Antibiotics are withheld until the appropriate sensitivities are confirmed
   d. Treatment includes joint irrigation
   e. Small joints are more commonly affected than large joints

Extended matching items questions (EMIs)

1. Theme: Clinical presentation

A chondromalacia
B degenerative meniscus
C osteochondritis dissecans
D chronic osteitis
E osteoarthritis
F separation of articular cartilage
G fibrous ankylosis
H synovial chondromatosis
I septic arthritis
J rheumatoid arthritis

Which of the diagnoses listed above most closely fits the clinical presentations described below:

1. An 8-year-old boy complaining of intermittent pain and swelling has occasional inability to fully extend the knee to different extents on different occasions.
2. A 70-year-old patient with various other joint problems has symmetrical genu valgus and knee pain with a moderate effusion.

3. A 65-year-old man with a year-long history of knee pain has well-localised medial joint line tenderness, a small effusion and loss of full range of movement. His knee X-ray shows no abnormalities.

2. Theme: Clinical presentation

A torn medial meniscus
B ruptured patellar tendons
C rectus femoris tear
D posterior cruciate ligament tear
E fractured femoral condyle
F avulsion of tibial tuberosity
G stellate fracture of patella
H medial collateral ligament tear
I anterior cruciate ligament tear
J tibial plateau fracture

Which of the diagnoses listed above most closely fits the clinical presentations described below:

1. A 50-year-old pedestrian suffers a direct blow to the knee in a fall on the pavement. There is superficial grazing and bruising over the patella and moderate swelling in the joint.
2. A sportsman suffers a twisting injury to the knee in a rugby tackle. The knee has become immediately very swollen and painful.
3. A 30-year-old marine jumping over a combat wall lands on his feet but is unable to weight-bear because of pain on the lateral side of the upper tibia. He has local swelling and a haemarthrosis.

Constructed response questions (CRQs)

CRQ 1

A 30-year-old fisherman twists his knee in a fall on a riverbank. He was able to limp back to his car, but on examination at the casualty department the next day, he has a moderate effusion in the knee joint with well-localised tenderness at the medial joint line. The range of movement is limited by pain but full extension is not possible on passive manipulation.

a. What is a likely diagnosis?
b. What is the term used to describe the loss of full extension in the knee?
c. You decide to manipulate the knee further. What special test might you do to confirm the diagnosis?

d. As the patient is more comfortable now the knee is moving normally again, he is keen to go home. You decide to investigate the injury as an out-patient. What investigation would you arrange?

e. The result of this investigation confirms the diagnosis. What procedure would be appropriate next and why?

CRQ 2

> The same patient attends your surgery 25 years later. He is now aged 55 and has had a year-long history of increasing pain on the medial side of his knee at the site of his previous injury. There is diffuse tenderness around the joint, a small swelling, loss of full range of movement and some crepitus in the joint. He reminds you that he is a farmer and wishes to continue working.

a. What is the likely diagnosis at this stage?

b. How would you visualize this?

c. Your investigation shows abnormalities limited to the medial compartment. Is there a connection between this and his previous surgery?

d. You discuss treatment options with him. What medical (non-operative) things may be helpful?

e. He returns 6 months later. His symptoms have not been improved, the pathology remain limited to the medial compartment. What surgical procedure is considered in this situation?

Objective structured clinical examination questions (OSCEs)

OSCE 1

Study the photograph of an X-ray of a patient's knees (Fig. 100).

a. What abnormalities can be seen here?

b. What is the diagnosis?

c. The patient is otherwise well but you have to consent her for surgery. What complications should she be made aware of?

OSCE 2

a. Study this diagram of the extensor mechanism of the knee and indicate which sites of extensor mechanism injury are associated with which age groups (Fig. 101).

b. In a patient with a transverse fracture of the patella, what would you expect to find on attempting active extension of the knee?

c. How should the fracture be treated?

d. You discover that there is an extensive tear in the quadriceps expansion on the medial side. How should this be treated?

e. How is the patient managed next?

Viva questions

1. Describe the management of a suspected case of acute septic arthritis in an adolescent's knee.

2. What are the principles of management for a patient with a depressed fracture of the lateral tibial condyle?

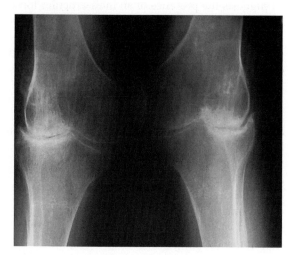

Fig. 100

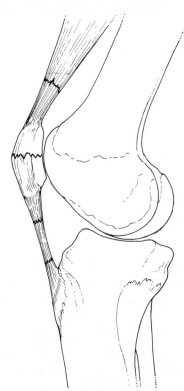

Fig. 101

Self-assessment: answers

Multiple choice answers

1. a. **True.** Medial joint line pain suggests medial meniscus pathology and, in a patient of this age, a cleavage lesion caused by degeneration within the meniscus is common. The tear is horizontal in contrast to the vertical orientation of acute tears.
   b. **True.** Chondromalacia patellae is one cause of anterior knee pain commonly found in teenage girls.
   c. **True.** Locking is a mechanical block to full extension and is classically caused by a displaced meniscal tear or an intra-articular loose body as found in osteochondritis dissecans.
   d. **False.** Pain in relation to the tibial tuberosity is associated with Osgood–Schlatter's disease which is found in adolescent boys especially.
   e. **False.** Acute infective synovitis presents dramatically with a painful swelling from pus within the joint. Intermittent effusions are more likely to be associated with an inflammatory cause such as rheumatoid arthritis or Reiter's syndrome.

2. a. **True.**
   b. **False.** Movement is restricted by acute pain.
   c. **False.** 'Best-guess' antibiotics should be prescribed as soon as specimens have been taken for bacteriological examination.
   d. **True.** Thorough irrigation of the joint often using the arthroscope will reduce the infection.
   e. **False.** The knee and hip are the most common sites of acute septic arthritis.

EMI answers

1. Theme: Clinical presentation

1. C. A loose body in the joint produced by osteochondritis dissecans causes intermittent locking in different degrees of flexion and extension.
2. J. Genu valgus is characteristically seen in rheumatoid arthritis together with a knee effusion. Other joint problems are often seen symmetrically in the body.
3. B. A degenerative meniscus causes joint effusion and pain and may limit knee movement.

2. Theme: Clinical presentation

1. G. A direct blow to the patella will produce a stellate fracture rather than disruption of any other part of the extensor mechanism.

2. I. A swollen knee developing immediately after a sports injury is most likely to be a haemarthrosis due to an anterior cruciate ligament tear.
3. J. A direct injury passing axially through the lower limb will produce a fracture at either the calcaneum or in this case at the tibial plateau. The hip and vertebral bodies are other areas which may be damaged in this type of injury.

CRQ answers

CRQ 1

a. Displaced medial meniscus tear (bucket handle tear).
b. Locking.
c. McMurray's test; this may 'unlock' the knee or produce locking.
d. Arthroscopy.
e. Arthroscopic repair of a peripheral tear is possible as both sides of the tear are vascularised
   For tears in other areas, the displaced portion can be removed arthroscopically while the remainder of the meniscus is retained to aid in weight-bearing.

CRQ 2

a. Osteoarthritis.
b. Plain X-ray
   Weight-bearing AP views.
c. Increased point loading to absence of the medial meniscus particularly if he had a total menisectomy.
d. NSAIDs
   Walking stick
   Weight reduction
   Intra-articular steroid injection.
e. High tibial (valgus) osteotomy — the result may be unpredictable so a total knee replacement may be considered if he will reduce his activity appropriately.

OSCE answers

OSCE 1

a. Bilateral genu valgus
   Marginal erosions
   Joint space narrowing
   Generalised osteopaenia
   Irregular joint surfaces.
b. Rheumatoid arthritis.
c. Wound infection and breakdown; loosening of components and instability.

OSCE 2

a. Tibial tuberosity avulsion — teens
   Patellar tendon tear — young adults
   Transverse fracture of patella — middle age
   Quadriceps tendon tear — elderly.
b. Pain on attempted extension of the knee. Unable to extend the knee.
c. Open reduction and internal fixation with lag screws or tension band wire.
d. Surgical suture.
e. The knee is protected for 3–4 weeks with a range of motion exercises only before starting a course of quadriceps-strengthening exercises.

Viva answers

1. When septic arthritis of the joint is suspected by the clinical examination, the diagnosis can be confirmed by a raised plasma viscosity and a polymorphonuclear leucocytosis. The joint should be aspirated. The presence of opaque synovial fluid or pus confirms the diagnosis and specimens should be sent for bacteriological examination. Arthroscopic lavage with large volumes of fluid is urgently necessary. While results are awaited, 'best-guess' antibiotics should be commenced, such as Flucloxacillin and Fucidin.

2. The extent of displacement of a depressed fracture of the lateral tibial plateau must be assessed by tomography or CT scan. Significantly depressed fragments require elevation and bone grafting. Buttress plate fixation may be required for large fragments. Postoperatively the knee may require protection in a splint until healing has occurred. Weight-bearing should be limited. Physiotherapy will be necessary to maintain quadriceps function.

10 Foot and ankle disorders

Chapter overview

Developmental degenerative and inflammatory conditions are often seen in the feet, presenting as bunions, hallux valgus, hallux rigidus, gout or rheumatoid arthritis. In addition, the feet are involved in the serious changes of progressive peripheral vascular disease. Fractures of the foot and ankle are commonly seen in the Accident and Emergency department, where it is important to be able to differentiate between those which will require further investigation and operative treatment and those which can be managed conservatively.

10.1 Clinical examination

Learning objectives

You should:

- remember to examine the patient's shoes and watch them walking
- observe the patient barefoot from behind both fully weight-bearing and standing on tiptoe
- examine the various joints individually: ankle, subtalar, midtarsal, metatarsophalangeal and interphalangeal.

Examination of the foot and ankle must include an examination of the patient walking and standing. It is import-

ant to remember to examine the patient's shoes for signs of wear on the sole and of damage to the uppers.

The patient's feet are observed while walking. With the patient standing with the feet together, the posture of the foot is examined. Looking from behind, the alignment of the calcaneum can be seen and any degree of calcaneovalgus noted. The posture of the longitudinal arches can be observed. If apparently absent, the arch will often reconstitute when the patient stands on tiptoe. With the patient seated and the foot cradled on the examiner's knee, the peripheral pulses, capillary circulation and peripheral sensation can be examined. Movements of the foot and ankle should be examined in turn. Movement occurs in the following joints:

- ankle
- subtalar
- midtarsal
- metatarsophalangeal
- interphalangeal.

At the ankle joint, only flexion and extension is possible. Subtalar movement is assessed by cupping the heel in the palm of the hand and inverting and everting the foot.

With the calcaneum immobilised on the talus, inversion and eversion at the midtarsal joint can be elicited. Flexion and extension are possible at the metatarsophalangeal and interphalangeal joints.

10.2 Foot disorders

Learning objectives

You should:

- be able to examine the foot for hallux valgus and deformity and differentiate this from hallux rigidus
- differentiate the pathology and management of the common form of hallux valgus in a middle-aged woman from that seen in an adolescent girl
- recognise the deformity of claw toes in the rheumatoid foot and know the different ways of managing this condition
- be able to recognise critical limb ischaemia in the lower limb.

Bunions and hallux valgus

This is the most commonly occurring deformity in the foot, but it is not always symptomatic. Two distinct groups of patients usually present.

The adolescent girl. There is a strong family history of hallux valgus. The underlying abnormality is varus deformity of the first metatarsal.

The middle-aged woman. There is forefoot splaying because of ligamentous laxity. Constricting footwear may provide an additional deforming force. There may be degenerative changes in the first metatarsophalangeal joint and abnormalities of the adjacent toes. Hallux valgus is often seen in association with rheumatoid arthritis in this age group.

Clinical features

- **Listen** — Patients complain of rubbing or pressure over the first metatarsophalangeal joint and that their shoes feel tight.
- **Look** — There is a prominent exostosis at the first metatarsal head covered with a protective bursa. This may become inflamed or even infected. The big toe is displaced laterally, pronated and crowds the second toe so that one may override the other. There may be callosities to see.
- **Feel** — If inflamed the bunion may be painful to touch.
- **Move** — Once established the valgus deformity cannot be corrected.

Diagnosis

Weight-bearing radiographs will show the extent of the deformity, the degree of subluxation of the joint and any secondary arthritic degeneration (Fig. 102).

Management

Initially all patients should consider accepting the deformity and adapting their footwear to accommodate it. If this is not acceptable to the patient, surgery can be discussed.

Adolescents. Management is usually with surgery. An osteotomy of the first metatarsal, which realigns the first ray and narrows the forefoot (Fig. 103), will correct the valgus deformity of the big toe but it may recur if the foot is still squashed into pointed shoes.

Adults

Orthoses. Comfortable, wide shoes that accommodate the splayed forefoot are the easiest solution. The shoe uppers should be soft over the bunion and have moulded insoles to support the metatarsal heads.

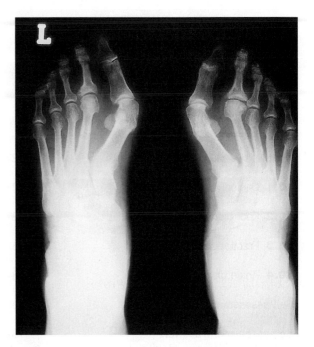

Fig. 102 Radiograph of the feet showing bilateral hallux valgus deformity. On the right there has been a previous excision of the exostosis but the underlying metatarsus primus varus remains.

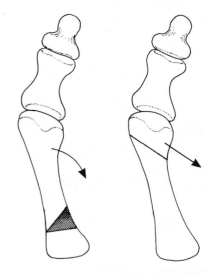

Fig. 103 Two types of osteotomy of the first metatarsal which will correct the underlying varus deformity and allow the big toe to become straighter.

Surgery

- realignment of the hallux can be achieved in patients with mild disease by a capsulorrhaphy of the first metatarsophalangeal joint and release of the adductor hallucis; an excision of the exostosis at the first metatarsal head can be included
- arthrodesis of the first metatarsophalangeal joint is indicated in more severe disease with secondary arthritis.

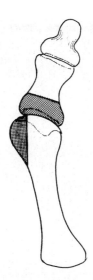

Fig. 104 Keller's arthroplasty of the first metatarsophalangeal joint.

- excision arthroplasty is suitable for older people who are less active; the base of the proximal phalanx and the exostosis are removed (Keller's operation; Fig. 104); the alignment is corrected but the big toe is now floppy and fails to provide a strong 'push off' when walking.

Complications

- local pressure effects
- bursitis.

Complications of surgery

- infection
- poor wound healing
- hallux varus or hallux erectus deformity from overcorrection
- recurrence
- altered sensation.

Hallux rigidus

Some forgotten minor trauma may be the precipitating cause of this condition, which affects men more than women. There is osteoarthritis of the first metatarsophalangeal joint, which causes pain and stiffness of the big toe (hallux rigidus). The changes are isolated and not part of widespread osteoarthritis.

Clinical features

- **Listen** — pain on walking, especially up hills
  — patients notice reduced stride length
  — women complain of pain when wearing high-heeled shoes

- **Look** — dorsal osteophyte
- **Feel** — local tenderness
- **Move** — first metatarsophalangeal joint is stiff
  — dorsiflexion is painful, resisted and limited.

Diagnosis

The familiar radiological features of osteoarthritis are present: sclerosis, joint space narrowing, osteophyte formation (Fig. 105).

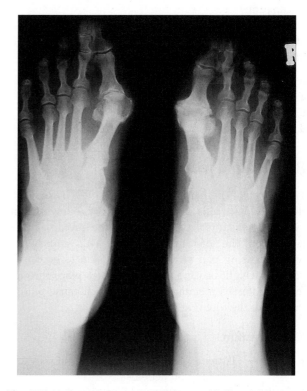

Fig. 105 Hallux valgus on the left foot and hallux rigidus on the right with radiological features of joint space narrowing, sclerosis and osteophyte formation.

Management

Conservative. A carbon fibre insole or rigid sole with a rocker bottom allows the patient to roll over the metatarsophalangeal joint. Low heels are comfortable.

Operative. Arthrodesis of the joint in slight dorsiflexion and adduction provides pain relief but may not accommodate varying shoe heel heights. Interposition arthroplasty has been used, but silicone joints tend to break down with time and cause an inflammatory synovitis. Excision of osteophytes is used if symptoms are only mild.

Complications of surgery

- choice of footwear is restricted
- silicone synovitis.

Fasciitis

Fasciitis is pain at the origin of the plantar fascia where it arises from the calcaneum.

Clinical features
The main clinical features are pain on walking and localised tenderness at the calcaneum.

Diagnosis
X-ray examination sometimes shows a spur on the calcaneum.

Management
Management includes:

- heel pad
- steroid injection
- AFO (ankle-foot orthosis) to wear at night
- Achilles tendon stretching

Rheumatoid feet

The foot, like the hand and wrist, is often involved in rheumatoid arthritis. Ligamentous laxity following synovitis allows dorsal dislocation of the proximal phalanges on the metatarsal heads. This causes the weight-bearing pad of thick plantar skin to be drawn distally; weight-bearing, therefore, takes place through the unprotected metatarsal heads, which cause pain in the sole of the foot (Fig. 106).

Clinical features

- **Listen** — Patients classically complain that they are 'walking on pebbles'.
- **Look** — There are pressure signs over the dorsum of the proximal interphalangeal joints of the toes. The metatarsal heads can be seen prominently in the sole.
- **Feel** — The metatarsal heads can be easily felt.

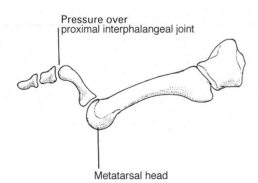

Pressure over proximal interphalangeal joint

Metatarsal head

Fig. 106 Mechanism of metatarsophalangeal joint displacement in rheumatoid arthritis.

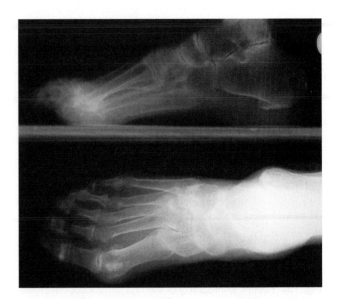

Fig. 107 This true lateral view of the foot shows the extent of the dislocation of the metatarsophalangeal joint. The metatarsal heads are touching the ground but the toes are displaced upwards and do not contribute to weight-bearing.

- **Move** — Eventually the toes cannot be corrected to their normal straight alignment.

Diagnosis
Radiological examination shows the extent of joint subluxation and of bone destruction (Fig. 107).

Management
Conservative. Wide, deep shoes with soft uppers and moulded insoles accommodate the foot comfortably.

Operative. In more severely affected patients, a forefoot arthroplasty is required. The metatarsal heads are excised, the toes realigned and the weight-bearing pad of skin, which has been drawn distally, is replaced under the metatarsal heads by excising a proximal ellipse of normal skin.

Complications
Persisting painful pressure areas in the sole are usually the result of failure to remove sufficient length from the distal metatarsals. Wound healing is occasionally prolonged.

Peripheral vascular disease

Usually the cause of peripheral vascular disease (PVD) is proximal large-vessel atheroma, but sometimes distal small-vessel disease due to diabetes is the cause. In these patients the condition is often complicated by persisting infection and ulceration, although either type of PVD may give rise to peripheral gangrene.

Clinical features

- **Listen** — In large-vessel disease, the patient complains of intermittent claudication and eventually of severe constant ischaemic pain in the limb.
- **Look** — There are peripheral trophic changes, including thinning of the skin and loss of skin hair. The skin is pale and ulceration and incipient or frank gangrene may be apparent (Fig. 108).

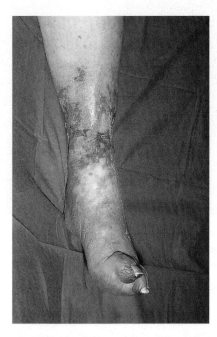

Fig. 108 Peripheral vascular disease showing rubor, trophic changes and incipient gangrene in the toes and forefoot.

- **Feel** — The leg feels cold below the knee and peripheral pulses are absent
- **Move** — Elevation of the limb produces further pallor but dependency causes rubor due to reactive hyperaemia (Buerger's test).

In diabetes, the proximal findings are not seen but peripheral infection, ulceration and dry or wet gangrene of individual toes may be present.

Diagnosis

The diagnosis can be confirmed and the level of critical ischaemia demonstrated by a non-invasive vascular assessment (NIVA). This includes:

- thermography
- arterial pressure studies
- skin pO_2
- blood glucose.

Management

Prevention. The control of diabetes mellitus and care of the feet to avoid infection are important in diabetics. Patients with proximal atheroma are investigated by anteriogram of the affected limb, and the circulation to the foot may be improved initially by a sympathectomy or in later cases by an appropriate bypass graft.

Surgery. Toes affected by dry gangrene can be allowed to demarcate and separate. In the presence of intractable pain and progressive wet gangrene, an amputation is required. Diabetic patients are well served by a below-knee amputation, which usually heals more reliably than a midtarsal amputation especially in the presence of co-existing large-vessel disease. The majority of patients with large-vessel disease can be treated by a below-knee rather than an above-knee amputation (Fig. 109). Well-supervised prosthetic fitting and physiotherapy are required post-operatively.

Complications

- advancing gangrene
- death.

Complications following surgery

- stump breakdown occurs if the limb has been amputated too distally
- phantom limb pain.

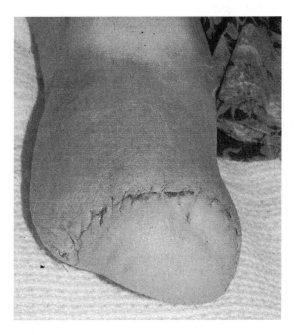

Fig. 109 A right below-knee amputation with a long, posterior myocutaneous flap to provide good wound healing and weight distribution.

10.3 Fractures

Ankle fractures

Injuries to the ankle are frequently seen. They are usually caused by twisting forces or angulating forces. Falls from a height often cause more severe injuries involving the distal tibial plafond, the calcaneum and, more proximally, the vertebral column or base of skull. At the ankle, a combination of ligamentous and bony injury are seen.

The ligaments involved are:
On the lateral side:

- inferior tibiofibular ligament
- anterior and posterior talofibular ligaments
- calcaneofibular ligament

On the medial side:

- deltoid ligament

The bony margins involved are:

- medial malleolus
- lateral malleolus
- posterior surface of the tibia.

The forces that give rise to the injury can be grouped as:

- pronation and external rotation
- pronation and abduction
- supination and external rotation
- supination and adduction.

Clinical features

There is pain and swelling over one or both sides of the ankle with bruising and sometimes fracture blisters. If there is associated dislocation of the joint, there will be gross deformity, stretching of the overlying skin and loss of normal peripheral circulation and sensation. In this circumstance an attempt at reducing the dislocation should be made immediately without waiting for X-ray confirmation.

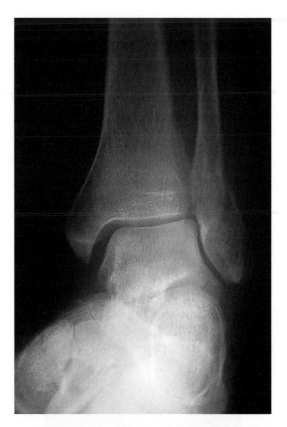

Fig. 110 Fracture of the lateral malleolus of the ankle of a young man with lateral displacement of the talus.

Diagnosis

A lateral and an antero-posterior radiograph centred on the ankle mortice are required to assess the injury and to demonstrate any lateral displacement of the talus (Fig. 110).

Management

Conservative. Dislocation should be reduced urgently to reduce pain, relieve pressure on the peripheral vessels and nerves and to prevent ischaemia of the overlying skin. Manipulation under anaesthesia in such a way as to reverse the direction of the injuring forces will correct a displaced fracture. An above-knee plaster or patella-bearing cast is required for those injuries where rotatory control is necessary; in other patients, a well-moulded below-knee plaster is sufficient. After initial swelling has settled, partial weight-bearing can be allowed. Radiological follow-up is necessary to ensure that the fracture does not redisplace while in plaster. Immobilisation is required until the fracture heals, usually between 6 and 8 weeks.

Operative. Open reduction and internal fixation is indicated for unstable fractures. This is best done before swelling develops and must not be done through very swollen tissues because of the risk of wound dehiscence. This technique restores the anatomical position of neck of the bone. Osteochondral fractures can also occur, which may eventually become loose bodies in the joint.

Clinical features

Clinical presentation is with pain, swelling and bruising. If a portion of the fractured talus is displaced, it may cause pressure effects on the overlying skin.

Diagnosis

Radiological examination shows the site of the fracture but CT will give more detail.

Management

Displaced fractures require open reduction and internal fixation if avascular necrosis of the proximal fragment is to be avoided. Even with adequate treatment, there is still a substantial risk of this happening.

Complications

- avascular necrosis of the body of the talus due to its retrograde blood supply being cut off by the fracture
- osteoarthritis of the subtalar, talonavicular or ankle joints
- formation of loose bodies from osteochondral fractures.

Calcaneum

A fall from a height is the usual cause of this injury and if present fractures in other sites must be sought, especially in the vertebrae, pelvis and base of the skull.

Clinical features

These include:

- pain
- deep bruising
- inability to bear weight
- fracture blisters
- swelling.

The heel may appear wider and shorter than the opposite one.

Diagnosis

Lateral and axial radiographs (Fig. 112) are required. Fractures are usually described as:

- extra-articular
- intra-articular

A CT scan will show the fracture pattern more precisely. 'Beak' fractures at the insertion of the Achilles tendon and fractures of the sustentaculum tali are usually then seen to be part of a more extensive intra-articular fracture.

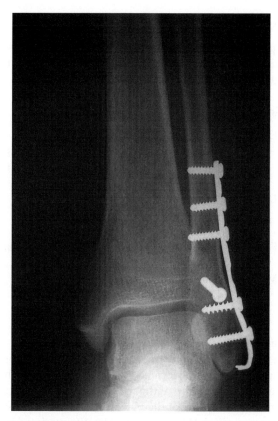

Fig. 111 The fracture has been treated with a neutralisation plate on the fibula, which restores it to normal alignment and length and reduces the displacement of the talus.

the articular surfaces and, by providing rigid fixation, allows early active mobilisation.

Lag screws are inserted across the fractures and the fibula is further kept out to length and stabilised by a neutralisation plate (Fig. 111). Tension band wiring may be used in porotic bone in preference to screws to avoid cutting out.

Complications of conservative treatment:

- malunion
- talar shift leading to
- secondary osteoarthritis.

Complications of operative treatment:

- infection
- wound dehiscence
- non-union.

Foot fractures

Talus

Forced dorsiflexion injuries to the foot can result in a fracture of the talus through either the body or the

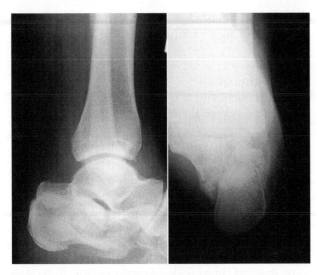

Fig. 112 Fracture of the calcaneum.

Management

Elevation and exercise of the ankle and subtalar joints is appropriate management for many of these fractures. In some cases, open reduction and internal fixation with a bone graft is possible, but adequate fixation is technically difficult and wound breakdown is common. After either procedure weight-bearing is prohibited for at least 8 weeks.

Complications

- persisting pain
- subtalar arthritis, requiring subsequent fusion of the subtalar joint.

10.4 Ankle disorders

Learning objectives

You should:

- be able to examine the calf and Achilles tendon and recognise the features of an Achilles tendon injury

Achilles tendon injury

Rupture of the Achilles tendon usually occurs in patients in middle age during the course of some strenuous activity such as running or playing squash.

Clinical features

- **Listen** — A sudden movement of the ankle is followed by acute severe pain. Patients frequently think they have been hit in the back of the calf.
- **Look** — The gap in the tendon may be visible beneath the skin before swelling develops.
- **Feel** — Palpation reveals a gap in the tendon at the ankle.
- **Move** — There may be loss of normal plantar flexion when the calf is squeezed (Symons' test).

Diagnosis

The clinical features are usually convincing, but sometimes tenderness is located in the mid-calf, in which case a partial rupture of the medial head of the gastrocnemius or a rupture of the plantaris tendon are possible diagnoses. Clinical findings must be differentiated from those of deep venous thrombosis.

Management

Conservative. An equinus above-knee cast is worn for the first 4 weeks before changing to a cast in plantigrade. After a further 4 weeks, a heel raise is fitted to the patient's ordinary shoes and exercises are begun.

Operative. Operative repair achieves a quicker result but the outcome in the long term is only marginally better than with conservative treatment.

Complications

- re-rupture
- poor spring during toe-off
- scar sensitivity after operative repair
- stiffness.

Self-assessment: questions

Multiple choice questions

1. Below-knee amputation:
   a. Walking requires less energy following this than following an above-knee amputation
   b. Is recommended for those patients who have 50° fixed flexion of the knee
   c. Is best performed utilising a long posterior myocutaneous flap
   d. Plaster of Paris is an accepted type of post-operative dressing
   e. Requires 3 months of healing before a prosthetic limb is applied

2. Symptoms from hallux valgus in a middle-aged woman may be treated satisfactorily by:
   a. Fusion of the first metatarsophalangeal joint
   b. Plaster splintage for 6 weeks
   c. Tendon transfer
   d. Proximal hemiphalangectomy of the proximal phalanx
   e. Amputation of the second toe

Extended matching items questions (EMIs)

1. Theme: Clinical presentation

A   Achilles tendon rupture
B   metatasalgia
C   phantom pain
D   dry gangrene
E   fractured lateral malleolus
F   peripheral vascular disease
G   fractured medial malleolus
H   metatarsophalangeal joint subluxation from rheumatoid arthritis
I   calcaneal fracture
J   hallux rigidus

Which of the diagnoses listed above most closely fits the clinical presentations described below:

1. A 49-year-old man playing squash suddenly experiences sharp ankle pain. He can weight-bear but can only walk with difficulty.
2. A 50-year-old woman with generalised joint pain has pressure effects from her shoes over the dorsum of all her toes. She says that her feet feel as though they are walking on pebbles.
3. A 45-year-old woman complains of pain in the first metatarsophalangeal joint. This is worst when walking uphill or wearing high heels.

2. Theme: Investigations

A   Symon's test
B   Buerger's test
C   skin pO_2 measurement
D   lateral X-ray
E   thermography
F   MRI scan
G   venogram
H   Doppler measurements
I   AP X-ray
J   CT scan

Which of the investigations listed above would be most appropriate for the clinical presentations described below:

1. A patient with night pain in both feet has no palpable pulses below the popliteal arteries.
2. A 50-year-old man complains of sudden painful loss of plantar flexion at the ankle.
3. A 20-year-old with severe heel pain and swelling has a fractured calcaneum which may require operative management.

Constructed response questions (CRQs)

CRQ 1

A 20-year-old youth is admitted in police custody to the Accident and Emergency department with a history of having jumped from a first-floor window. He is complaining of *bilateral* foot and ankle pain and swelling and cannot weight-bear.

a. What would you expect to find on physical examination?
b. How would you investigate the patient at this stage?
c. On the left side the fibula is fractured at the ankle joint. What other deformity should be looked for on the AP X-ray?
d. X-ray of the opposite foot shows an intra-articular fracture of the calcaneum with many fragments. What further information is needed?
e. What ways of treating this are possible?

CRQ 2

A 58-year-old woman complains of pain in her feet at the end of a long day standing at work. She says her shoes are rubbing and she has difficulty getting the shoes she likes to fit. She has no discomfort on walking.

a. What diagnosis do you suspect?

b. Visual examination shows pressure effects over the first metatarsal head and the characteristic deformity of the joint. How would you like to proceed with your examination?

c. As long as her foot can be made comfortable she is keen to have surgery. What would you recommend?

d. Her teenage daughter is concerned that her feet may suffer the same way. X-ray examination shows an underlying bony deformity. What may this be?

e. What operative treatment might be appropriate for her?

Objective structured clinical examination questions (OSCEs)

OSCE 1

Study the picture of a radiograph of a young man's ankle fracture (Fig. 113).

a. How would you describe the fractures?

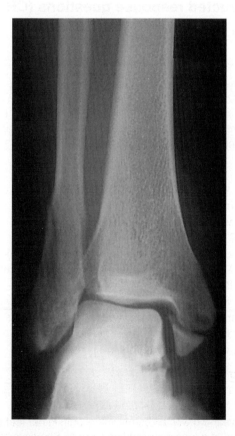

Fig. 113 Ankle injury in a young man.

b. What direction has the injury enforced been applied?

c. The fracture is unstable and lateral migration of the talus can be seen. How should this fracture be treated?

d. Postoperative management is essential to avoid prolonged stiffness. What would you ask the patient to do?

OSCE 2

Study the clinical photograph of an ankle and foot of a 70-year-old man with a long history of smoking and cardiovascular disease (Fig. 114).

a. What features of peripheral vascular ischaemia should be looked for?

b. What other body systems may be affected in a patient with peripheral vascular disease?

c. What other systemic disease would you want to know about?

d. How would you investigate the patient further?

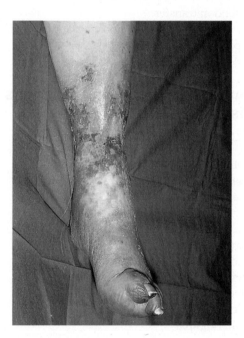

Fig. 114

Viva questions

1. Describe the advantages and disadvantages of open reduction and internal fixation of ankle fractures.

2. Describe the clinical findings to be seen on examination of the rheumatoid foot.

Self-assessment: answers

Multiple choice answers

1. a. **True.**
   b. **False.** The presence of an uncorrectable fixed flexion deformity of the knee precludes a below-knee amputation, instead an above-knee amputation is necessary.
   c. **True.** The provision of a posterior myocutaneous flap allows the anterior suture line to be more proximal and away from the stump end.
   d. **True.** Postoperative oedema in the stump is best controlled by a light plaster of Paris dressing.
   e. **False.** Early temporary prosthetic fitting is encouraged to allow the patient to stand upright and begin mobilising as soon after surgery as possible.

2. a. **True.** This operation maintains the length of the first ray and controls the position of the hallux.
   b. **False.** The deforming forces have produced an established deformity that will not be corrected by splintage.
   c. **False.** This operation may be more appropriate in younger patients.
   d. **True.** This operation corrects the valgus deformity but shortens and weakens the big toe.
   e. **True.** In some patients, more space can be made for the deformed hallux by amputating the adjacent toe.

EMI answers

1. Theme: Clinical presentation

1. A. A rupture of the Achilles tendon classically presents in this fashion in this age group.
2. H. Subluxation of the metatarsophalangeal joints produces clawing of the toes, which rub on the shoes. The prominent metatarsal heads are painful to walk on.
3. J. In hallux rigidus, flexion of the metatarsophalangeal is painful.

2. Theme: Investigations

1. H. Doppler measurements are regularly carried out and should be done in the absence of peripheral pulses.
2. A. When examining a patient with a suspected rupture of the Achilles tendon, Symon's test should be carried out. This involves squeezing the calf and observing the foot move into plantar flexion if the Achilles tendon is intact.
3. J. A fractured calcaneum often requires further imaging to determine the best line of management. A CT scan would be appropriate.

CRQ answers

CRQ 1

a. Bruising
   Swelling
   Deformity
   Fracture blisters
   The heel may be appear wider than normal when viewed from behind.
b. AP and lateral X-rays of the foot and ankle with axial view of the heel if clinically suspect.
c. Talar shift.
d. CT scan.
e. Internal fixation with bone graft may be required to restore normal anatomy of the subtalar joint.

CRQ 2

a. Hallux valgus.
b. Examine her shoes to see if they are obviously tight or too small in the forefoot area.
c. Keller's procedure and bunionectomy.
d. Varus deformity of the first metatarsal (metatarus primus varus).
e. An osteotomy of the first metatarsal will correct the hallux valgus deformity by altering the alignment of the metacarpal.

OSCE answers

OSCE 1

a. Bimalleolar fracture.
b. Supination, external rotation injury.
c. Open reduction and internal fixation using a lag screw or fully threaded cancellous screw in the medial malleolus and a third tubular neutralisation plate to control the length and position of the lateral malleolus (see Fig. 115).
d. Elevate the limb
   Early active mobilisation
   No weight-bearing until the fracture is healed.

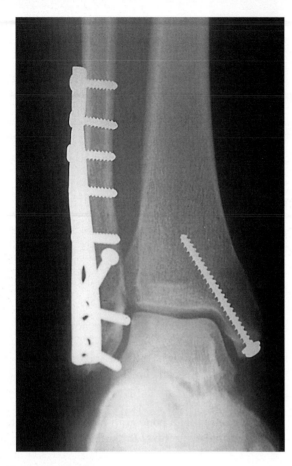

Fig. 115 The fracture has been treated by internal fixation with a fully threaded cancellous screw to the medial malleolus and neutralisation plate to the fibula.

OSCE 2

a. Peripheral trophic changes
   Changes in the skin
   Loss of skin hair
   Pale, thin, ulcerated skin
   Frank gangrene.

b. Coronary artery occlusion
   Vertebrobasilar insufficiency
   Renal failure.
c. The presence of diabetes mellitus.
d. Thermography
   Pressure studies
   Skin pO_2 measurements.

Viva answers

1. The advantages of open reduction and internal fixation of an ankle fracture are:

   * anatomical reduction
   * early mobilisation
   * the avoidance of malunion, which would lead to point loading and osteoarthritic degeneration of the joint.

   The disadvantages of surgically correcting a fracture are:

   * risk of infection
   * delayed or non-union
   * implant failure
   * it may be necessary to remove the fixation devices later because of local pressure effects or persisting pain.

2. The rheumatoid foot classically shows hallux valgus and dorsal dislocation of the metatarsophalangeal joints. Examination of the sole shows the metatarsal heads to be prominent and covered only by superficial skin. The thick weight-bearing pad of skin has been pulled distally. The metatarsophalangeal joints may have subluxated or be dislocated, and passive reduction may be impossible. There may be callosities or pressure effects over the dorsum of the proximal interphalangeal joint of these toes. Peripheral circulation and sensation should be examined. The presence of vasculitis in the toes should be noted.

11 The ear

Chapter overview

The ear is divided into three parts — the external, middle and inner ear. The external and middle ears function to channel and amplify sound waves into the cochlea of the inner ear, where they are converted into electrical impulses which travel along the cochlear part of the vestibulo-cochlear (eighth) nerve.

Any dysfunction of the external or middle ears causes a conductive loss, dysfunction of the inner ear a sensory loss, and of the eighth nerve a neural loss.

Examination of the tympanic membrane is performed with an otoscope, while hearing is tested with a pure tone audiogram and balance function with a caloric test (among others).

Hearing loss may be treated surgically or with a hearing aid if conductive or by a variety of electronic aids if sensorineural.

Each part of the ear and surrounding structures has disease processes particular to it.

11.1 Anatomy and physiology

Learning objectives

You should:

- understand the basic anatomy of the ear — external, middle and inner

- know the two functions of the ear — *hearing* and *balance*

- know the five presenting complaints of ear disease.

The ear is subdivided into three parts (Fig. 116):

- external
- middle
- inner.

External ear

The external ear is composed of the auricle and the external auditory canal, and extends to the tympanic membrane. The ear canal skin covers bone medially and cartilage laterally. Epithelial migration of the skin of the ear canal is from medial to lateral. Laterally the skin contains hair follicles and ceruminous glands. The tympanic membrane has an upper thin part, the pars flaccida, and a lower thicker part, the pars tensa (Fig. 117). The malleus handle is embedded in the substance of the tympanic membrane and the long process of the incus may be seen deep to the tympanic membrane postero-superiorly.

Middle ear

The middle ear is connected to the nasopharynx via the Eustachian tube and also posteriorly to the mastoid air cells. The ossicular chain comprises three ossicles, the

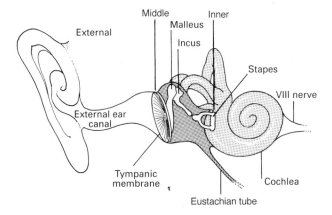

Fig. 116 Anatomy of the ear.

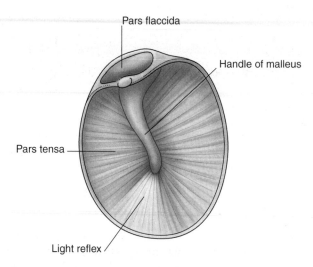

Pars flaccida

Handle of malleus

Pars tensa

Light reflex

Fig. 117 The left tympanic membrane.

malleus, incus and stapes. They transmit vibration from the tympanic membrane to the inner ear. The stapedius and tensor tympani muscles are attached to the stapes and malleus, respectively. The facial nerve lies in a narrow bony tunnel (Fallopian canal) in the temporal bone and may be damaged by disease of the surrounding bone.

Inner ear

The inner ear comprises the cochlea, concerned with hearing, and the semicircular canals, utricle and saccule, concerned with balance. These structures relay neural impulses to the central auditory and central vestibular systems, respectively. The central vestibular system also receives and coordinates proprioceptive and visual information.

Common presenting complaints are:

- hearing loss
- tinnitus
- vertigo
- aural discharge
- otalgia.

11.2 Clinical examination

Learning objectives

You should:

- know how to use an otoscope to examine the tympanic membrane
- know the difference between conductive and sensorineural hearing loss

- understand how tuning fork tests can tell us which type of hearing loss a patient has
- be aware of the basic tests of hearing and balance — *audiometry* and *caloric tests*
- understand the basic functioning of a hearing aid.

Ear examination involves inspection of the surrounding skin as well as of the ear canal and tympanic membrane with a battery-powered otoscope.

Initially the ear is inspected for surgical scars, both postaural and endaural.

To straighten the ear canal for otoscopic examination in adults, gently pull the auricle up and back. In children, gently pull the auricle straight back and if necessary slightly downwards. The otoscope should be held like a pen. This initially feels awkward but allows easier, more gentle inspection. Remember that in some patients not all of the tympanic membrane can be seen. In particular the antero-inferior part of the tympanic membrane may be obscured by a prominent anterior canal wall. The pneumatic attachment to the otoscope can be used to assess the mobility of the tympanic membrane (Seigeloscopy).

A 512 Hz tuning fork is used for Rinne and Weber hearing tests.

Investigations

Tests of hearing

Assessment of hearing is made initially by noting the patient's response to a normal conversational voice. Hearing loss caused by disease of the external or middle ear is termed conductive hearing loss, that caused by disease of the inner ear is termed sensory hearing loss and that caused by the disease of the auditory nerve is termed neural hearing loss. In practice, it is often difficult to distinguish the last two types of hearing loss and they are commonly referred to as sensorineural or perceptive hearing loss.

Tuning fork tests
The 512 Hz tuning fork is struck on the tester's knee or elbow, and air and bone conduction hearing is tested.

The Rinne test compares air conduction with bone conduction in the test ear. The tuning fork is placed lateral to the ear to test air conduction and on the mastoid process to test bone conduction. In the normal ear, air conduction should be greater than bone conduction. This is called a positive Rinne test. It may also indicate sensorineural hearing loss. If bone conduction is greater than air conduction, a negative Rinne test, conductive hearing loss is present in the test ear.

A false negative Rinne occurs in the test ear when this ear has a severe sensorineural hearing loss. This is because bone conduction is heard in the opposite ear when the tuning fork is applied to the mastoid of the ear with the sensorineural loss. The introduction of a blocking sound to the non-test ear (masking) is required.

The Weber test compares bone conduction in both ears. The tuning fork is placed in the midline of the skull. If the sound is heard in midline the test is normal. In an abnormal test, the sound lateralises to the side of conductive hearing loss and away from the side of sensorineural loss.

Audiometric tests

These may be subjective or objective.

Subjective. Pure tone audiometry measures hearing over a range of frequencies in each ear by air and bone conduction. Speech audiometry tests speech reception thresholds and speech discrimination.

Objective. Impedance audiometry detects middle ear disease such as otitis media with effusion and can also assess the condition of the ossicular chain. Evoked response audiometry measures evoked potentials from brain stem, mid-brain and auditory cortex. These may be used to determine auditory thresholds, and brain stem audiometry is a useful screening test for retro-cochlear disease such as acoustic neuroma.

Tests of balance

Maintenance of balance involves integration of information provided by the inner ears, the eyes and the proprioceptive organs. This integration occurs in the central vestibular system. Disruption of the integrity of the vestibular system results in vertigo, which is a hallucination of movement of self or of surroundings.

The labyrinths send nerve impulses to the brain stem and their function is analogous to that of a twin-engined aeroplane. Loss of function of one end organ can be compensated by central mechanisms, but acute loss is characterised by vertigo and nystagmus. Compensation occurs rapidly in the young, but in the elderly complete compensation may not be achieved.

The integrity of the vestibular apparatus may be tested in various ways. In the Hallpike test, the patient sits on an examination couch in the erect position. The patient's head is then brought briskly to hang over the end of the couch and the eyes are examined for nystagmus. The patient returns to the original position and the test is repeated with the head rotated to the left and again with the head rotated to the right. The fistula test is performed by applying positive pressure to the column of air in the ear canal, either by digital pressure on the tragus or using a pneumatic otoscope. If a fistula to the inner ear is present, the patient will complain of imbalance or vertigo and nystagmus may be observed.

Caloric stimulation of the inner ear by irrigation of the ear canal by warm (44°C) or cold (30°C) air or water results in nystagmus, which may be measured to assess the integrity of the labyrinth being stimulated.

Imaging

The middle and inner ears as well as the posterior cranial fossa may be imaged by conventional CT scanning and MRI scanning.

Aids to hearing

A hearing aid has three components: a microphone, an amplifier and an earphone. Sound is conducted to the ear via an ear-mould or very occasionally through the skull via a bone vibrator. 'In the ear' aids and 'in canal' aids are available commercially and 'in the ear' aids are now being introduced in the UK through the NHS. Larger body-worn aids are sometimes helpful for those who have difficulty manipulating the small controls of conventional hearing aids. All hearing aids have an O/T/M switch. O is for off; M is for microphone and T is for switching the microphone to the telecoil for use with an induction loop system. Frequency adjustment may also be made with the H (high) and L (low) tone screw.

Even the most sophisticated hearing aid is essentially an amplifier. Patients with conductive hearing loss do well with properly adjusted hearing aids, but patients with poor speech discrimination tend to do less well. Patients fitted with hearing aids should be reviewed routinely to identify problems as they arise. Other devices such as telephone amplifiers, loud doorbells and flashing alarm lights can improve the quality of life of the hard of hearing. Cochlear implants are appropriate only for patients who are profoundly deaf in both ears. Cochlear implantation is now being undertaken in both adults and children.

11.3 Diseases of the ear

Learning objectives

You should:

- be aware of the treatment of external otitis and foreign bodies in the external ear

- know the symptoms and treatment of acute otitis media and otitis media with effusion

- know that cholesteatoma is squamous epithelium in the middle ear; how it presents; the complications and the treatment

- know that presbycusis is the high-tone sensorineural hearing loss of old age and be aware of the other main causes of hearing loss

- understand the symptoms and treatment of Menières disease.

The external ear

Infection

Infection is also known as external otitis, often called swimmer's ear, and is caused by opportunistic bacteria or fungi. This condition is treated by local debridement and ear drops, which usually contain a steroid in combination with an antibacterial or antifungal agent.

Obstruction

Osteomas (solitary benign bony tumours) and exostoses (diffuse, usually multiple, bony swellings) narrow the ear canal. They may not produce symptoms, but if they result in wax impaction and external otitis they need to be surgically removed.

Foreign bodies in the ear canal usually occur in toddlers. If not easily removed, referral to an otologist is required and occasionally general anaesthesia is needed. More damage may be done to the ear by unskilled attempts at removal than by the presence of the foreign body itself.

Wax impaction can obstruct the ear. The wax may be softened by use of bicarbonate, olive oil or almond oil ear drops. Once soft, wax may be removed by syringing, but if perforation of the tympanic membrane (current or healed) is suspected, a wax curette should be used. Occasionally wax removal under magnification using the operating microscope is necessary.

The middle ear

Infection

Acute otitis media is most common in young children and it is usually caused by *Haemophilus influenzae* infection. It presents with otalgia, hearing loss and, if the tympanic membrane ruptures, discharge. It is usually preceded by an upper respiratory tract infection and antibiotics are usually given. Tympanic membrane perforations following this condition usually heal spontaneously. Should the perforation fail to heal spontaneously, surgical repair of the tympanic membrane (myringoplasty) may be undertaken. If the ossicular chain has been damaged, it may be repaired by ossiculoplasty. Myringoplasty has a very high success rate —

usually over 90%. Temporalis fascia is the most commonly used graft material. Ossiculoplasty results are much less predictable as the grafts or prostheses used to reconstruct the ossicular chain are subject to infection, migration and extrusion.

Otitis media with effusion is common in children. It is associated with a conductive hearing loss and may present as slow speech development, poor performance at school and disruptive behaviour. Fluid accumulates in the middle ear space as a result of Eustachian tube blockage. The fluid is usually sterile. The condition is usually self-limiting but if persistent may require myringotomy, possibly with the insertion of a grommet to maintain ventilation. Sometimes adenoidectomy is required in addition. Depending on the design, grommets tend to extrude spontaneously in six to twelve months. Occasionally grommets require to be removed surgically.

Chronic suppurative otitis media is associated with tympanic membrane perforation and aural discharge. There may be associated external otitis. Gram-negative organisms are usually involved. It may respond to medical therapy, but if cholesteatoma is present, surgery is usually required.

Cholesteatoma results from the presence of keratinising squamous epithelium in the middle ear. It presents as a chronic, smelly aural discharge. The epithelium invades the underlying bone and may result in complications such as intracranial infection, labyrinthitis and facial nerve paralysis. Mastoid surgery is required to remove disease and to prevent development of complications. Such surgery may result in the creation of a mastoid cavity, which will require periodic debridement by the otologist throughout the patient's life. Nowadays it is sometimes possible to remove cholesteatoma without the creation of a mastoid cavity (intact canal wall procedure).

Hereditary disease

Otosclerosis results in fixation of the stapes footplate, with resultant conductive hearing loss. The inner ear is sometimes involved with associated sensory hearing loss. The condition is familial and is transmitted by autosomal dominant inheritance with incomplete penetrance. The incidence is likely to be similar in both sexes, but because of hormonal influences it presents twice as commonly in females. Treatment is by hearing aid or operation (stapedotomy), which replaces the immobile stapes with a prosthesis. Stapedotomy is generally a very successful operation resulting in elimination of the conductive hearing loss (closure of the air–bone gap on the audiogram). Occasionally damage to the inner ear occurs, resulting in sensorineural hearing loss, tinnitus and vertigo. These risks need to be explained to the patient. Because of them, stapedotomy is not undertaken in an only hearing ear.

Tumours

Tumours of the external, middle and inner ears are uncommon. Glomus tumours involving the middle ear or the base of the skull may present as unilateral pulsatile tinnitus. They are treated by surgery, sometimes preceded by embolisation.

Trauma

Minor trauma results from foreign bodies being inserted into the ear canal in an attempt to remove wax. This usually results in further wax impaction.

The inner ear

Hearing loss of old age

Presbycusis is the hearing loss of old age. Higher frequencies of hearing tend to be affected first and patients have difficulty hearing female voices and background noise. There is associated deterioration of the central auditory system. A hearing aid is usually helpful but requires quiet surroundings to function best.

Noise-induced hearing loss

Noise-induced hearing loss may result from industrial or recreational noise exposure. Initially the hearing loss is often reversible, but with repeated exposure, permanent damage occurs. The loss is often greatest initially at 4 and 6 kHz. Avoidance of hazardous noise exposure is best, but if this is not possible adequate hearing protection should be worn.

Trauma

Trauma to the temporal bone may result in conductive, sensory or mixed hearing loss with or without facial paralysis. The inner ear is well protected in the petrous temporal bone and fractures of this bone usually result from considerable force, often associated with loss of consciousness.

Drugs

Ototoxic drugs, e.g. aminoglycosides, may affect the auditory, vestibular or both parts of the inner ear. Most ototoxic drugs induce permanent changes in the inner ear, but a few drugs such as aspirin and quinine result in reversible damage.

Sudden hearing loss

Sudden sensorineural hearing loss results from viral or vascular damage to the inner ear. Hearing loss may be temporary, but in some patients it is permanent and profound.

Tumour

Acoustic neuroma, more properly termed vestibular schwannoma, commonly presents with unilateral tinnitus and hearing loss. Imbalance is common but true vertigo is unusual. Any unexplained, progressive unilateral or asymmetrical sensorineural hearing loss should be investigated for possible acoustic neuroma. MRI scan of the posterior fossa and internal auditory meatus is the definitive investigation. Ideally acoustic neuromas are detected when small and are treated surgically by removal with minimal morbidity. The approach to the tumour may be neurosurgical, otologic or combined. In elderly unfit patients with minimal symptoms, slowly growing tumours may best be left untreated. Serial MRI scans allow tumour growth to be assessed over time.

Menière's disease

Menière's disease is characterised by fluctuating sensory hearing loss, tinnitus and vertigo. There is often an associated feeling of fullness in the affected ear. The aetiology is unknown. The disease is usually unilateral, but with time the other ear may become affected. There is no clear evidence that the natural course of the condition is affected by medical therapy. Various operations are described for severe, intractable disease. Destructive operations, such as labyrinthectomy and division of the vestibular nerve are effective in controlling symptoms. Labyrinthectomy, by definition, destroys the hearing function of the inner ear and is only undertaken when the affected ear has very poor hearing. Non-destructive procedures include decompression and shunting of the endolymphatic sac, but the efficacy of such procedures remains in doubt.

Vertigo

Vestibular neuronitis presents as acute vertigo with no associated hearing loss or tinnitus. It is self-limiting over a period of days or weeks.

Benign positional vertigo results from semicircular canal dysfunction and is characterised by episodic vertigo consequent upon adopting a given head position. It may occur after head injury and is usually self-limiting after some months.

11.4 Miscellaneous conditions

Learning objectives

You should:

- be aware of Bell's palsy and know that it is a diagnosis of exclusion

- be aware of Ramsay–Hunt syndrome and its clinical presentation

- know what tinnitus means and that unilateral tinnitus requires investigation

- understand that pain in the ear may be referred from elsewhere.

Diseases of the facial nerve

Bell's palsy is an isolated, idiopathic lower motor neurone paralysis of the facial nerve, which is suspected to be caused by herpes viral infection. The eye becomes vulnerable if it does not close completely and tear production may be diminished. The patient should be advised about the need for eye protection. Patients with incomplete Bell's palsy recover spontaneously and require no treatment. Those with complete paralysis require investigation and possibly steroid therapy. Other diseases that may result in lower motor neurone facial paralysis, such as cholesteatoma, acoustic neuroma and parotid malignancy, must be excluded.

Ramsay–Hunt syndrome results from herpes zoster involvement of the inner ear. It is characterised by hearing loss, vertigo and facial nerve palsy. Recovery of the facial nerve palsy may be incomplete. Systemic anti-herpetic therapy may be helpful in relieving symptoms.

Trauma to the facial nerve may occur at any point along its course. A stab of the cheek may result in peripheral division of the nerve, while fractures of the temporal bone may damage it more proximally. Early surgical repair with grafting, if indicated, offers the best chance of recovery in a facial nerve which has been divided.

Tinnitus

Tinnitus, commonly described as buzzing or hissing noises in the ears or head, is common and usually associated with hearing loss. Resolution of the hearing loss may improve the tinnitus because of the masking effect of previously unheard sounds. Bilateral tinnitus is rarely of serious significance and patients should be reassured. Unilateral tinnitus requires further investigation. Background noise or a masker often helps to suppress the tinnitus. Anxiety and depression should be treated appropriately.

Referred otalgia

Pain felt in the ear in the absence of any ear disease is very common. Although the teeth and temporomandibular joints are common sources, disease of the tongue and throat must be excluded. Occasionally pain is referred from the thyroid (de Quervain's thyroiditis) or trachea.

Self-assessment: questions

Multiple choice questions

1. Recognised complications of acute otitis media include:
   a. Tympanic membrane perforation
   b. Facial nerve paralysis
   c. Temporal lobe abscess
   d. Sensorineural hearing loss
   e. Recurrent tonsillitis

2. Conductive hearing loss is a symptom of:
   a. Clinical otosclerosis
   b. Menière's disease
   c. Cholesteatoma
   d. Bell's palsy
   e. Acoustic neuroma

Extended matching items questions (EMIs)

1. Theme: Diagnosis

A vestibular neuronitis	F otitis externa
B Bell's palsy	G presbycusis
C otosclerosis	H tympanosclerosis
D Menière's disease	I cholesteatoma
E otitis media with effusion	J glomus tumour

Match the clinical finding below to the most appropriate diagnosis from the list above:

1. A patient presents with a discharging ear and a facial palsy.
2. A patient presents with conductive hearing loss in both ears, although her tympanic membranes look normal.
3. A patient complains of recurrent vertigo, hearing loss and tinnitus.

2. Theme: Diagnosis

A unilateral otitis media with effusion
B aural discharge
C sensorineural hearing loss
D impedance audiometry
E tinnitus
F pure tone audiometry
G vertigo
H caloric testing
I facial palsy
J brain-stem audiometry

Which of the above most accurately matches the questions below:

1. Nasopharyngeal carcinoma may present with which ear problem?
2. Disorders of the semicircular canals will mainly cause which of the above?
3. Which of the above tests the function of the semicircular canals?

Constructed response questions (CRQs)

CRQ 1

> Olivia is a 3-year-old girl who appears to be having problems with her hearing. She also has recurrent episodes of pain in her ears with occasional slight discharge. Her parents are concerned and take her to you, their GP.

a. Which two main diagnoses will you be considering?
b. Apart from her hearing, what other developmental problems might she have because of her ear disease?
c. You treat her conservatively for 3 months, but her problems become more severe. You refer her to the local ENT department. Which two surgical procedures may be considered?
d. When she is 16 years old she returns to your surgery complaining of recurrent discharge from her right ear. She has also failed a hearing test for the Royal Air Force and is concerned as this is her chosen career. Which two diagnoses are most likely, given her history?
e. Name *one* surgical procedure to deal with *one* of your diagnoses above.

CRQ 2

> A 43-year-old schoolteacher complains of tinnitus and mild hearing loss affecting the left ear for several months. She has also noticed slight unsteadiness when getting up to go to the bathroom in the dark. Her ears look normal on examination. Using the 512 Hz tuning fork, the Rinne test is positive on both sides and the Weber test lateralises to the right ear. You are concerned that she may have a vestibular schwannoma (acoustic neuroma).

a. Which type of hearing loss does this patient probably have?

b. Which other physical examinations would you perform?

c. Which audiological tests might be appropriate?

d. Which radiological tests are appropriate?

e. Assuming that she has a vestibular schwannoma, what treatment would you offer and what complications would you discuss?

Objective structured clinical examination questions (OSCEs)

OSCE 1

Look at the photograph (Fig. 118).

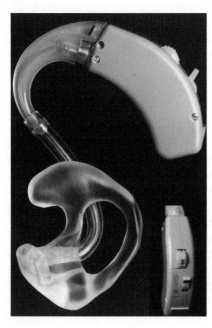

Fig. 118

a. What is this device?

b. Look at the controls. What does O stand for? What does T stand for? What does M stand for?

c. Hearing aids sometimes whistle when fitted incorrectly. What is this whistling noise caused by?

d. What is the name given to the hearing loss suffered by many elderly people?

e. Which frequencies are mainly affected in this type of hearing loss — high, middle or low?

f. Name three other aids that may help a person with hearing loss.

OSCE 2

Look at Figure 119. This shows the ear of a 52-year-old woman complaining of right otalgia and facial weakness. She has Ramsay–Hunt syndrome.

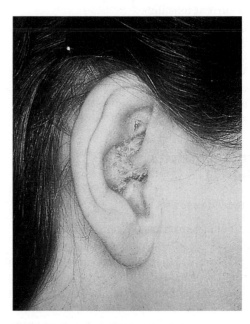

Fig. 119 (Reproduced courtesy of Mr R S Dhillon FRCS.)

a. What abnormalities do you see?

b. What has caused these lesions?

c. What other symptoms may this patient have?

d. What treatment would be appropriate?

e. Which long-term problems may the patient have?

Viva questions

Discuss the following:

1. management of Bell's palasy
2. otitis externa

Self-assessment: answers

Multiple choice answers

1. a. **True.** Rupture of the tympanic membrane in acute otitis media is often associated with bloodstained purulent discharge and relief of pain.
   b. **True.** Facial nerve paralysis may occur when the bony covering of the nerve in its passage through the middle ear is thin or absent.
   c. **True.** Possible, but extremely rare. Intracranial complications are much more likely to occur when cholesteatoma is present.
   d. **False.** Conductive hearing loss is a feature of acute otitis media. Sensorineural hearing loss implies involvement of the labyrinth.
   e. **False.** Acute otitis media results from infection ascending from the nasopharynx. Recurrent tonsillitis may occur in association with acute otitis media but is not a complication.

2. a. **True.** Progressive conductive hearing loss is the cardinal feature of clinical otosclerosis.
   b. **False.** Menière's disease is characterised by a fluctuating, progressive sensory hearing loss.
   c. **True.** Cholesteatoma damages and frequently destroys parts of the ossicular chain. Hearing may be preserved by transmission of sound through the cholesteatoma. The conductive hearing loss may, therefore, be greater following surgery to eradicate cholesteatoma.
   d. **False.** Bell's palsy is not associated with hearing loss.
   e. **False.** Acoustic neuroma is characterised by a neural (retrocochlear) hearing loss that is unilateral. The patient often notices tinnitus before hearing loss.

EMI answers

1. Theme: Diagnosis

1. I   Discharge from the ear and a facial palsy suggest a cholesteatoma that has eroded the bone overlying the facial nerve and caused the nerve to stop functioning. A Bell's palsy is a viral infection that affects the nerve causing a palsy — it is not associated with an aural discharge.
2. C   Otosclerosis is a condition that affects the bone around the footplate of the stapes in the oval window. There is overgrowth of the bone, which fixes the footplate in position therefore stopping effective transmission of sound to the cochlea giving a conductive hearing loss. Otitis media with effusion and tympanosclerosis may also cause a conductive loss, but the tympanic membrane will not look normal.
3. D   This trio of symptoms is classic for Menière's disease, which presents with episodic attacks of vertigo, a low-frequency hearing loss and tinnitus. A vestibular schwannoma (acoustic neuroma) may present in the same way and an MRI scan of the internal auditory canals is usually required to make a diagnosis. Vestibular neuronitis (a presumed viral infection of the vestibular nerve) causes vertigo without other symptoms.

2. Theme: Diagnosis

1. A   Nasopharyngeal carcinoma may cause obstruction of the lower end of the Eustachian tube in the nasopharynx and the consequent development of an effusion. A unilateral effusion (particularly if the patient is of Chinese origin) necessitates examination of the nasopharynx and possible biopsy.
2. G   The semicircular canals are involved with balance. Dysfunction causes vertigo and imbalance.
3. H   A caloric test is performed by putting warm then cool water, or air, into the ear canals and measuring the nystagmus caused. The different temperatures of the water cause heating and cooling of the fluid in the semicircular canals and consequently it flows around them. If they are functioning normally this will cause nystagmus.

CRQ answers

CRQ 1

a. Recurrent acute otitis media or otitis media with effusion (glue ear).
   Recurrent acute otitis media is more likely to cause pain in the ears as it involves infection in the middle ear space, but otitis media with effusion may also cause discomfort. Both will cause reduction of hearing.
b. Speech and language delay
   Behavioural problems
   Poor coordination/clumsiness/imbalance.
   If hearing is affected, children do not develop language as well as they should as they cannot hear

the words to repeat. Behavioural problems arise often due to boredom as the child cannot hear what is going on around them. Imbalance appears to arise due to an effect of the effusion on the vestibular system.

c. Grommet insertion
   Adenoidectomy.
   Insertion of a grommet allows the middle ear pressure to return to normal with resolution of the effusion. Adenoidectomy removes the excess tissue causing obstruction to the Eustachian tubes in the postnasal space. This allows air to pass up the tube and equalise middle ear pressure.

d. Chronic suppurative otitis media (perforated eardrum)
   Cholesteatoma.
   Longstanding ear disease as a child may predispose to a chronic perforation with consequent discharge and hearing loss. Cholesteatoma arises if the attic area of the tympanic membrane is retracted and squamous epithelium becomes trapped. This causes a smelly discharge and hearing loss (usually due to erosion of the long process of the incus).

e. Myringoplasty
   Mastoidectomy.
   Myringoplasty is the term given to repair of the tympanic membrane (usually with temporalis fascia). Mastoidectomy usually involves drilling out the mastoid bone and opening the middle ear and mastoid spaces to the outside. This stops the cholesteatoma spreading intracranially.

CRQ 2

a. A left sensorineural loss.
   The presence of unsteadiness suggests a possible peripheral vestibular disorder. The tuning fork tests suggest either a left sensorineural hearing loss or a mild right conductive loss. Given that the patient complains of left-sided hearing loss, it is most likely to be sensorineural.

b. Examination of the trigeminal and facial nerves
   Look for nystagmus
   Test balance and cerebellar function.
   Cranial nerves V and VII should be examined as these may be involved in cerebello-pontine angle lesions such as vestibular schwannoma. Evidence of spontaneous, gaze and positional nystagmus should be looked for. Cerebellar and posterior column function should be tested.

c. Pure tone audiometry
   Speech audiometry
   Brain-stem evoked responses.
   Pure tone audiometry is essential to confirm the hearing loss, and speech audiometry may also be useful. Brain-stem responses (to see if there is a

delay on one side suggestive of a schwannoma) are still occasionally performed, but their reliability is limited.

d. MRI of posterior fossa and internal auditory meatus
   CT of posterior fossa and internal auditory meatus.
   MRI scanning of the posterior fossa and internal auditory meatus is now the standard investigation for suspected cases of vestibular schwannoma. CT scanning will show larger tumours but will miss smaller ones.

e. Craniotomy and removal of tumour
   Complications are of hearing loss, possible facial nerve damage, vertigo and CSF leak among others. In a younger patient removal of the tumour is appropriate, but in elderly or frail patients annual scanning may be performed to monitor the tumour, which is usually very slow growing. The main complications of removal of a vestibular schwannoma relate to the surrounding nerves, the auditory and facial, with possible deafness and facial palsy, vertigo due to the surgery involving the vestibular nerve, CSF leak through the craniotomy and a variety of complications common to all intracranial procedures.

OSCE answers

OSCE 1

a. A hearing aid.
   A hearing aid is made up of a microphone, an amplifier and a speaker. The speaker is attached to the ear mould, which should fit snugly into the ear.

b. O for off
   T for telecoil or telephone
   M for microphone.
   The T setting is used when an induction loop facility is available. This transmits radio signals from the sound source (such as a microphone in church or the sound track of a film in the cinema) directly to the hearing aid so reducing the problem of background noise. The M setting allows normal use.

c. Feedback.
   If the ear mould is loose and allows sound to escape from the ear canal this may be picked up by the microphone and a feedback loop set up causing whistling.

d. Presbycusis.
   Presbycusis is the symmetrical, high frequency sensorineural hearing loss found in the elderly. The prefix presby- means old (as in presbyopia).

e. High.
   The higher frequencies are lost first, possibly because the first turn of the cochlea is nearest to the stapes and receives most noise trauma over a

lifetime. It is this part of the cochlea that deals with the higher frequencies.

f. Flashing doorbell
Flashing/amplified telephone
Vibrating alarm clock
Subtitles on television
Flashing smoke alarm
Spectacles to allow lip-reading
Hearing dog for the deaf.

There are many aids that a person with hearing difficulties may find useful. A hearing therapist and the social work department of the local council should be approached for advice.

OSCE 2

a. Vesicles and crusting on the pinna.
Vesicles and crusting of the pinna associated with pain is very typical of Ramsay–Hunt syndrome (herpes zoster oticus).
b. Herpes zoster virus.
The lesions and the facial palsy are caused by the herpes zoster virus.
c. Hearing loss and vertigo.
She may suffer from a variety of cranial nerve disorders secondary to a neuritis caused by the virus. Facial palsy, hearing loss and vertigo are due to involvement of the VII and VIII nerves. Involvement of IX leads to vesicular eruptions on the palate and of X to vocal cord palsy.
d. Analgesia
Bed rest if vertigo is severe.
Antiviral therapy such as Aciclovir. Systemic antiviral therapy, such as Aciclovir, may shorten the attack, though whether it is useful in promoting recovery of facial nerve function is less certain.
e. Facial palsy
Hearing loss
Neuralgia.
In contrast with Bell's palsy when 90% of patients will recover facial function, only about 60% do so after Ramsay–Hunt syndrome. Post-herpetic neuralgia may be troublesome and the hearing may not recover.

Viva answers

1. Bell's palsy is a diagnosis of exclusion and other causes of lower motor neurone facial palsy such as cholesteatoma and parotid malignancy must be excluded. If the paralysis is incomplete and does not progress, prognosis is excellent and no specific treatment beyond reassurance and eye protection is required. If the face is totally paralysed, a course of steroids for 5 to 10 days is usually given. In 90% of all patients with Bell's palsy, good facial function will be regained. Aberrant reinnervation may result in synkinesis and mass movement.

2. Otitis externa results from infection of the skin of the ear canal by opportunistic bacteria such as *Pseudomonas* and *Proteus* spp. and sometimes by fungi such as *Candida albicans* and *Aspergillus niger*. The infection tends to occur more commonly in swimmers and during warm humid weather. The mainstay of treatment is debridement of the ear canal with the removal of debris and instillation of appropriate medication, which is usually antibiotic and steroid-containing ear-drops. If the condition is chronic or recurrent, underlying causes such as more generalised skin problems or diabetes mellitus should be considered.

12 The nose and paranasal sinuses

Chapter overview

The nose functions to allow the passage of air to the lungs and to the olfactory mucosa for smell. It warms, cleans and humidifies the air as it passes. The paired paranasal sinuses (frontal, maxillary, anterior and posterior ethmoid, and sphenoid) surround the nose, with all but the sphenoid and posterior ethmoid sinuses draining to the middle meatus, the key area in the treatment of sinus disease.

Nasal obstruction, discharge, sneezing, loss of sense of smell, and facial pain are common symptoms of sinonasal disease. These problems are often associated with anatomical abnormalities such as deviation of the nasal septum, or with mucosal inflammation such as is found with allergic rhinitis.

Epistaxis (nose bleed) is usually trivial and easily controlled but can be life threatening, especially in older patients.

12.1 Anatomy and physiology

Learning objectives

You should:

- understand the basic anatomy and functions of the nose — *smell* and *breathing*
- know the names of the paranasal sinuses and where they drain.

The nose

The external nose (Fig. 120)
The upper one-third of the external nose is bony and is covered by mobile thin skin. The lower two-thirds is cartilaginous and is covered by tightly adherent skin that contains multiple sebaceous glands.

The nasal cavities
These pass in an antero-posterior (not superior) direction in the skull for 6 to 7 cm in the adult. They are divided by a bony and cartilaginous nasal septum (Fig. 121), which is rarely absolutely in the mid-line. The major features of the lateral nasal wall (Fig. 122) are the superior, middle and inferior turbinates, which contain erectile tissue. The cavities are lined by respiratory epithelium that is thick over the turbinates and thinner over the septum. The nose has a rich blood supply from both the external and internal carotid arterial systems. Some nasal venous drainage passes intracranially to the cavernous sinuses.

Function
Besides being the olfactory organ, the nose warms and humidifies the inspired air. Particulate matter is trapped anteriorly at the nasal vestibule by the nasal vibrissae. Smaller particles adhere to the mucus blanket that lines

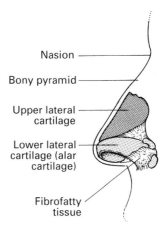

Nasion

Bony pyramid

Upper lateral cartilage

Lower lateral cartilage (alar cartilage)

Fibrofatty tissue

Fig. 120 The external nose.

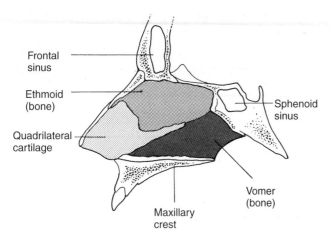

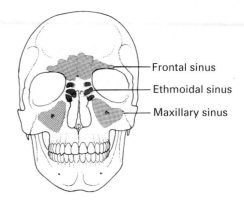

Fig. 121 The nasal septum.

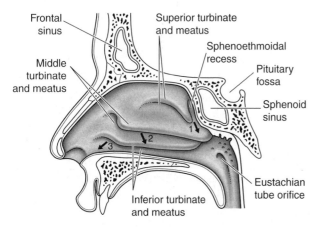

Fig. 122 Structure of the lateral wall of the nasal cavity, showing the superior (1), middle (2), and inferior (3) meatuses.

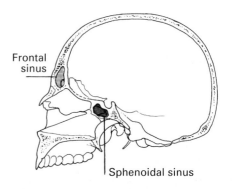

Fig. 123 The paranasal sinuses.

the nasal mucosa and are transported posteriorly by mucociliary activity and swallowed. The olfactory epithelium is located high in the nasal cavity below the cribriform plates. Nasal obstruction from any cause results in reduced air flow and reduced sense of smell. Nasal obstruction may also result in loss of vocal resonance. Excess nasal patency also alters voice quality.

Paranasal sinuses

These are paired structures (Fig. 123) comprising:

- anterior group: frontal, maxillary and anterior ethmoid sinuses; these all drain to the middle meatus below the middle turbinate
- posterior group: posterior ethmoid and sphenoid sinuses, draining to the sphenoethmoidal recess.

Not all paranasal sinuses are present at birth. They tend to enlarge rapidly in late childhood and at puberty as the facial bones grow anteriorly and inferiorly from the skull base. In humans, the paranasal sinuses have no known function.

12.2 Clinical examination

Learning objectives

You should:

- know the common presenting features of nasal disease
- be aware of the methods available to examine the nose
- know how to differentiate a polyp from a turbinate
- be aware of the two methods of testing for allergy — *skin prick testing* and *RAST*.

Clinical features

Obstruction

This is the most common problem and may be unilateral or bilateral. The cause may be structural or related to mucosal swelling. Common causes of nasal obstruction include deviation of the nasal septum, mucosal inflammation (rhinitis), nasal polyps and, more rarely, neoplasia.

Discharge

This may be clear or coloured, unilateral or bilateral, anterior or posterior (catarrh). Unilateral bloodstained nasal discharge suggests a foreign body in a toddler or a neoplasm in the elderly.

Sneezing

This results from nasal mucosal irritation and is a common feature of allergic rhinitis.

Pain

Facial discomfort and pain may be secondary to sinus obstruction and inflammation.

Anosmia

Anosmia is commonly secondary to nasal obstruction. In the absence of nasal obstruction, alteration of smell may result from disease in the anterior cranial fossa.

Cosmesis

Cosmetic nasal deformities are common and include humps, sagging of the nasal dorsum and deviation of the nose. Complaints about nasal size are also common. Nasal appearance is often racially determined and complaint thresholds vary from culture to culture. Some patients present with complaints about nasal function when their main concern is cosmetic.

Investigations

The exterior and interior of the nose must be carefully examined in all patients with nasal complaints. The external nose should be examined for deviation, scars and skin abnormalities. Standard anterior rhinoscopy using a nasal speculum allows a very limited assessment of the nasal cavities and this examination is best undertaken nowadays with a rigid or flexible endoscope, which allows an assessment of the nasopharynx.

In children, the internal nose can be inspected by tilting the nasal tip with the examiner's thumb: instruments tend to frighten children.

The anterior end of the inferior turbinate is often mistaken for a nasal polyp; gentle probing will elicit discomfort from a turbinate but not from a polyp.

Gentle stimulation of the locally anaesthetised nasal septal mucosa will often allow identification of a bleeding spot in Little's area.

Physical examination may be supplemented by imaging including CT and MRI scanning. Allergy testing by skin prick or RAST (radioallergosorbent test) is helpful in patients suspected of having allergic rhinitis. Mucociliary clearance testing and rhinomanometry are becoming used more routinely.

12.3 Infection and inflammation

Learning objectives

You should:

- know the symptoms and signs of acute and chronic sinusitis and be aware of the appropriate treatment
- be aware of the causes and presentation of atrophic rhinitis
- know the causes and presentation of allergic rhinitis
- be aware of the treatment of allergic and vasomotor rhinitis.

Rhinitis

The most common cause of rhinitis is the common cold, caused by viral infection. This condition is characterised by nasal obstruction, nasal discharge and sneezing. It is usually self-limiting within 4 to 5 days but may be complicated by secondary bacterial infection. It is most common in young children who have not yet developed immunity to the causative viral agents. Symptoms tend to be more severe and longer lasting in smokers, who have impaired mucociliary function.

Sinusitis

Acute sinusitis may be a complication of the common cold as ventilation of the paranasal sinuses may be impaired by swollen mucosa and thick secretions. Steam inhalations and local or systemic decongestants produce symptomatic relief. Secondary bacterial infection may be treated with broad-spectrum antibiotics. Occasionally, maxillary sinusitis is associated with infection of the apices of the premolar and molar teeth, which protrude into the sinus cavity. Such infections are commonly caused by anaerobic organisms. Typically acute sinusitis of rhinogenic origin is associated with pain located over the affected sinus, nasal obstruction and sometimes purulent nasal discharge. Medical treatment is by decongestants, analgesics and antibiotics. Occasionally, surgical intervention is required to drain the maxillary or frontal sinuses if pain is severe or complications such as orbital cellulitis or intracranial spread of infection threaten.

If acute sinusitis does not resolve adequately, *chronic* sinusitis may develop with further damage to the mucosal lining of the involved sinuses. Medical treatment to improve sinus drainage and reduce infection may help, but surgical intervention is sometimes necessary. Nowadays this is commonly accomplished by functional endoscopic sinus surgery (FESS), rather than by older operations, which were designed to remove damaged mucosa and to provide large drainage channels from the sinuses to the nasal cavity.

Nasal vestibulitis

Inflammation of the nasal vestibules may be secondary to infected anterior nasal discharge or may result from infection of the hair follicles, usually by *Staphylococcus aureus*. In children, vestibulitis is sometimes associated with a foreign body or more rarely with unilateral choanal atresia. Careful examination of the nose is required. Pus should be sent for culture and sensitivity testing, followed by appropriate antibiotic treatment. Diabetic and immunosuppressed patients are more prone to recurrent infection of the hair follicles in the nasal vestibules (furunculosis).

Atrophic rhinitis

This rare condition appears to be associated with poor hygiene and malnutrition. It is characterised by nasal crusting and often with foetor (ozaena). Medical treatment involves removal of the crusts and application of nasal douches and drops. Surgical treatment to reduce the size of the nasal cavities is sometimes needed.

Allergic and non-specific (vasomotor) rhinitis

Allergic rhinitis may be either seasonal or perennial. In the UK, common seasonal allergens include tree and grass pollen in spring and summer, respectively. Mould spores may cause allergies in the autumn. In North America, ragweed pollen is a potent source of allergic symptoms in the late summer.

Perennial allergic rhinitis commonly results from exposure to animal dander, feathers and the house dust mite. Some patients develop nasal symptoms resulting from ingested allergens such as eggs, milk products and various nuts. Allergic rhinitis is common, affecting up to one in five of the population. It results from a type 1 hypersensitivity reaction in which an IgE and allergen complex binds to mast cells. These cells degranulate, releasing inflammatory mediators including histamine.

The nasal mucosa may also react to non-specific stimuli, such as changes in temperature and humidity, and to stress and hormonal changes such as those occurring at puberty and during pregnancy. This type of non-allergic rhinitis is known as *non-specific* or *vasomotor* rhinitis and is mediated by the autonomic innervation of the nasal mucosa.

In both allergic and non-specific rhinitis, nasal obstruction, clear nasal discharge and bouts of sneezing occur.

Nowadays, the mainstay of treatment of both types of rhinitis is the use of steroid nasal sprays. These may be used long term, but after symptom control is established a minimum maintenance dose of the spray should be employed. In allergic rhinitis, topical and systemic antihistamine therapy may help as may topical sodium cromoglycate. Surgery in the form of turbinate reduction may help nasal obstruction but does not benefit other manifestations of allergic and vasomotor rhinitis.

Prolonged use of topical nasal decongestants may itself result in nasal inflammation, producing a condition known as rhinitis medicamentosa. This is treated by stopping the use of the topical decongestant and substituting a steroid nasal spray. Compliance is better if one nostril is treated at a time. Systemic decongestants may also help.

12.4 Nasal septum

Learning objectives

You should:

- be aware of the management of septal haematoma and nasal fracture

- know the term used for the procedure to straighten the nasal septum — *septoplasty*

- be aware of the symptoms and causes of septal perforation.

Trauma

Injuries to the nose may result in damage to nasal soft tissues, cartilage and bone. Patients presenting with nasal injuries should be assessed for associated damage to the head, neck and facial bones. If a nasal septal haematoma is present, it should be drained, the nose packed to prevent reaccumulation of blood and systemic antibiotics given. If the nasal bones are fractured, the nose should be re-examined after a few days when the bruising and swelling has settled to assess any residual cosmetic deformity. This should be corrected by nasal manipulation within 10 to 14 days of the injury; otherwise the bones will heal and the deformity will require formal correction by rhinoplasty. Septal deviations resulting from injury may require surgical correction. Untreated, a septal haematoma may form an abscess with the risk of intracranial spread of infection. Later resorption of the septal cartilage may cause a saddle nose deformity.

Deviation

This may result from differential nasal growth or from trauma. It may involve bone or cartilage of the septum or both. Cartilaginous septal deviations may result in deviation of the external nose. Asymptomatic septal deformities require no treatment, but if there is compromise of function or cosmesis, surgical correction by submucosal resection of the septum, or septoplasty or septorhinoplasty is indicated.

Perforation

Perforations are commonly asymptomatic and are seen as an incidental finding. If symptomatic they may produce bleeding, crusting and whistling. They usually result from trauma, often surgical, but may be caused by nose picking and cocaine abuse. Rare infections such as tuberculosis or syphilis may result in septal perforation.

If asymptomatic, perforations require no treatment. Small to medium-sized perforations can be closed surgically or more simply by the placement of a silastic obturator. Large septal perforations may not be amenable to any form of therapy.

12.5 Epistaxis

Learning objectives

You should:

- know the usual site of bleeding within the nose — *Little's area*

- understand the reasons that posterior epistaxis may result in life-threatening haemorrhage

- be aware of the various ways that epistaxis can be controlled

- be aware of the investigations and management that are appropriate for a patient with severe epistaxis.

Nose bleeds usually result from disruption of blood vessels in the anterior portion of the septum (Little's area). This area is the site of a rich vascular anastomosis and is relatively easily traumatised. Bleeding is readily controlled by sitting the patient up with the head slightly forward and pinching the tip of the nose. Blood loss from such bleeding is usually not severe. Cautery of the bleeding area can be carried out under local anaesthesia using silver nitrate sticks or electrocautery.

Potentially more serious nose bleeding results from rupture of larger unsupported posteriorly placed vessels. This type of nose bleed tends to occur in elderly patients who are hypertensive and have arterial disease. Blood loss may be extremely rapid and the patient must be assessed clinically for shock. Blood loss in this situation is often underestimated as the patient swallows a great deal of blood. Measurement of pulse and blood pressure is essential and intravenous infusion and blood transfusion are often necessary. The exact site of a posterior nose bleed is often difficult to determine even with adequate illumination and suction. If a bleeding point can be identified with a nasal endoscope, it may be cauterised under endoscopic control. Most such bleeding is controlled by anteriorly placed nasal packing, but occasionally postnasal packing is required. The latter usually requires general anaesthesia. Compressive balloons are available to control bleeding and in an emergency a Foley catheter may be used as a posterior pack. If anterior packing is to be in place for more than 48 hours, systemic antibiotics should be given. The presence of a posterior pack mandates the use of antibiotics.

Underlying causes of severe or continuous bleeding should be sought. Coagulation disorders and patients on anticoagulant therapy may present with severe nose bleeds. Associated conditions such as hypertension need to be controlled. If conservative measures do not control the bleeding, arterial ligation may be necessary. Vessels commonly ligated are the anterior ethmoid and maxillary arteries or occasionally the external carotid artery. The sphenopalatine artery may also be ligated endoscopically.

12.6 Nasal obstruction

Learning objectives

You should:

- understand the term choanal atresia and its management

- know what a polyp is and where it comes from

- understand why a unilateral polyp requires further investigation

- be aware of the significance of a unilateral nasal discharge in a child — *foreign body*

- know what a rhinolith is.

Choanal atresia

Choanal atresia results from failure of breakdown of the bucco-nasal membrane. If bilateral it presents as an acute respiratory obstruction in the neonate, as neonates are obligate nasal breathers. Unilateral cases present later in infancy or childhood with unilateral purulent nasal discharge and obstruction.

Diagnosis

Diagnosis is confirmed by failure to pass a soft catheter through the nostril and can be definitively imaged by CT scanning, which helps to differentiate bony from membranous atresia.

Management

Bilateral atresia in neonates requires establishment of an oral airway as an emergency followed by urgent surgical correction of the atresia. Surgery may be delayed in unilateral cases.

Polyps

Nasal polyps are made up of redundant oedematous mucosa and usually arise from the ethmoid sinuses. Most commonly they are bilateral and present in the middle meatus causing nasal obstruction. Occasionally they arise from the maxillary sinus in which case they pass posteriorly and are known as antrochoanal polyps. They are often associated with non-allergic asthma and aspirin intolerance but do not occur in children except in association with cystic fibrosis. Typically polyps have the appearance of skinned green grapes and are insensitive to probing, unlike inferior turbinates for which they are often mistaken.

Unilateral nasal polyps should be regarded with suspicion. In infants, a polypoid nasal mass may be a congenital abnormality such as a meningoencephalocoele. In adults, unilateral polyps may result from neoplastic growth.

Large polyps require surgical removal possibly with surgery to the associated sinus. Small polyps may be managed by use of local steroid sprays.

Foreign bodies

These are usually seen in toddlers and occasionally in mentally disturbed patients. Inert foreign bodies such as small pebbles or metal ball-bearings may produce few symptoms. Other materials such as foam, wool or vegetable matter result in a brisk inflammatory reaction which produces a purulent, often blood stained, nasal discharge. This can result in vestibulitis of the ipsilateral nasal skin.

Unless the foreign body can be easily and safely removed, referral to a rhinologist is indicated. Inhalation of the foreign body during manipulation is a risk and in young children general anaesthesia is sometimes required.

Rhinoliths result from accumulation of calcium and magnesium salts around a foreign body. They may reach a very large size and produce obstruction and discharge. General anaesthesia is often required for their removal.

Self-assessment: questions

Multiple choice questions

1. Causes of recurrent maxillary sinusitis include:
   a. Apical dental infections
   b. Repeated epistaxes
   c. Recurrent bouts of otitis media
   d. Deviation of the nasal septum
   e. Nasal foreign body

2. Allergic rhinitis:
   a. Is caused by a type 1 hypersensitivity reaction
   b. Is best treated by turbinate surgery
   c. Is commonly complicated by profuse nose bleeds
   d. Increases the risk of development of nasal carcinoma
   e. Produces symptoms mainly in elderly people

Extended matching items questions (EMIs)

1. Theme: Anatomy

A sphenoid sinus	F frontal sinus
B pituitary fossa	G middle turbinate
C middle meatus	H nasal septum
D anterior ethmoid sinus	I Little's area
E inferior meatus	J inferior turbinate

Which of the anatomical areas above most accurately answers the questions below:

1. The anterior ethmoid and maxillary sinuses drain into this area.
2. The nasolacrimal duct drains here.
3. This is the usual site for minor epistaxis to start.

2. Theme: Diagnosis

A vasomotor rhinitis	F vestibulitis
B allergic rhinitis	G anosmia
C nasal polyp	H sinusitis
D choanal atresia	I orbital cellulitis
E atrophic rhinitis	J rhinolith

Which of the diagnoses above most accurately fits the conditions below:

1. This presents with nasal crusting and a bad smell from the nose.
2. May occur because a foreign body has been left in the nose for a long time.
3. May occur as a complication of acute ethmoiditis.

Constructed response questions (CRQs)

CRQ 1

> Jamie is a 25-year-old veterinary surgeon. He has problems with nasal obstruction every summer, which is accompanied by itching of his eyes and palate.

a. What is the correct name for the problem Jamie has, and what is he probably allergic to?
b. Name two tests that could be performed to determine what he is allergic to.
c. Which two groups of drugs might be useful in managing this condition?
d. When his symptoms are particularly bad he sometimes also becomes short of breath. What may he be suffering from, and what treatment should you give him?
e. Jamie also has a severe allergic reaction when he comes into contact with cats. Because of his job, it is impossible for him to avoid cats. What type of treatment can we offer him that may permanently resolve this problem?

CRQ 2

> Jill is a 30-year-old woman with a long history of asthma. She has no history of nasal trauma but has noticed increasing bilateral nasal obstruction and loss of her sense of smell. She comes to see you, her GP.

a. Which diagnoses will you consider the most likely?
b. You look in her nose with a torch and see something that looks swollen. How can you differentiate an inferior turbinate from a nasal polyp?
c. She appears to have polyps in both nostrils. How would you treat her initially?
d. After three months of treatment, Jill still has a very poor nasal airway. You refer her to the ENT department of your local hospital and it is decided that she needs surgery. Which surgical procedures might be used to deal with her polyps?
e. Jill asks you about the risks of the operation. What would you tell her?

Objective structured clinical examination questions (OSCEs)

OSCE 1

Look at Figure 124. This patient has had an epistaxis.

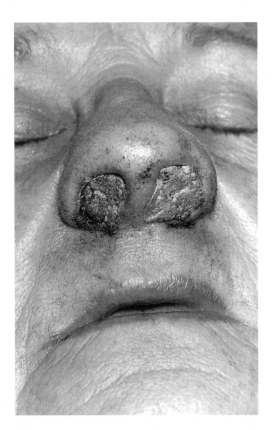

Fig. 124

a. What has this patient had done to stop the bleeding?
b. Name two other methods that are available to try to stop bleeding from the nose.
c. In the elderly population, which two common drugs may make this condition more severe?
d. Elderly patients are more prone to arterial bleeding in the nose than younger people. Apart from drugs, why is this?
e. Name three blood tests that you would perform on this patient and state why they would be relevant to the current problem.

OSCE 2

Look at Figure 125. This patient has recently been struck in the face with an iron bar and has had his nose broken.

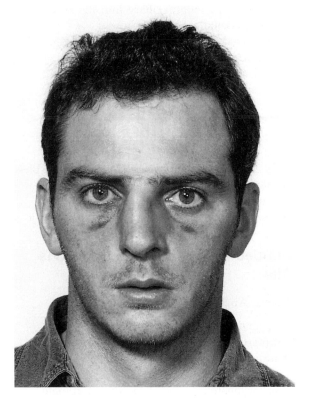

Fig. 125

a. Which clinical examinations would you perform to rule out other associated injuries?
b. He may require to have his nasal bones manipulated. What would make you decide that this was necessary?
c. For how long after the injury will it be possible to manipulate the nasal bones?
d. If the nasal bones are not manipulated within this period, what treatment may he eventually require?

Viva questions

Discuss the following:

1. deviated nasal septum
2. foreign body in the nose.

Self-assessment: answers

Multiple choice answers

1. a. **True.** Apical dental infections are usually caused by anaerobic organisms and the roots of the premolar and molar teeth may project into the antrum with minimal or absent bony covering.
   b. **False.** Epistaxis may be a feature of recurrent maxillary sinusitis, but it is not a cause.
   c. **False.** Otitis media, particularly in children, may be associated with sinus infections, but it is not causative.
   d. **True.** Deviations of the nasal septum may be sufficiently severe to cause impaired drainage of the maxillary sinus, resulting in recurrent infections.
   e. **True.** Nasal foreign bodies are most common in children and the mentally retarded and may result in obstruction of the maxillary sinus ostium producing chronic recurrent infections.

2. a. **True.** This results in degranulation of mast cells with release of histamine and other chemical mediators, which result in the classic symptoms of allergic rhinitis.
   b. **False.** The most appropriate treatment is avoidance of the allergen if possible. Topical nasal steroid sprays are the mainstay of treatment nowadays. Turbinate surgery should be limited to those patients in whom there is an irreversible turbinate hypertrophy.
   c. **False.** Mucosa tends to be swollen by oedema rather than by engorgement with blood.
   d. **False.** There is no association between allergic rhinitis and the development of nasal carcinoma.
   e. **False.** Allergic rhinitis tends to be less troublesome in the elderly. Symptoms tend to be maximal in the teens and twenties.

EMI answers

1. Theme: Anatomy

1. C The middle meatus is the area under the middle turbinate. The frontal, maxillary and most of the ethmoid sinuses drain into it. The sphenoid sinuses drain into the sphenoethmoidal recess at the back of the nose.
2. E The nasolacrimal duct is the only structure to drain into the inferior meatus.
3. I Little's area is the name given to the anterior part of the nasal septum. A number of veins and small arteries are found in the mucosa, which

may bleed as it is an area frequently traumatised by picking the nose. Older patients may have arterial bleeding that is usually more posteriorly sited and more severe.

2. Theme: Diagnosis

1. E Atrophic rhinitis may be related to poor living conditions with atrophy of seromucinous glands in the nasal mucosa, though the exact cause is uncertain. This leads to excessive patency of the nasal airway with consequent drying of the mucosa, crusting and infection. Surgical removal of the inferior turbinates may rarely cause this problem.
2. J A rhinolith (stone in the nose) is a concretion of calcium and magnesium salts that can form around a foreign body in the nose if left for months or years.
3. I Orbital cellulitis is an infection of the orbital contents usually occurring by venous spread through the lamina papyracea from infection in the ethmoid sinuses. It mainly affects young children but can occur at any age.

CRQ answers

CRQ 1

a. Seasonal allergic rhinitis
   Grass pollen.
   Seasonal allergic rhinitis occurs only during the period when the allergen is in the air, as opposed to a perennial rhinitis, which is present all year. Seasonal rhinitis is caused by tree pollen in the spring, grass pollen in the summer, and moulds and spores in the autumn and winter.
b. Skin prick test
   Radio allergosorbent test (RAST).
   The skin prick test is a cheap and rapid method of demonstrating atopy. A standard battery of allergens is used consisting of a positive (histamine) and negative (saline), dog, cat, grass and house-dust mite. Most atopic patients will react to one or more of these. The RAST is a blood test that measures the level of IgE circulating in the blood, which reacts with the various allergens tested against. It is more expensive but may be useful in testing for food allergies.
c. Antihistamines
   Intranasal steroids.
   Antihistamines are rapid acting and reduce nasal itch and discharge, but are less effective at relieving

nasal blockage. Intranasal steroids are slow acting but more effective at clearing the nose.

d. Asthma (or bronchial hyperreactivity).
Provide a bronchodilator (e.g. Sabutamol) and possibly an inhaled steroid.
Allergic asthma and allergic rhinitis have the same underlying causes and often coexist.
Bronchodilators and inhaled steroids may be necessary to relieve bronchoconstriction.

e. Immunotherapy (desensitisation).
Immunotherapy involves injecting increasing amounts of an allergen subcutaneously until the patient becomes desensitised. It can offer extremely effective and long-lasting relief of symptoms.

CRQ 2

a. Nasal polyposis
Inferior turbinate hypertrophy
Septal deviation.
Nasal polyposis and non-allergic asthma often coexist, though the reason for this is not clear. Inferior turbinate hypertrophy may be the result of allergic rhinitis with swelling of the mucosa. Patients with turbinate hypertrophy often complain that the obstruction switches from side to side — this is the turbinate cycle. Deviation of the nasal septum is very common, even without a history of trauma, though it would not usually present at this age if there were no other factors involved. A minor septal deviation may not cause obstruction until there is a minor mucosal swelling. The combination may result in symptomatic obstruction.

b. Touch it with a blunt instrument. Nasal polyps have no sensation.
A swollen inferior turbinate may look quite like a polyp and they are often confused by the inexperienced. Touching a polyp will cause no pain but your patient will let you know if you touch a turbinate!

c. Intranasal steroids.
Intranasal steroids are the mainstay in the treatment of bilateral simple polyps. Occasionally systemic steroids are required. Remember, unilateral polyps require urgent assessment and biopsy as they may be malignant. It is very rare for bilateral polyps to be malignant.

d. Simple nasal polypectomy
Bilateral ethmoidectomies — either intranasal or external.
A simple nasal polypectomy may be performed under local or general anaesthesia, but the polyps are very likely to recur. Endoscopically controlled intranasal ethmoidectomies are now commonly performed, and seem to lead to fewer recurrences of polyps. (Remember, the polyps arise in the ethmoid sinuses).

e. Haemorrhage
CSF leak
Damage to the orbit
Recurrence of polyps
Sense of smell may not return.
The area of the cribriform plate is very thin and can be traumatised when removing polyps. This may lead to a CSF leak. The lamina papyracea is also thin and separates the orbit from the nose. If it is breached there will be bruising around the eye, and occasionally damage to the globe or optic nerve. Any operation to deal with polyps does not cure the problem it simply debulks the volume of disease and improves the access for intranasal steroids. Polyps may therefore recur. The olfactory area in humans is very small and polyps or mucosal oedema will easily obstruct the passage of air to this narrow area. No guarantees can be given that smell will improve, though postoperatively it sometimes does.

OSCE answers

OSCE 1

a. The nose has been packed.
A long gauze pack, impregnated with antiseptic, has been inserted to put pressure on the bleeding vessel and allow a clot to form within it.

b. Cautery
Diathermy
Arterial ligation
Arterial embolisation.
Chemical cautery using a silver nitrate stick is often successful in stopping bleeding from the anterior septum. Bipolar diathermy can be used for more serious bleeds. The sphenopalatine artery can be clipped within the nose under endoscopic control. The internal maxillary artery can be clipped by exposing it behind the posterior wall of the maxilla, and the external carotid artery can be tied off in the neck. The anterior and posterior ethmoidal arteries can be clipped as they pass through the medial wall of the orbit.

c. Warfarin
Aspirin.
Warfarin reduces the ability of the blood to clot, and aspirin inhibits the ability of platelets to aggregate. Both may cause bleeding to be prolonged.

d. Arteriosclerosis.
Arteriosclerotic changes in vessel walls reduce their ability to contract and close when damaged. Bleeding may therefore be prolonged.

e. Full blood count — to assess blood loss and give a baseline haemoglobin, and measure platelet numbers
   Group and save/crossmatch — in case of further bleeding
   Coagulation screen/INR — to detect abnormal clotting
   Liver function test — to estimate any liver dysfunction that may affect clotting
   Arterial blood gases — if respiration compromised by nasal packing.
   A full blood count will give an estimate of the baseline haemoglobin, but if bleeding has been brisk, the patient will not have had time to haemodilute, so this must be treated with caution. An INR should be requested if a patient is on warfarin to ensure that their results are within the therapeutic range. Occasionally warfarin may need to be stopped for a few days.

OSCE 2

a. Examine skull and cervical spine for injury
   Assess dental occlusion
   Feel for a step in the infraorbital rim
   Test sensation over the cheek.
   A history of the nature of the injury should be obtained. Significant head and cervical spine injury must be excluded as a priority. The most likely associated injuries are those to the maxilla or zygoma. Problems with dental occlusion and a palpable step in the inferior orbital rim are features of a fracture of the maxilla. Loss of sensation over the cheek suggests damage to the infraorbital nerve, which is a feature of an orbital blow-out fracture where pressure on the eye has caused the floor of the orbit to fracture and orbital contents to prolapse into the maxillary sinus.
b. Cosmetic appearance
   Nasal obstruction.
   The reasons for reducing any facial fracture are to achieve restoration of function and/or to improve cosmesis. If there is no significant deformity and the patient is able to breathe comfortably through both nostrils, reduction is unnecessary.

c. Approximately 2 weeks.
   Fracture reduction should take place within 2 weeks of injury. Up to 10 days after injury the fractured nasal bones can be easily manipulated, but they become progressively more 'sticky' and after 2 weeks will be virtually immobile.
d. Septorhinoplasty or rhinoplasty.
   If reduction is delayed, definitive treatment usually involves a rhinoplasty, which entails osteotomies to refracture the nasal bones. They can then be manipulated into position.

Viva answers

1. Deviation of the nasal septum most commonly results from injury. In children and adolescents deviations may become more marked with growth. The condition may cause no symptoms and may be found incidentally at examination. Nasal septal deviation is a common cause of nasal obstruction, which may be unilateral or bilateral. It may contribute to recurrent sinus infection because of compromise to aeration and drainage of the sinuses. The caudal end of the septum is commonly dislocated into the nasal vestibule, while further back the septal cartilage lies obliquely producing obstruction on the opposite side. If symptoms are severe, surgery in the form of submucosal resection of septal cartilage or nasal septoplasty is indicated.

2. Foreign bodies in the nose most commonly occur in toddlers who place beads, pieces of paper, peanuts, etc. in their noses. The child usually presents with a unilateral foul smelling, occasionally bloodstained discharge with excoriation of the skin of the nasal vestibule. The child will rarely admit to placing a foreign body in the nose and several weeks normally elapse prior to presentation. Removal of the foreign body may be achieved in the cooperative child using local analgesia with appropriate lighting and forceps. In an uncooperative child general anaesthesia will be required.

13 The throat

Chapter overview

The term 'throat' covers the oropharynx, hypopharynx and larynx and therefore the functions of swallowing, breathing and voice. Common symptoms in this area are pain in the throat, difficulty swallowing, changes in the voice and airway obstruction.

Pharyngitis and tonsillitis may be viral or bacterial and are usually treated supportively or occasionally with antibiotics. Painless difficulty in swallowing may suggest more serious disease. The cause of a change in voice may range from an entirely benign process such as laryngitis to malignant disease in the neck or chest. Hoarseness for more than 3 weeks should therefore be investigated.

Airway obstruction in children may be caused by infection as in croup or supraglottitis, or result from a congenital disease such as laryngomalacia. In adults malignancy must be considered.

13.1 Clinical examination

Learning objectives

You should:

- know how to examine the mouth and neck, and be aware of the techniques of examination of the larynx and pharynx

- be aware of the use of endoscopic equipment and MRI and CT scanning in the examination of the head and neck.

Common symptoms are:

- sore throat
- difficulty in swallowing
- changes in the voice
- airway obstruction.

With a good source of illumination, tongue depressors, gauze swabs (to gently draw the tongue forwards) and appropriate mirrors, the entire oral cavity, pharynx and larynx can be examined. Mucosal surfaces should be carefully inspected and, if necessary, palpated. Palpation is particularly important in assessing oral cavity lesions. Fibre-optic telescopes, both rigid and flexible, may be necessary to examine those patients in whom mirrors do not give an adequate view. Examination of the neck includes inspection and palpation in a systematic fashion. The entire neck should be exposed, which may necessitate the removal of high-necked shirts.

Imaging techniques, including plain and contrast radiology, CT and MRI scanning are useful adjuncts to physical examination.

13.2 Sore throats

Learning objectives

You should:

- be aware that most sore throats have a viral cause

- know the symptoms of bacterial tonsillitis

- know the indications for and complications of tonsillectomy.

Pharyngitis

Throat infections are usually caused by viruses and are associated with other upper respiratory tract symptoms. Bacterial infection, commonly streptococcal, may be primary or secondary. Infected sore throats should be treated with oral analgesics, plentiful oral fluids and, if severe, bed rest. Antibiotics are given only if bacterial infection is suspected. Other types of infection include *Candida* spp., which may occur in diabetic or immuno-compromised patients and is sometimes seen in patients who use steroid inhalers for asthma. It presents as fluffy white patches on the fauces and responds to topical antifungal agents.

Tonsillitis

Bacterial tonsillitis is characterised by:

- sore throat lasting for a week
- dysphagia (difficulty swallowing)
- odynophagia (pain on swallowing)
- fever
- cervical lymphadenopathy
- malaise.

If recurrent attacks significantly interfere with school or work, tonsillectomy should be considered. Tonsillectomy is generally not indicated for less than three or four attacks of tonsillitis per year.

Complications of tonsillectomy

- reactionary haemorrhage occurs in the first 24 hours following tonsillectomy.
- Secondary haemorrhage usually occurs a week or so following surgery and is associated with separation of slough from the tonsillar bed.

13.3 Disorders of swallowing

Learning objectives

You should:

- know the definition of dysphagia (*difficulty in swallowing*) and odynophagia (*pain on swallowing*)
- be aware of the progression of severity of dysphagia, which ranges from difficulty with solids to semi-solids to liquids
- know the term *globus* for a sensation of a lump in the throat without dysphagia
- be aware that dysphagia may be a presenting feature of carcinoma of the pharynx or oesophagus.

Clinical features

Organic dysphagia may arise acutely from foreign body impaction, but this history may be difficult to elicit from young children. More characteristically, dysphagia presents as a progression of difficulty in swallowing solids to difficulty with semi-solids and then to difficulty swallowing liquids. It is usually associated with weight loss. If associated with hoarseness, cervical lymphadenopathy and otalgia cancer should be suspected. Dysphagia associated with aspiration of liquids suggests neuromuscular disease. The sensation of a lump in the throat without dysphagia is termed globus pharyngis. The need to swallow twice, particularly if associated with regurgitation of undigested food following a meal, suggests a pharyngeal pouch.

Diagnosis

A limited examination of the hypopharynx can be undertaken using the laryngeal mirror or fibre-optic endoscope. A barium swallow will usually define a lower lesion.

Classification

- Intrinsic lesions, e.g. neoplasia, diverticulum, stricture, achalasia
- Extrinsic lesions, e.g. goitre, mediastinal masses
- Generalised disease, e.g. scleroderma, dermatomyositis
- Neuromuscular disorders, e.g. myasthenia gravis, motor neurone disease, disseminated sclerosis.

13.4 Change in the voice

Learning objectives

You should:

- be aware of some of the causes of hoarseness — *laryngitis, nodules, polyps, cancer*
- understand why a patient who is hoarse for 3 or more weeks must have their larynx examined
- be aware of the role of the speech therapist.

Dysphonia is an alteration in the quality of the voice. Aphonia is absence of voice. The most common cause is acute laryngitis associated with viral infection and is self-limiting. The inflammation is exacerbated by smoking, alcohol and voice abuse. If these factors are not corrected, chronic laryngitis may develop.

Voice abuse may lead to nodules (singer's or screamer's nodules) at the junction of the anterior third and posterior two-thirds of the true vocal cord. It may also result in polypoid changes in the vocal cords and frank polyps may form. Speech therapy is essential to correct poor vocal habits. Surgical removal is indicated for lesions that do not resolve with conservative therapy. Hoarseness may result from neoplastic disease of the larynx and a patient with hoarseness persisting for more than 3 weeks should have their larynx examined by indirect laryngoscopy.

The voice quality in unilateral vocal cord palsy is variable depending on the position of the paralysed cord in relation to its mobile partner. If there is a significant gap between the vocal cords on phonation, the voice is weak and breathy. The patient may also have difficulty with aspiration of liquids. In bilateral cord palsy, the voice may be good, but the airway is often inadequate. Vocal cord palsy may be idiopathic or result from damage to the laryngeal nerve supply anywhere between the brain stem and the mediastinum.

13.5 Airway obstruction

Learning objectives

You should:

- know the definition of the terms stertor, snoring, stridor and wheeze, and where in the airway they are produced

- be aware of the causes of sleep apnoea

- understand the presentation of supraglottitis and the need for urgent treatment to establish an airway

- be aware that carcinoma of the larynx occasionally presents as an acute airway obstruction.

Stertor is the name given to the sound resulting from obstruction of the airway above the larynx. The sound is characterised by a snuffling, snorting quality. Snoring results from vibration of the tissues of the soft palate and pharynx. Complete or partial airway obstruction during snoring may result from collapse of the hypopharyngeal airway and also from posterior displacement of the base of the tongue. During sleep, the airway may become periodically completely obstructed causing sleep apnoea. In young children in whom the tonsils may be relatively large and the pharynx relatively small, this is a recognised cause of sleep apnoea, which is an indication for tonsillectomy in the young child. In older children and young adults, infectious mononucleosis may result in marked tonsillar hypertrophy, again with the risk of airway obstruction. Tumours of the tongue base and pharynx rarely become large enough to produce airway obstruction — dysphagia is a more common presenting feature.

Airway obstruction resulting from laryngeal disease may present at any age. Congenital abnormalities of the larynx may result in stridor at birth. Laryngomalacia, a condition in which the laryngeal cartilages are soft and floppy, is a common cause of stridor in the first year of life. Acute supraglottitis (epiglottitis) results from *H. influenzae* infection and presents with airway obstruction and drooling in the young child. The onset is rapid and the child sits in an upright position struggling for breath. This is an acute emergency. The child requires immediate transfer to hospital where the airway is usually established by passage of a nasotracheal tube in a setting where facilities for bronchoscopy and tracheostomy are available.

Bilateral paralysis of the vocal cords is a rarer cause of airway obstruction at all ages. Carcinoma of the larynx occasionally presents as airway obstruction. This is particularly true where the tumour involves the supraglottis or subglottis. Such patients are occasionally misdiagnosed as having asthma. The noisy breathing in this condition is stridor not wheeze!

Self-assessment: questions

Multiple choice questions

1. Hypopharyngeal diverticulum:
   a. Is associated with achalasia of the oesophagus
   b. Is a premalignant condition
   c. Is uncommon in people over age 50 years
   d. Tends to regress with time
   e. Is associated with iron-deficiency anaemia

2. A 6-month-old baby has had mild inspiratory stridor for the last 2 months. Possible causes include:
   a. Subglottic stenosis
   b. Acute epiglottitis
   c. Croup
   d. Tonsillar hypertrophy
   e. Laryngomalacia

Extended matching items questions (EMIs)

1. Theme: Terminology

A odynophagia
B laryngitis
C hoarseness
D stridor
E stertor
F tonsillitis
G vocal cord palsy
H dysphagia
I laryngomalacia
J pharyngitis

Which of the diagnoses above most appropriately fits the descriptions below:

1. Vocal abuse commonly presents with this symptom.
2. This word describes pain on swallowing.
3. This describes the sound made when the laryngeal airway is narrowed.

2. Theme: Diagnosis

A post-cricoid web
B unilateral quinsy
C laryngeal nodules
D Epstein–Barr virus
E pharyngeal pouch
F Reinke's oedema
G bilateral abductor palsy of the vocal cords
H infectious mononucleosis
I laryngitis
J adenoid hypertrophy

Which of the answers above match the questions below:

1. Paterson–Brown Kelly syndrome (Plummer–Vinson syndrome) is associated with which abnormality?
2. This disease may require emergency tonsillectomy to protect the airway.
3. This problem may result in aspiration pneumonia.

Constructed response questions (CRQs)

CRQ 1

> Thomas is 6 years old and has been suffering from recurrent sore throats. His mother brings him to your surgery and wonders whether he should have his tonsils removed.

a Which four questions would you ask her?
b. He has been having episodes of tonsillitis for 3 years. How many attacks per year would he have to suffer before you would consider tonsillectomy?
c. Name two postoperative complications that Thomas might suffer.
d. Name three reasons (other than recurrent tonsillitis) why a patient may require a tonsillectomy.

CRQ 2

> Nelly is an 85-year-old female patient with increasing dysphagia of 8 months' duration who feels generally lethargic and has lost 5 kg in weight over the last few months. Clinical examination of the head and neck reveals no abnormalities. Her full blood count shows that she is anaemic with a haemoglobin of 8.7 g/dl and the film shows a microcytic picture.

a. Which radiological investigation would you request?
b. Your investigation reveals that she has a post-cricoid web. What will you do next?
c. Will correcting her anaemia with ferrous sulphate therapy cause the web to resolve?
d. In a patient with a post-cricoid web, what would you be concerned about?
e. If this more serious condition had developed, how would you treat her?

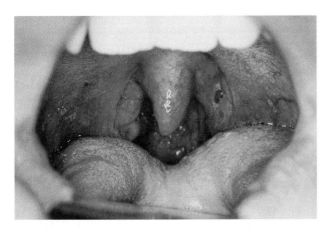

Fig. 126

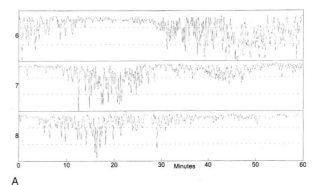

A

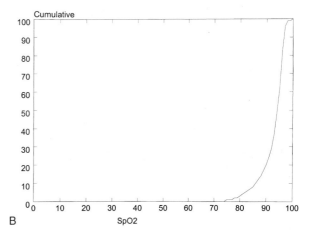

B

Fig. 127

Objective structured clinical examination questions (OSCEs)

OSCE 1

Look at Figure 126. Note particularly the swelling lateral to the right tonsil. This tissue is firm, reddened, swollen and painful. A needle mark can be seen in the anterior pillar on the right.

a. What disease process does it show?
b. Give two symptoms the patient might be complaining of that would make you decide to admit her?
c. What treatment would you give soon after admission?
d. Which factors in her history would help you decide whether she requires a tonsillectomy, and when would you perform it?
e. Following tonsillectomy, how long will you tell her to stay off work and how long will her throat be painful?

OSCE 2

Look at Figures 127A and B. They show some of the results of a sleep study performed on a 3-year-old child. **A.** shows the oxygen saturation during 3 hours of sleep where the top line of each section is a saturation of 100% and the bottom line a saturation of 70%. The average oxygen saturation curve is shown in **B**. His parents tell you that he snores and seems to struggle to breathe at night.

a What do you notice about the oxygen saturation values shown in A?
b The average value for oxygen saturation shown in B is approximately 92%. What is the range of normal values?
c What is the name for the problem this child is likely to be suffering from?
d What symptoms may he have because of this?
e What operative procedures may benefit him?

Viva questions

Discuss the following:

1. Treatment of chronic laryngitis.
2. Aetiology of vocal cord paralysis.

Self-assessment: answers

Multiple choice answers

1. a. **False.** The two conditions are quite distinct.
   b. **False.** Malignancy in hypopharyngeal diverticulum has been reported only extremely rarely.
   c. **False.** This disease tends to occur in people over the age of 50.
   d. **False.** The diverticulum tends to enlarge with time.
   e. **False.** The Plummer–Vinson syndrome, not hypopharyngeal diverticulum, is classically associated with iron-deficiency anaemia.

2. a. **True.** Subglottic narrowing may be congenital or acquired. Acquired cases usually result from prolonged endotracheal intubation. Most congenital cases are self limiting as the child grows.
   b. **False.** Acute epiglottitis develops rapidly, usually in a period of hours. It would not cause symptoms for 2 months.
   c. **False.** Acute laryngotracheo-bronchitis develops rapidly and is associated with a characteristic cough.
   d. **False.** Tonsillar hypertrophy may cause airway obstruction producing stertor. Stridor results from narrowing of the laryngeal or tracheal airway.
   e. **True.** This is a common cause of stridor in this age group.

EMI answers

1. Theme: Terminology

1. C   Vocal abuse (shouting or other misuse of the voice) may cause trauma to the vocal cords and consequent formation of swelling or nodules presenting with hoarseness. These are called singer's nodules, or screamer's nodules in young children. Patients may also have laryngitis, but this is a diagnosis not a symptom.
2. A   Odynophagia is pain on swallowing. Dysphagia is difficulty swallowing.
3. D   Stridor is caused by air flowing through a narrowed laryngeal or tracheal airway and is often louder on inspiration than on expiration. Stertor is caused by the vibration of tissues above the larynx, and snoring by tissues in the oro- and nasopharynx. Wheeze arises in the bronchioles and is usually expiratory.

2. Theme: Diagnosis

1. A   Paterson–Brown Kelly syndrome is usually seen in women in their 40s, often with a microcytic hypochromic anaemia. Such patients, who may suffer from dysphagia, should have their haemoglobin checked and may require endoscopy and biopsy as it can be a premalignant condition.
2. H   Any condition that causes bilateral swelling of the tonsils, or causes them to be pushed medially as with bilateral quinsies, may cause obstruction of the airway. Epstein–Barr virus causes infectious mononucleosis (glandular fever).
3. E   A pharyngeal pouch is an outpouching of mucosa from the pharynx in which food and liquid may collect. This may then be regurgitated into the larynx later and aspirated into the lungs causing pneumonia.

CRQ answers

CRQ 1

a. How often is he getting these attacks?
   How long has he been having these problems?
   How severe are the symptoms?
   Can he eat and drink during an attack?
   Does he get a fever?
   Has he lost time from school?
   Do the tonsils look any different during an attack?
   The important questions to ask are to determine how often the tonsillitis occurs and how severe the symptoms are, measured by time lost from school, inability to eat and so on. The appearance of the tonsils during an attack confirms that the problem is indeed tonsillitis. It is by judging the severity of the problem that a decision can be made that the risk of an operation is worthwhile.
b. 3–4 times per year.
   5–6 attacks in one year only, or 3–4 attacks over two or more years are usually regarded as indications for tonsillectomy.
c. Reactionary haemorrhage
   Secondary haemorrhage
   Throat pain
   Ear pain
   Infection of tonsil bed.
   Secondary tonsillar haemorrhage is common following tonsillectomy (5–10% of patients). Throat pain is universal and many patients complain of pain referred to the ear.

d. Obstructive sleep apnoea
   Recurrent quinsy (peritonsillar abscess)
   Biopsy of tumour
   Airway management in glandular fever (rare).
   Children suffering from obstructive sleep apnoea
   frequently benefit from removal of tonsils and
   adenoids to increase the potential airway. Following
   one peritonsillar abscess there is only a 20% chance
   of recurrence, therefore tonsillectomy is not usually
   advised. A further abscess requires tonsillectomy as
   subsequent infection becomes much more likely.
   Tonsillitis may precipitate attacks of nephritis and
   psoriasis in susceptible individuals or cause
   rheumatic fever. This is probably due to a common
   antigen on the streptococcus and on the affected
   tissue, which is then attacked by the immune system.

CRQ 2

a. A barium swallow.
   A barium swallow will often show a lesion in the
   pharynx or upper oesophagus to give a diagnosis
   and to guide direct endoscopy.
b. Direct endoscopy under general anaesthesia with
   possible biopsy.
   This patient requires an endoscopy to rule out
   malignancy. The web seen on barium swallow is
   often found to be a simple mucosal fold, but this
   may be difficult to identify. Direct endoscopy is,
   however, mandatory.
c. Yes, if it is minimal.
   Correction of the anaemia with appropriate therapy
   (usually iron or vitamin B12 depending on the cause
   of the anaemia) will cause an early web to resolve.
d. That she may have developed a post-cricoid
   carcinoma.
   Post-cricoid carcinoma is a potentially lethal
   condition associated with a post-cricoid web.
e. If limited, with radiotherapy.
   If more extensive by laryngo-pharyngo-
   oesophagectomy and stomach pull-up.
   Early limited post-cricoid carcinoma may be
   successfully treated with radical radiotherapy. More
   extensive tumours require removal of the larynx,
   pharynx and oesophagus and replacement by
   pulling the stomach up through the chest and
   connecting it to the oropharynx.

OSCE answers

OSCE 1

a. Quinsy/peritonsillar abscess.
   The photograph shows a right-sided peritonsillar
   swelling. Note that the tonsil itself looks normal,
   but is pushed medially, i.e. the swelling is lateral to
   the tonsil, not in the tonsil itself. 4 ml pus were
   drained from this abscess through a needle that was
   inserted through the anterior pillar. Some quinsies
   drain up to 10 ml pus or more.
b. Unable to eat
   Unable to drink
   Severe pain.
   If a patient can eat and drink, they can normally be
   managed with oral antibiotics as an out-patient. If
   they cannot drink because of pain and swelling,
   they require intravenous fluid therapy. They may
   also have marked trismus (limited mouth opening).
c. Intravenous fluids
   Intravenous antibiotics
   Drainage of abscess
   Analgesia.
   A patient may put up with several days of pain and
   inability to swallow before presenting and therefore
   need fluid therapy. Drainage of the peritonsillar
   abscess usually results in rapid resolution of
   symptoms.
d. If she has had a previous quinsy, then she should
   have a tonsillectomy. Tonsillectomy is usually
   performed 6 weeks after the acute infection to allow
   inflammation to settle and reduce bleeding during
   the procedure. Occasionally the tonsils are removed
   during the acute episode to drain the pus.
   After one quinsy, 80% of patients will not have a
   recurrence, therefore tonsillectomy is not usually
   indicated. A second quinsy means that the patient is
   at higher risk of further recurrences and
   tonsillectomy should be performed. Tonsillectomy is
   only rarely performed during the acute infection
   due to the risk of increased bleeding, but may be
   necessary in patients who cannot tolerate drainage
   under local anaesthesia (particularly children,
   though quinsy is unusual in this group)
e. 2 weeks off work
   At least 7–10 days sore throat.
   Many patients (and doctors!) underestimate the
   discomfort they will suffer after tonsillectomy.
   Swallowing is painful for at least a week despite
   regular analgesia, and at least 14 days off work or
   school should be anticipated.

OSCE 2

a. There are dips in the level of oxygen saturation.
   The oxygen saturations can be seen to fall to below
   70% on occasion. This is abnormal. Normal
   saturation levels never fall below 90%.
b. 95–100%
   The average oxygen saturation in this study is 92%;
   this is well below normal.

c. Obstructive sleep apnoea.
Obstructive sleep apnoea suggests an abnormality in the airway. In children, this is usually due to enlarged tonsils and adenoids. Central sleep apnoea (when there is a reduced respiratory drive) is much less common. A full examination must be performed before surgery, however, to determine the site of any obstruction.

d. Snoring
Daytime sleepiness
Poor concentration
Pulmonary hypertension
Failure to thrive
Bed wetting
Headache
Bagginess under eyes.
These children wake frequently throughout the night to improve their airway and therefore suffer from a very poor quality of sleep.

e. Tonsillectomy
Adenoidectomy.
Removing the tonsils and adenoids should enlarge the airway sufficiently to cure the obstruction if preoperative examination has confirmed that this is the problem.

Viva answers

1. Chronic laryngitis may result from infection in the upper or lower aerodigestive tracts and this should be sought out and eliminated. Other causes of chronic laryngeal inflammation include irritation by noxious substances, such as may occur in industrial environments. Vocal abuse in the form of overuse or incorrect use of the voice is a common associated factor in the development of chronic laryngitis. Gastro-oesophageal reflux with spillover of acid into the larynx may result in chronic laryngitis.

2. Vocal cord palsy may result from disease anywhere from the brain stem to the mediastinum. Because of its longer course in the thorax, the left recurrent laryngeal nerve is more vulnerable. Intrathoracic disease, such as mediastinal lymphadenopathy and aortic aneurysm, may result in left vocal cord palsy. In the neck, malignant disease, particularly of the thyroid gland and occasionally in the larynx itself, may result in cord palsy. Brain-stem disease such as infarct or tumour is usually associated with other neurological features.

14 Head and neck neoplasia

14.1 Clinical examination

Learning objectives

You should:

- remember that most malignant tumours of the head and neck are squamous cell carcinomas

- know the functions that these tumours may impair — *breathing, swallowing* and *speech*

- be aware of the methods used to diagnose these tumours

- be aware of the treatment for these tumours — surgery, *radiotherapy* and occasionally *chemotherapy*.

Chapter overview

Most cancers of the head and neck are squamous cell carcinomas and are often, though not always, linked to excessive consumption of alcohol and tobacco. If presenting in the glottis (the vocal cords) they are often found early as they cause hoarseness and the cure rate is high. Other sites in the larynx present later with poorer results. The usual treatment is radiotherapy or laryngectomy. Tumours of the oral cavity present earlier the further anterior they arise. Posterior tumours may produce few symptoms and present later. Pharyngeal tumours may present with referred pain to the ear or dysphagia. They often present late and have a poor prognosis. The tonsil may be the site for extranodal lymphoma. Nasopharyngeal carcinoma is commonest amongst the Chinese population and is linked to the Epstein–Barr virus. It may present with a unilateral otitis media with effusion and is treated with radiotherapy.

Presentation

Most malignant tumours of the mucosal surfaces of the head and neck are squamous cell carcinomas. Adenocarcinomas and lymphomas are less common. Squamous cell carcinomas spread by metastasising locally to the regional cervical lymph nodes. These tumours may disrupt breathing, swallowing and speech, are often painful and may alter the patient's appearance. Most squamous cell carcinomas of the mucosal surfaces of the head and neck in western countries are associated with tobacco and alcohol abuse. In the Indian subcontinent betel nut chewing is a predisposing factor. The Epstein–Barr virus has been implicated in the development of nasopharyngeal carcinoma and Burkitt's lymphoma and may possibly predispose to other head and neck cancers too. Exposure to radiation may result in the development of malignancy many years later. Premalignant conditions include leucoplakia (white mucosal patches), erythroplakia (red mucosal patches) and erosive lichen planus.

Diagnosis

In the clinical examination the oral cavity should be examined in a systematic fashion, with careful inspection of the floor and roof of the mouth. When a laryngeal mirror is used, the tongue is pulled very gently to avoid pressure on the undersurface of the tongue from the lower teeth.

A flexible rhinolaryngoscope allows ready examination of the nasopharynx, larynx and hypopharynx.

The regions of the neck are examined in a systematic fashion. To palpate the deep cervical lymph nodes, place the examining fingers deep to the anterior border of the sterno-mastoid muscle: warn the patient that this may be slightly uncomfortable.

The clinical examination is supported by endoscopy and biopsy.

Management

Most squamous cell cancers of the head and neck are treated primarily by surgery, radiation or a combination of both. Chemotherapy is best used in the context of controlled clinical trials. Occasionally, patients present with such advanced disease that no curative treatment is possible. Such patients require physical and psychological support, often best provided in hospice care.

14.2 The larynx

Learning objectives

You should:

- know the definitions of stridor and wheeze

- know the presenting sign of squamous carcinoma of the glottis — *hoarseness*

- be aware of the methods of treatment for laryngeal cancer — *radiotherapy* and/or *laryngectomy*

- be aware of the methods used to rehabilitate speech postoperatively.

It is important to distinguish between stridor, which arises from large airway obstruction, and wheeze, which originates in the smaller airways. Stertor is the term used to denote noisy breathing resulting from partial airway obstruction above the larynx.

Benign tumours

These are best treated with a carbon dioxide laser. Multiple treatments may be required.

Malignant tumours

Squamous cell carcinoma of the larynx most commonly affects the glottis (vocal cords) and presents with hoarseness. Any patient whose hoarseness persists for more than 3 weeks should be examined by indirect laryngoscopy. Early glottic disease has a good progno-sis. The true vocal cords have no lymphatic drainage and 95% of patients with squamous cell carcinoma limited to the glottis can, therefore, be cured by radical radiotherapy. Cancers involving the area of the larynx above the vocal cords (supraglottis) and below the vocal cords (subglottis) have a much poorer prognosis as they present later and spread to cervical lymph nodes is more common because of the rich lymphatic drainage from these areas. Patients with very large tumours may present with stridor and dysphagia. Such patients may require urgent tracheostomy prior to definitive therapy.

Management

A few patients with laryngeal carcinoma may be suitable for partial laryngectomy, but in the UK most laryngeal cancers are treated with radical radiotherapy. Once a radical course of radiotherapy has been completed, further radiotherapy cannot be given because of the risk of damage to normal tissue.

Total laryngectomy is reserved for patients with very large tumours at presentation and those who fail to respond to radiotherapy. Total laryngectomy involves the creation of an end tracheostome, which is brought out to the surface of the skin. The pharyngeal mucosa is reconstituted over a nasogastric tube and healing occurs in non-radiated patients within 7 to 10 days. Healing takes about twice as long in patients who have previously undergone radiotherapy.

Following total laryngectomy, about one in five patients develops oesophageal speech, which involves vibration of a segment of the reconstituted pharynx and upper oesophagus by swallowed air. Alternative methods include various hand-held battery-powered devices that are held against the neck skin and produce vibration in the pharyngo-oesophageal segment.

14.3 The oral cavity

Learning objectives

You should:

- know that anterior tumours present earlier and with less chance of metastasis than posterior ones

- know the usual presentation of carcinoma of the tongue — *an ulcer on the lateral border*

- be aware of the techniques available to reconstruct the oral cavity and oropharynx

- be aware of the use of the laser within the oral cavity.

Most malignancies are squamous cell carcinomas and the prognosis tends to be worse the further back in the mouth the tumour is sited. Neoplasms presenting anteriorly in the oral cavity are readily seen, whereas those more posteriorly placed often grow large, producing relatively few symptoms and metastasise early to the cervical lymph nodes. As well as tobacco and alcohol exposure, poor dental hygiene and teeth with sharp irregular edges are thought to promote malignant change in the oral epithelium. In the Indian subcontinent, betel nut quid, which contains tobacco, is an important causative factor.

Squamous carcinomas of the lip are usually treated by surgical excision. They present early and usually have a good prognosis.

Carcinoma of the tongue usually presents as an ulcerated lesion on the lateral border. The ulcer is initially painless, but when superinfection and deeper invasion occur, pain is experienced either locally or referred to the ipsilateral ear. Tumours arising in the posterior third of the tongue and in the area of the retromolar trigone (posterior to the third molar tooth) often present late with cervical metastases, so the prognosis is poorer.

Management

Small malignancies of the oral cavity do well with either surgery or radiotherapy. Larger tumours do poorly no matter what modality of treatment is employed. With improved reconstructive techniques, large oral cavity defects can be closed providing adequate rehabilitation of speech and swallowing. Free radial forearm flaps and pectoralis major myocutaneous flaps are routinely used in this type of reconstruction. If the mandible is involved by tumour, to a limited degree marginal mandibulectomy may be possible, preserving the integrity of the mandibular arch. If full thickness bone of the mandible is removed, this can be replaced by bone from the radius in association with a forearm flap.

Carcinoma of the buccal mucosa, often associated with pipe smoking, may be treated by vaporisation using a carbon dioxide laser. An alternative approach uses excision of the mucosa in association with split skin grafting. Metastatic cervical lymph node disease is usually managed by neck dissection, but small nodes may respond to radiotherapy. When surgery is performed, the primary tumour and the neck dissection specimen are removed in continuity.

14.4 The pharynx

Learning objectives

You should:

- know that pharyngeal tumours often present late with cervical node involvement

- be aware that hypopharyngeal tumours may require excision by laryngopharyngectomy and oesophagectomy
- know that non-Hodgkin's lymphoma may present in the tonsil
- be aware of the term angiofibroma and in whom it presents — *adolescent boys*
- know that nasopharyngeal carcinoma is common among the Chinese and how it may present — *cervical lymphadenopathy* and *unilateral otitis media with effusion.*

Oropharynx

The oropharynx and hypopharynx have a rich lymphatic supply and squamous cell cancers in these areas commonly present with cervical lymphadenopathy. Tumours in this area have a large space in which to grow before symptoms are apparent. Referred otalgia may be a presenting complaint. Patients with tumours in this area often have a high alcohol intake and are heavy smokers who often take little care of themselves. The extent of disease is assessed (usually under general anaesthesia), by inspection and palpation. Imaging with MRI and CT is helpful in determining the exact extent of tissue involvement.

Management

Treatment involves surgery, radiotherapy or a combination of both. Following surgery, reconstruction is by local or distant flaps.

Hypopharyngeal tumours may require laryngopharyngectomy with or without oesophagectomy, and reconstruction is by an interposed viscus, such as stomach, colon or jejunum.

The oropharynx is the most common site of presentation of extranodal lymphoma. These are usually non-Hodgkin's lymphomas and present as mass lesions usually in the area of the tonsil. Staging studies need to be undertaken. If localised, they respond to radiotherapy.

Nasopharynx

Benign tumours

Angiofibroma of the nasopharynx is a rare tumour, which typically presents in adolescent males with nasal obstruction and epistaxis. Although histologically benign, they are often locally aggressive, extending laterally into the infratemporal fossa and occasionally through the skull base to the intracranial cavity.

CT, MRI and angiography are all used to define the extent of tumour.

They are usually removed surgically, sometimes with immediate preoperative embolisation to reduce vascularity. For those lesions that cannot be surgically removed safely, radiation is an alternative treatment.

Malignant tumours

Carcinoma of the nasopharynx has its highest incidence in south-east Asia, particularly in the Chinese population of Hong Kong. The Epstein–Barr virus has been implicated in the development of this tumour. The viral genome is incorporated into the DNA of the normal cell, which may become malignant in response to other environmental agents. Because the tumour has a large space in which to grow undetected, presentation is late and variable.

Clinical features

- cervical lymphadenopathy
- otitis media with effusion (indicating obstruction of the Eustachian tube)
- facial pain and altered facial sensation (indicating fifth nerve involvement)
- Horner's syndrome (indicating invasion of the sympathetic chain).

Diagnosis

Diagnosis is made by examination and biopsy. Submucosal lesions can be difficult to detect clinically and may even be missed by biopsy. The extent of the tumour is defined by CT or MRI scanning. Epstein–Barr virus antibody titres may be used to follow the response to treatment and to detect recurrence of disease.

Management

These tumours are treated by radiotherapy. The prognosis is poor, only about one-third of patients surviving for 5 years.

14.5 The nose and paranasal sinuses

Learning Objectives

You should:

- be aware of the variety of benign and malignant tumours that affect this area
- know that the maxillary sinus is the sinus most frequently affected by malignancy, usually squamous carcinoma

- be aware of the presentation of Wegener's granulomatosis
- understand the significance of a unilateral nasal polyp.

Benign tumours

Benign tumours are:

- osteoma
- papilloma: squamous or transitional cell.

Squamous papillomas are common in the nasal vestibule and are treated with cautery or excision. Inverting papilloma, although histologically benign, behaves aggressively and requires extensive removal of the lateral nasal wall. About 10% of inverting papillomas are associated with squamous cell carcinoma.

Osteomas of the fronto-ethmoid complex often present with symptoms of obstruction of the fronto-nasal duct. They are slow growing but if symptomatic require removal.

Malignant tumours

Malignant tumours include:

- squamous cell carcinoma (most common)
- adenocarcinoma
- transitional cell carcinoma
- anaplastic tumours and lymphoma
- olfactory aesthesioneuroblastoma
- minor salivary gland tumours
- melanoma.

Wegener's granulomatosis is a systemic disease associated with necrotising granulation of the nose. Death is usually caused by associated renal disease.

Lethal mid-line granuloma is a T cell lymphoma and is treated by radiotherapy.

Clinical features

The maxillary sinus is most commonly involved in malignancy. The patient presents with features resulting from the tumour breaching the walls of the antrum. Diplopia indicates orbital involvement; ill-fitting teeth or dentures indicate extension to the oral cavity. Nasal obstruction results from a breach of the medial wall of the antrum. A bleeding polyp in an elderly patient should be regarded with suspicion.

Diagnosis

The extent of disease is defined by CT scanning and a tissue diagnosis obtained by biopsy.

Management

Treatment involves radical radiotherapy followed by surgery. Functional and cosmetic rehabilitation is usually provided by prostheses. The prognosis is poor with a 66% mortality by 5 years.

14.6 The salivary glands

Learning objectives

You should:

- know that 80% of salivary gland tumours involve the parotid and that 80% of these are benign
- be aware that the smaller salivary glands are more likely to be affected by malignancy
- be aware of the names of the common salivary gland tumours
- know that facial nerve paralysis often suggests malignancy in a parotid tumour
- know that the treatment of most parotid tumours is by parotidectomy, either total or superficial.

Of all salivary gland neoplasms, 80% occur in the parotid and of these 80–90% are benign. Generally speaking, however, the smaller the salivary gland the more likely it is that a tumour involving the gland will be malignant. In the submandibular gland, about 50% of tumours are malignant and in the minor salivary glands about 90% are malignant.

Benign tumours

- pleomorphic adenoma
- monomorphic adenoma
- Warthin's tumour.

Malignant tumours

- adenoid cystic carcinoma
- squamous cell carcinoma
- pleomorphic carcinoma.

Tumours of intermediate malignancy

- mucoepidermoid tumour
- acinic cell tumour.

Pleomorphic adenoma

This presents as a slowly growing painless lump usually below and a little behind the earlobe. It should not be mistaken for an upper cervical lymph node. It does not invade the facial nerve but if present for many years may undergo malignant change.

Fine needle aspiration cytology may help in establishing a histological diagnosis.

Treatment is by superficial or total parotidectomy, depending on the part of the gland involved, taking care to preserve the facial nerve.

Warthin's tumour

This parotid tumour usually occurs in older men and is often bilateral. Clinically it feels soft. Histological examination reveals lymphoid tissue.

Malignant tumours

These tend to grow rapidly, invade the facial nerve and are usually painful. Adenoid cystic carcinoma is the most common. This tumour spreads by invasion of the perineural spaces. Local spread is to the cervical lymph nodes and distant spread is commonly to the lungs.

CT and MRI scan show the extent of disease.

Treatment involves parotidectomy with facial nerve excision if necessary.

Self-assessment: questions

Multiple choice questions

1. Nasopharyngeal carcinoma:
   a. Is most common in people from south-east China
   b. Presents early with nasal pain
   c. Is treated by wide surgical excision
   d. Is monitored by measurement of Epstein–Barr virus antibodies
   e. Is curable in 90% of patients

2. Carcinoma of the hypopharynx:
   a. Is usually an adenocarcinoma histologically
   b. May present with referred otalgia
   c. Is best treated by chemotherapy
   d. Is often disseminated widely throughout the body at time of presentation
   e. Is curable in 90% of patients

Extended matching items questions (EMIs)

1. Theme: Management

A radiotherapy
B oesophagectomy
C laryngectomy
D maxillectomy
E parotidectomy
F radical neck dissection
G glossectomy
H chemotherapy
I tracheostomy
J biopsy

Which of the procedures above most appropriately matches the descriptions below:

1. This procedure is designed to remove a tumour that has spread to the cervical lymph nodes.
2. Excision of the tongue.
3. This operation may be performed as a superficial or total procedure depending on the location of the tumour.

2. Theme: Disease processes

A inverting papilloma
B squamous cell carcinoma
C adenocarcinoma
D leucoplakia
E pleomorphic adenoma
F Warthin's tumour
G Wegener's granulomatosis
H Epstein–Barr virus
I adenoid cystic carcinoma
J lymphoma

Which of the disease processes above best match the descriptions given below:

1. This disease often presents with involvement of the kidneys and lungs.
2. This is the commonest tumour found in the parotid gland.
3. This is the commonest malignant tumour of the maxillary sinus.

Constructed response questions (CRQs)

CRQ 1

> You are an ENT surgeon seeing a patient whom a GP colleague has referred urgently to you. Colin is a 57-year-old alcoholic who has smoked 100 g tobacco per week in 'roll-ups' for at least 40 years. He has recently been losing weight and complains of a pain in his left ear.

a. You think that he may have cancer. Which two sites are the most likely given his symptoms?
b. Name two procedures that you want to perform on the day that you see him.
c. Name two investigations that you would book to be done urgently.
d. Unfortunately Colin continues to lose weight rapidly and starts coughing up blood. What other pathology may he be suffering from?
e. Colin can no longer swallow food or liquid, including his own saliva. He is also in pain. What methods do we have to palliate symptoms in patients such as Colin?

CRQ 2

> Rhoda is a 60-year-old woman who has noticed a slowly growing mass in her right cheek, just below and behind her ear. It is painless and she has no evidence of a facial palsy.

a. What is the most likely diagnosis?
b. How could a histological diagnosis be made without performing an open biopsy?

c. Is the facial nerve likely to be involved?
d. What treatment should Rhoda receive?
e. What complications of your treatment should Rhoda understand before you start?

Objective structured clinical examination questions (OSCEs)

OSCE 1

Look at Figure 128.

a. Which procedure has this patient undergone?
b. For which two reasons might we perform this procedure?
c. Which two complications of this procedure might your patient suffer?
d. Three weeks after the operation you are called to see the patient at 4 a.m. He is having great difficulty breathing. What is likely to be wrong, and what would you do about it?
e. Give three symptoms that a patient with laryngeal cancer might present with?

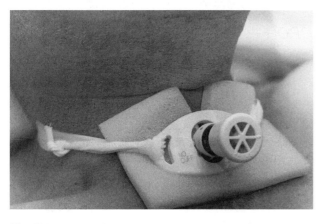

Fig. 128

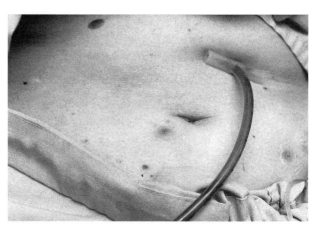

Fig. 129

OSCE 2

The patient in Figure 129 has a carcinoma of the hypopharynx and has had treatment with radiotherapy. This is a view of her abdomen.

a. What is the name of the procedure that has been performed?
b. What is the function of this device?
c. What symptoms may this patient have that require such a device?
d. Why might she have such symptoms?
e. Describe briefly how most of these devices are inserted.

Viva questions

1. Give an account of the therapeutic modalities currently used in the treatment of squamous cell malignancies of the mucosal surfaces of the head and neck.

2. Many head and neck cancers are diagnosed late; why is this?

Self-assessment: answers

Multiple choice answers

1. a. **True.** Nasopharyngeal carcinoma is the most common malignant tumour in men from the Hong Kong area of China.
   b. **False.** Pain is a late feature.
   c. **False.** Radical radiotherapy is the mainstay of treatment.
   d. **True.** Antibodies to specific parts of the Epstein–Barr virus are a sensitive measure of the presence of active tumour.
   e. **False.** Overall survival in all series is much less than 90%.

2. a. **False.** Like most carcinomas of the mucosal surfaces of the head and neck, squamous cell carcinoma is the most common variant.
   b. **True.** Involvement of the superior laryngeal branch of the vagus nerve results in otalgia.
   c. **False.** Surgery and radiotherapy are the mainstays of treatment.
   d. **False.** Early metastases are to the cervical lymph nodes. Widespread dissemination throughout the body is a late feature.
   e. **False.** These tumours are commonly far advanced at the time of presentation and 5-year survival rates are generally less than 50%.

EMI answers

1. Theme: Management

1. F   A radical neck dissection involves removal of the sternocleidomastoid muscle and the internal jugular vein along with all the associated lymph nodes. Together with treatment of the primary tumour this may be curative as head and neck tumours tend to metastasise late to the liver or lungs.
2. G   The prefix gloss- refers to the tongue (as in glossopharyngeal, glossitis, etc).
3. E   Many parotid tumours lie superficial to the facial nerve and thus only this part of the parotid gland has to be removed. If the tumour is deep to the nerve then a total parotidectomy is performed.

2. Theme: Disease processes

1. G   Wegener's granulomatosis is a systemic vasculitis, which may present with crusting and bleeding from the nose. It is life threatening because of the necrotising glomerulonephritis

that also occurs, leading to eventual renal failure, and because of lung involvement. Blood testing often shows a positive cANCA (antineutrophil cytoplasmic antibody). It is *not* a type of cancer.

2. E   Pleomorphic adenoma is a benign parotid tumour, which makes up 80% of the tumours found in the gland. Warthin's tumour (monomorphic adenoma) is also benign but is much less common (8%). Adenoid cystic carcinoma is an aggressive malignant tumour that is fortunately unusual; 25% of patients present with a facial palsy as it often involves the facial nerve.

3. B   Squamous cell carcinomas make up the vast majority of head and neck cancers. Adenocarcinoma is sometimes found in the ethmoid sinuses but usually occurs in people who work with hard woods, such as carpenters and cabinet makers.

CRQ answers

CRQ 1

a. The hypopharynx
   The upper oesophagus
   The larynx
   The tonsil
   The base of the tongue.
   As he is complaining of ear pain, the area affected must be supplied by the glossopharyngeal or vagus nerves, which also send fibres to the ear (referred pain). Tumours involving the hypopharynx, tonsil and base of tongue and the larynx are the most likely to cause ear pain.
b. Indirect or endoscopic examination of the larynx
   Examination of the neck
   Chest X-ray.
   The immediate examination in out-patients is to see where his tumour is by examining the larynx, pharynx and mouth with an endoscope or a mirror. The neck is examined for enlarged cervical lymph nodes indicating possible spread of the tumour. The chest X-ray may show pulmonary metastases or a second primary lung tumour.
c. Barium swallow
   CT of neck and chest (or MRI).
   Direct laryngoscopy, oesophagoscopy and bronchoscopy with biopsy.
   A barium swallow allows tumour in the oesophagus to be seen and CT of the neck and chest may show

the extent of the tumour, involved lymph nodes and lung lesions. Direct endoscopy and biopsy are necessary for histological diagnosis.

d. Lung cancer.
   As Colin is a heavy smoker he may have a second primary bronchial tumour.

e. Stenting of tumour in oesophagus
   Palliative radiotherapy
   Gastrostomy tube for feeding
   Subcutaneous or rectal analgesia
   Psychological support.
   Palliative medicine is a specialty with its own experts who should always be consulted when dealing with such patients. The type of palliative therapy that is appropriate depends on the clinical problem, but radiotherapy to shrink the tumour and enteral feeding are frequently used.

CRQ 2

a. Pleomorphic adenoma.
   The mass involves the area of the right parotid gland. Over 80% of tumours in this area are pleomorphic adenomas. This is compatible with the age of the patient and the fact that the tumour has been enlarging slowly. Other salivary gland tumours are possible, as are tumours in adjacent structures, but a pleomorphic adenoma is the most likely in this area.

b. Fine needle aspiration cytology.
   Fine needle aspiration cytology (FNAC) is the most accurate way of obtaining a tissue diagnosis without performing an open biopsy.

c. No, not if the tumour is benign.
   It is very unusual for the facial nerve to be involved in a benign parotid tumour. Benign tumours grow slowly and the large motor fibres in the nerve can adapt to slowly increasing pressure. This is in contrast to malignant tumours, which invade the nerve early and may result in facial weakness or spasm when the tumour is relatively small.

d. Superficial parotidectomy.
   In an otherwise healthy 60-year-old, superficial parotidectomy is the most appropriate treatment. Most of the tumours arise superficial to the facial nerve but if left will gradually enlarge. There is also a small risk of malignant change.

e. Possible damage to the facial nerve
   Some loss of sensation in the side of the face postoperatively
   Frey's syndrome
   Recurrence of tumour.
   The main risk of superficial parotidectomy is damage to the facial nerve. In skilled hands this risk is small, but the course of the nerve is variable and the nerve is at risk even with small tumours. To

remove the tumour, the great auricular nerve must be divided, which leads to a localised loss of sensation of the side of the face in the area of the ear lobe. Some patients postoperatively become aware of sweating from the skin overlying the gland when eating or thinking of food (gustatory sweating). This results from aberrant innervation from nerve fibres that originally supplied the salivary gland tissue regrowing into the sweat glands of the overlying skin (Frey's syndrome).

OSCE answers

OSCE 1

a. Tracheostomy.
   This is a tracheostomy tube, which has been inserted into the trachea to create an airway as the normal airway has been obstructed (in this case due to a carcinoma of the base of the tongue and supraglottis).

b. To create an airway if obstructed
   For ventilation
   To reduce dead space
   To allow suction of bronchial secretions.
   Patients requiring ventilation in the intensive care unit often have a tracheostomy performed after 10 days or so to allow the oral endotracheal tube to be removed. This allows easier suction of secretions in the lungs, more comfort for the patient and prevents the formation of a subglottic stenosis, which may occur if an endotracheal tube is left in place for long periods. This is even more important in children.

c. Haemorrhage
   Displacement of tube from trachea and obstruction
   Crusting causing obstruction of tube
   Pneumothorax (rarely)
   Pulmonary oedema (very rarely).
   Haemorrhage is a particular risk when performing a tracheostomy in a child as the innominate vein may lie high in the neck and be traumatised. The domes of the pleura may lie higher than usual in patients with lung disease such as emphysema and if damaged will lead to pneumothorax. Pulmonary oedema can occur in patients who have longstanding laryngeal or tracheal obstruction. The pressures needed to move air in these patients suddenly fall when a patent airway is created, and fluid may then leak into the lungs.

d. There is probably crusting in the tube, or it has become displaced.
   Remove the inner tube and clean it. If this is ineffective remove and replace the entire tube.
   A tracheostomy is simply an opening into the trachea below the larynx. The normal airway

remains, though it may be partially or totally obstructed. Following laryngectomy the trachea is brought out on to the skin of the neck, the airway above it having been removed. These patients have no other route for breathing, a fact to be remembered if giving oxygen or nebulisers. Crusting of mucus within the tube is not uncommon, and may not be noticed until the tube is almost occluded. Most long–term tracheostomy tubes have an inner cannula that can be removed and cleaned. After 3 weeks it should be possible to change the tube safely as a track will have formed. In the first week after tracheostomy this may be much more difficult.

e. Hoarseness
   Stridor
   Breathing difficulty (dyspnoea)
   Dysphagia
   Haemoptysis
   Cervical node swelling
   Weight loss
   Otalgia.
   Hoarseness is an early sign of glottic carcinoma (involving the vocal cords). Patients who have been hoarse for more than 3 weeks should have their larynx examined. Stridor occurs when the tumour starts to limit the airway and may be associated with dyspnoea — at first with exercise and then also at rest. Dysphagia and referred otalgia occur if the tumour is invading the hypopharynx. Haemoptysis may occur from the ulcerated surface of the tumour itself, or from a second primary lung or oesophageal tumour. Enlargement of the cervical lymph nodes may suggest spread of tumour to the lymphatic system, although sometimes nodes become enlarged due to infection on the surface of the tumour. Weight loss may occur due to dysphagia, or to wider metastatic spread.

OSCE 2

a. Gastrostomy.
   A gastrostomy is an opening into the stomach. The tube can be placed further down the gastrointestinal tract into the duodenum or jejunum if required.
b. To allow feeding and drug administration
   The tube allows food and drugs to be given to the patient.
c. Dysphagia (or complete obstruction)
   Odynophagia.
   The ideal treatment for such a patient would be to allow food and drugs to be taken by mouth, but if this is not possible a gastrostomy may be necessary.
d. Obstruction by tumour
   Mucositis caused by radiotherapy.

Obstructing tumour may not be resectable or amenable to stenting. Radiotherapy frequently causes a marked mucositis, therefore during and after treatment, until the mucositis settles, a gastrostomy tube may be necessary to allow feeding and the administration of drugs. As the tumour shrinks and the mucositis settles, it may be possible to remove the tube.

e. A flexible endoscope is passed into the stomach. The light from the endoscope is seen through the anterior abdominal wall and the abdomen is punctured. The gastrostomy tube is then passed through. Gastrostomy tubes are usually inserted endoscopically, but if the tumour is so extensive as to completely occlude the pharynx or oesophagus, an open approach through the abdomen may be necessary.

Viva answers

1. Generally speaking, the therapeutic modalities available for treatment of squamous cell cancers of the mucosal surfaces of the head and neck include surgery and radiotherapy, with chemotherapy being reserved usually for advanced tumours in the context of controlled clinical trials. In early limited tumours, e.g. of the tongue, surgery or radiotherapy are equally effective and the choice often lies as to which modality produces less patient discomfort and most optimally preserves function. For example, early carcinoma of the vocal cord is treated by radiotherapy as this has a minimal effect on the voice.
   In more advanced tumours, surgery and radiotherapy are often combined, with surgery preceding radiotherapy in some circumstances and vice versa in others. Some patients present with malignancies at such an advanced stage that cure is not possible and palliative treatment only may be the best option for the patient.

2. Patients who develop squamous cell carcinomas of the mucosal surfaces of head and neck often smoke heavily and abuse alcohol. They tend to be self-neglectful and seek medical treatment late. Tumours in particular areas of the head and neck may grow large before producing symptoms. For example, the nasopharynx and hypopharynx are spaces in which tumours can develop undetected. Many such tumours are not painful in their early stages and symptoms such as hoarseness and dysphagia may be ignored for many months. Patients with head and neck cancers often have other diseases such as chronic bronchitis and cardiovascular disease, which to the patient produce more pressing symptoms than the apparently innocent features of head and neck cancer.

SECTION 3
Ophthalmology

3

15 History and examination

Chapter overview

This chapter describes the techniques used to obtain an accurate ocular history and how to tailor a systematic examination towards the presenting complaint. Emphasis in history taking is placed upon the complaints of red eye and visual disturbance. It is important to explore the patient's general health, as many eye conditions are associated with an underlying systemic disease.

A system for examining the eye is described, which should be altered depending on the differential diagnosis formulated from the history.

The nature of the chapter requires a broad understanding of ophthalmology and therefore cross-referencing with other chapters will be necessary.

15.1 History

Learning objectives

You should:

- understand how to take a systematic ocular history regarding the predominant complaint
- be able to explore in more detail some specific common ocular symptoms
- combine this information to create a differential diagnosis before examining the patient.

Asking a patient questions about their symptoms will help clarify the predominant complaint or suggest a likely diagnosis. This will help direct and tailor your examination.

Common to all ocular symptoms it is useful to clarify specific aspects of the presenting complaint and the history of the presenting complaint. These include:

- if this is the first episode or it is a recurrent condition
- if one or both eyes are affected
- the duration of symptoms
- if the symptoms are intermittent or constant
- if anything helps to relieve or aggravate the symptoms
- if the problem is getting better, staying the same or worsening
- whether there are any associated systemic or neurological symptoms (e.g. headache or nausea).

It is useful to explore some aspects of certain symptoms. This will help to create a differential diagnosis.

Examples in more detail include:

Red eyes

- both eyes affected suggests infective or allergic conjunctivitis
- purulent discharge may suggest bacterial conjunctivitis
- itch may suggest allergy
- photophobia suggests inflammation of the anterior segment (e.g. iritis or keratitis)
- a red eye with reduced visual acuity suggests more serious pathology (e.g. acute closed-angle glaucoma, iritis, corneal ulcer)

Visual disturbance

- both eyes affected suggests a postchiasmal neurological lesion
- one eye affected suggests pathology of the globe or optic nerve
- acute visual loss in a quiet white eye with temporal headache and scalp tenderness suggests temporal arteritis
- acute visual loss with a red eye and systemic upset such as vomiting may suggest acute closed-angle glaucoma
- gradual painless visual loss suggests either cataract or age–related macular degeneration

After taking the ocular history it is also important to explore the general medical history, drug history, family history and social history.

Once a clear and accurate history has been taken proceed with the examination.

15.2 Examination

Learning objectives

You should:

- be familiar with the full systematic ocular examination

- tailor the eye examination around the patient's main complaint identified in the history

- remember to spend a few moments observing the patient before starting the examination.

In examining an ophthalmic patient, a balance should ideally be achieved between a thorough systematic examination and a more concise examination orientated around the patient's main complaint or likely diagnosis identified in the history. With practice and greater experi-

ence, a swift smooth examination will be possible without missing important steps but while avoiding unnecessary time-consuming ones. It is important to take a few moments to observe the patient for clues that may help to identify the diagnosis before examining the patient.

The complete systematic examination should include:

- visual acuity
- external eye
- pupil responses
- ocular motility
- field of vision
- ophthalmoscopy.

Visual acuity

Vision is most commonly assessed using a standard Snellen chart (Fig. 130A). Each eye is tested in turn, testing the right eye first as routine. If the patient wears glasses, they should be worn for the test, and if the patient is unable to read the chart then they should be asked to look through a pin-hole aperture as this 'neutralises' any refractive error. The chart should be placed 6 m from the patient, who is asked to read the chart from the top covering the other eye with an occluder. If they are only able to see the top letter then the acuity is documented as 6/60 (a person with normal vision should be

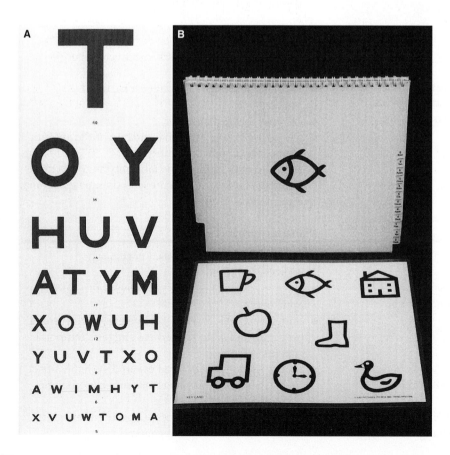

Fig. 130 Methods of testing visual acuity. **A.** The Snellen Chart. **B.** Kay's pictures.

able to see the top letter from 60 m away). If the chart can be read down to the bottom, then the acuity is 6/6, i.e. 'normal' vision. If the patient is unable to see the chart at all, then vision should be recorded progressively as the ability to count fingers (CFs), perceive hand movements (HMs), perceive light (PL) or not perceive light (NPL).

Near vision should also be tested. This can be done using a standard reading book, although if this is not available any text would do.

In younger children visual acuity assessment can be challenging. A variety of methods are employed depending on the child's age. In children less than 18 months preferential looking tests using simple patterns are used. Beyond 18 months, matching tests using shapes, pictures (see Fig. 130B) or letters (Sheridan Gardiner test) can be employed.

The external eye

The eye should be examined using a good light and magnification if possible (Fig. 131). Magnification can be obtained using the plus 10 dioptre lens in the ophthalmoscope.

Systematically examine:

- the skin around the eyes.
- the eyelids, remembering to evert the lid to examine the underside (see Fig. 132), and eyelashes.
- the 'white' of the eye, which includes the thin vascular conjunctiva and the underlying thicker tough sclera.
- the cornea. Loss of the bright corneal reflex is a useful sign of a corneal epithelial abnormality. A drop of fluorescein dye should be instilled into the conjunctival sac as this stains areas of epithelial loss bright green when viewed with a blue light or a bright white light. This helps to identify corneal foreign bodies or abrasions.
- the anterior chamber (the space between the cornea and iris/lens plane). The anterior chamber should be examined to assess its depth and the presence of any blood or pus.

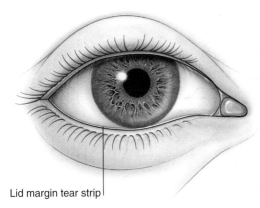

Lid margin tear strip

Fig. 131 Light reflex.

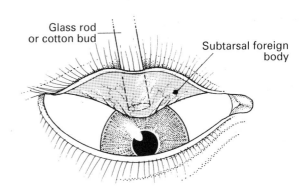

Glass rod or cotton bud

Subtarsal foreign body

Fig. 132 Everting the upper lid. Ask the patient to look downwards and evert the lid over a glass rod or cotton bud by pulling on the lashes.

Pupil responses

Spending a few moments carefully observing a patient's pupils and eyes before shining a pen torch will be rewarding, often revealing useful clues to the likely underlying pathology.

On observation

- The relative size of the pupils should be almost equal under all light conditions.
- If the pupils are markedly unequal in size (anisocoria) an efferent 'motor' pathology is likely to be present (see p. 280).
- If a mild ptosis is present on the same side as an excessively small pupil, a sympathetic palsy may be present suggesting a Horner's syndrome (see p. 281).
- If a dilated pupil is noted as an isolated finding, a parasympathetic palsy may be present such as in an Adie's pupil (see p. 281).
- If a more significant ptosis is present along with a 'down and out' ocular misalignment and a dilated pupil, a parasympathetic palsy is likely to be present due to a third nerve palsy (see p. 281).
- If the pupils are equal in size then an afferent 'sensory' problem may be present and an efferent 'motor' lesion is less likely.
- A slight degree of inequality in size of pupils is often seen even in normal eyes. This is called 'physiological' anisocoria and is not associated with any pathology.

After making careful initial observation examine the pupillary responses to light

- Using a bright pen torch, instruct the patient to fixate a target at least 6 m away.
- Ask the patient *not* to look at the pen torch or yourself as this may induce an accommodative miosis.

- Bring the bright pen torch in from the temporal side and examine the direct response in the right eye then the left eye.
- Repeat the sequence but this time observe the non-illuminated eye for the consensual response.
- If the direct response is less than the consensual response on the same side, an 'afferent pupillary defect' is said to be present (see Ch. 24 and Fig. 191).

Pupil response to accommodation

- The pupil response to accommodation is tested by asking the patient to look in the distance and then requiring them to fix on an object held at approximately 30 cm from their nose
- Both pupils should constrict when looking at the near object
- Light/near dissociation is said to be present when the near response is more pronounced than the light response.

Ocular motility

Any patient with a suspected squint or complaining of double vision should be examined by performing a cover test (Fig. 133) then asked to move the eyes into all nine positions of gaze (see Fig. 134).

Cover test

This is the basic examination for the patient with a squint. Only by carrying out this test can one determine whether a patient has a squint or not.

- Ask the patient to fix on an interesting target (e.g. a small picture or a letter) held 60–90 cm away. Look closely at the eyes to assess whether there is any obvious ocular misalignment before performing the cover test.

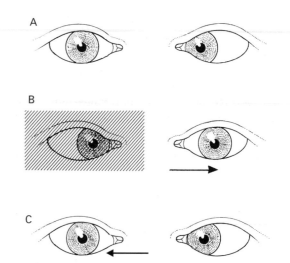

Fig. 133 The cover test. **A.** Patient fixating the target; the left eye appears convergent. **B.** The right eye is covered and the left eye moves out to take up fixation on the target confirming a left convergent squint. **C.** The cover is removed and the left eye becomes convergent again.

- Cover the left eye and observe the right eye for any movement. Then cover the right eye and observe the left eye.

In a non-squinting person, when either eye is covered the other eye does not move. In a person with a convergent squint, the squinting eye will move outwards from its in-turning position to a straight position (to take up fixation) when the other eye is covered. In a divergent squint, the diverging eye moves inwards to take up fixation.

Extraocular eye movements

- Request the patient to fixate and follow a pen torch. Ask the patient to report any double vision during the test. During the examination, observe for any limitation in eye movement and attempt to consider

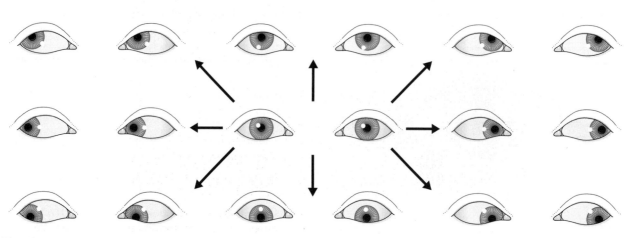

Fig. 134 The nine positions of gaze.

this in the context of a cranial nerve palsy or extraocular muscle limitation such as thyroid eye disease.

- Move the pen torch slowly from the primary position sequentially into all other 8 positions of gaze (see Fig. 134) always returning to the primary position after each movement. Try to maintain the pen torch reflexes on both corneas at all times.

The eyes must be examined in all nine positions of gaze in order to identify whether the squint is concomitant or incomitant (see Ch. 20).

- In concomitant squints, the deviation does not vary with different positions of gaze. Concomitant squints occur due to poorly understood anomalies of central neurological binocular control usually with full ranges of movement.
- In incomitant squints, the deviation increases or decreases depending on which direction the eyes are looking. Incomitant squints are usually caused by disease of the muscles or nerve supply to the muscles with the affected eye demonstrating a reduction in movement in one or more directions.

Field of vision

When assessing a patient's field of vision the examiner should compare their own field of vision with that of the patient's i.e. 'to confrontation'. By presenting targets within the four visual field quadrants, a gross assessment of the common neurological visual field defects can be made. Initially perform a simple binocular field examination using the palms of your hands as targets, then a more elaborate uniocular examination using counting fingers as a target. Any target presented should be placed midway between the examiner and patient. This is to ensure the same angle of field is being assessed in both the examiner and the patient. The examiner should sit approximately 1 meter from the patient with their eyes at the same height (see Fig. 135).

Before examining the patient's visual fields, observe for any clues that may assist in suggesting the likely field defect present.

- On observation, if the patient displays a right hemiparesis then a right hemianopia may also be present. If the patient has a dysphasia suggesting dominant left hemisphere pathology, the field defect is likely to be on the right side. After observation move onto the examination proper.
- With both the patient's eyes open ask the patient to fixate upon your nose. Emphasise to the patient to maintain fixation on your nose and avoid looking at the targets being presented.
- Present both your palms above the horizontal meridian in opposite quadrants. Ask the patient how many palms they see. If they only see one ask them to point to the one they do see. Repeat this for the lower quadrants.

Having formed a thesis as to what field defect the patient may have, go on to prove this by examining each eye in turn with the more visually challenging counting fingers stimuli.

- Ask the patient to cover their left eye with the palm of their left hand and close your right eye. Ask the patient to fixate your 'open' eye. This allows you to monitor the patient's fixation during the examination.
- Explain to the patient that you are going to hold up fingers and that you would like them to state how many fingers they see. Again emphasise that they are to maintain fixation on your open eye at all times and not to look directly at the fingers.

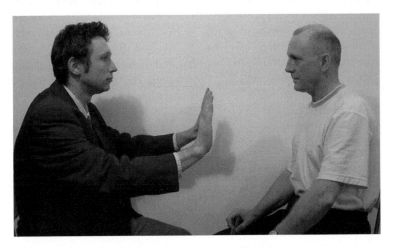

Fig. 135 Assessing a patient's field of vision. Sit opposite the patient with your eyes at the same level. Present targets equidistant in the middle of a quadrant avoiding the horizontal and vertical meridia.

- Initially present the fingers in the centre of the field. This allows you to confirm that the patient both understands the test and that their visual acuity is good enough to see counting fingers at 50 cm.
- Present one or two fingers briefly in the centre of each quadrant. Repeat any quadrants in which the patient's response is absent or incorrect until you are satisfied that the patient is responding consistently. Repeat for the patient's left eye.

This form of examination is useful for identifying gross neurological visual field defects such as hemi- and quadrantanopias (see Ch. 23). It is less appropriate for assessing subtle prechiasmal visual field defects such as in glaucoma where more sophistcated computerised field analysis is usually employed.

Ophthalmoscopy

Ophthalmoscopy is a difficult technique to master. Ideally the student should learn the technique in eyes with clear media and a dilated pupil in a darkened room. The general medical ward rarely affords such an opportunity and therefore the specific opportunities should be sought to learn the technique during medical diabetic clinics or ophthalmology attachments. As with any examination technique a system should be employed.

- The patient is asked to fixate a distant object of interest with the eyes in the primary position. Turn the ophthalmoscope on and set the lens to zero. Stand back from the patient, looking through the peep hole to observe the red reflexes of each eye through the pupil. This will allow an assessment of the clarity of the media. Initially examine the patient's right eye with your right eye then their left with your left.
- Turn the lens to +10 (the plus lenses are usually the black numbers) and move to within 10 cm of the patient's eye. The ophthalmoscope should now be focused on the front of the eye (the anterior segment) and by working backwards through the lenses (+9, +8, +7, etc.), by turning the lens rack knob, the focus moves progressively further posterior through the lens and vitreous humour onto the retina. By doing this it is possible to identify opacities in the media such as a cataract or a

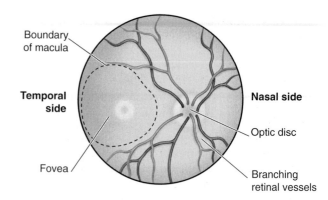

Fig. 136 Diagrammatic representation of the main structures at the posterior pole.

vitreous haemorrhage. This technique will also allow the examiner to focus on the retina even if the patient has a significant refractive error.
- By approaching the patient slightly from their temporal side, the optic disc (which is situated slightly nasal at the posterior pole) should come into view. If this is not initially visible then any V shape created by the branches of retinal vessels will point in the direction of the disc (see Fig. 136). Once the disc is seen, comment on the Margin, Colour and Cupping (MCC). After describing the optic disc examine the retinal vessels.
- The central retinal artery divides into superior and inferior divisions then each division divides again into nasal and temporal branches (see Fig. 136). Running with each of these branches is the returning venous blood in the retinal venules. The thin red arterioles run on top of the slightly fatter and darker-appearing venules. Examine each of the four main branches in turn then examine the peripheral retina.
- Adequate examination of the peripheral retina with the direct ophthalmoscope is difficult. The field of view with this instrument is very small while the peripheral retina is relatively very large. Ask the patient to look up, temporally, down and nasally to aid in making a gross examination of the periphery. Once this has been carried out finish by examining the macula.
- Ask the patient to look directly at the ophthalmoscope light source. The instrument should now be focused on the foveal region at the centre of the macula.

Self-assessment: questions

Multiple choice questions

1. In testing visual acuity with a Snellen chart, which statements are correct:
   a. Testing is normally performed with the patient situated at 6 m from the Snellen Chart
   b. The patient should observe the chart using a 'pin-hole' if they have forgotten their glasses
   c. If the patient cannot see the top line of the chart then visual acuity of no perception of light is recorded
   d. Always record distance visual acuity with the patient wearing reading glasses
   e. It is the best means of assessing vision in very young children

2. Regarding the examination of pupil responses which statements are accurate:
   a. The direct light response requires cerebral function
   b. Pupil diameter generally diminishes with age
   c. Inequality of pupil size (anisocoria) always represents pathology
   d. An absent direct pupil response of the right eye always represents disease of the right optic nerve
   e. It is important that the patient does not accommodate while testing the light responses

Extended matching items questions (EMIs)

1. Theme: History

A left-sided cerebrovascular accident of the postchiasmal visual pathway
B left retinal detachment
C acute closed-angle glaucoma affecting the right eye
D dense cataract of the left eye
E primary open-angle glaucoma of the left eye
F right-sided cerebrovascular accident of the postchiasmal visual pathway
G primary open-angle glaucoma of the right eye
H giant cell arteritis causing a left anterior ischaemic optic neuropathy
I space occupying lesion of the right occipital lobe
J chiasmal compression from a pituitary tumour

Match the most likely diagnosis above with the history from below:

1. Painless sudden onset flashing lights with a dark shadow in the peripheral visual field of the left eye of a 25-year-old short-sighted male.

2. Painless acute onset right-sided visual field loss affecting both eyes in a 65-year-old male with a past medical history of hypertension and hypercholesterolaemia.
3. Acute onset complete loss of vision in the left eye of a 82-year-old female with associated temporal headache, shoulder pain and weight loss.

2. Theme: History

A subconjunctival haemorrhage
B bilateral anterior uveitis
C acute closed-angle glaucoma of the right eye
D anterior uveitis of the right eye
E acute closed-angle glaucoma of the left eye
F rubeotic glaucoma of the right eye
G primary open-angle glaucoma of the right eye
H chemical conjunctivitis
I bacterial conjunctivitis
J allergic conjunctivitis

Match the most likely diagnosis above with the history from below:

1. A 63-year-old woman with a painful firm left red eye and reduced visual acuity with cloudy cornea. The pupil is mid-dilated and unreactive. She is long-sighted with a history of similar episodes, which normally resolve spontaneously.
2. A 6-year-old boy with an 18-month history of intermittently bilateral itchy red eyes. The symptoms are worse in spring and summer. He has a past medical history of asthma and eczema.
3. A 27-year old male presents with a 1-week history of a photophobic, watering red right eye. He has previously had similar episodes, which, after having seen an ophthalmologist, settled with topical steroids. He has a past medical history of ankylosing spondylitis.

Constructed response questions (CRQs)

CRQ 1

A 73-year-old man attends complaining of visual disturbance.

a. What further questions regarding the nature of the visual disturbance would aid in identifying the cause?

Before examining the patient it is important to ask further questions not directly related to the presenting complaint.

b. What categories do these questions fall into?

The patient suggests that the visual disturbance is constant and worse on the right side.

c. Outline the steps of the standard systematic eye examination.
d. State the steps that are most relevant to this man's presenting complaint.

His visual acuity is 6/6 in both eyes but he still complains of right-sided visual disturbance.

e. Describe in detail the process of clinically assessing a patient's visual fields to confrontation.

CRQ 2

A 67-year-old woman presents to her GP complaining of double vision.

a. What questions might the GP ask regarding her symptoms that would help in identifying a possible aetiology?
b. What other information regarding the patient might help the GP in identifying a possible aetiology?
c. Describe how the GP might perform a clinical assessment of this patient's eye movements.
d. What clinical signs on observation might aid in suggesting a possible aetiology?

Objective structured clinical examination questions (OSCEs)

OSCE 1

A picture of the head of an ophthalmoscope is shown in Figure 137.

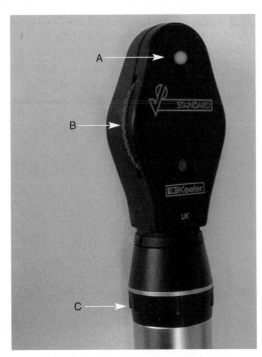

Fig. 137

a. What is the function of the different parts of the ophthalmoscope labelled A to C?
b. What structures of the eye may be examined with the ophthalmoscope?
c. Figure 138 shows a medical student claiming to be examining the optic disc of a patient.
What is wrong with the student's technique?

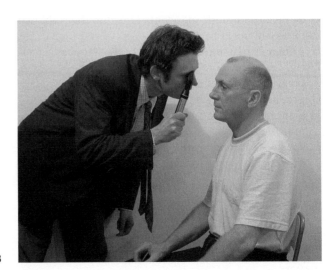

Fig. 138

OSCE 2

Figure 139 shows a medical student performing a visual field examination 'to confrontation'.

a. What types of visual field defects can reasonably be identified using such a technique and what defects require visual field plotting machines?
b. What does 'to confrontation' mean?

c. What steps must be performed before presenting a 'counting fingers' target to each eye?
d. What is wrong with this student's technique?

Viva questions

1. Describe the routine of ophthalmoscopy.

2. Describe the routine of examining the external eye structures.

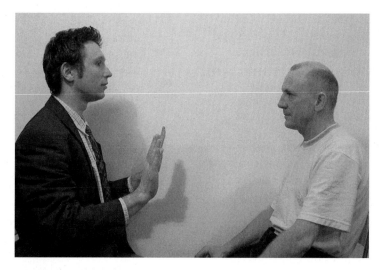

Fig. 139

Self-assessment: answers

Multiple choice answers

1. a. **True.** It is conventional to assess visual acuity from 6 m although any distance may be used. The distance is recorded in metres as the numerator of the visual acuity fraction.
   b. **True.** It is helpful to use a 'pin-hole' as this neutralises any refractive error.
   c. **False.** The patient may be able to see the top line from 3 m. If not then visual acuities of counting fingers (CF), hand movements (HM), perception of light (PL) and then no perception of light (NPL) may be recorded.
   d. **False.** The patient should wear their usual distance spectacles. The reading spectacles should be used to assess near vision using a reading chart or newspaper.
   e. **False.** A variety of different methods are employed to assess the vision of young children. The Snellen chart is not a suitable method of assessing children who are under 5 years of age.

2. a. **False.** The light reflexes are dependent on brainstem function. The pupil response to a near stimulus, however, requires the conscious cortical appreciation of an image to focus upon.
   b. **True.** Older patients generally have smaller pupils often making the pupil responses more subtle and difficult to interpret.
   c. **False.** Physiological anisocoria is present in a significant minority of the normal population.
   d. **False.** An absent direct light response may be due to either 'sensory' retinal or optic nerve pathology or 'motor' pathology of the sphincter muscle either neurological such as a parasympathetic palsy or direct muscle damage from blunt trauma. If a consensual response is seen in the fellow eye, this would suggest that the sensory function is intact.
   e. **True.** It is important to emphasise to the patient to fix on a distant target and avoid looking either at the pen torch or the examiner as they may induce accommodation and therefore miosis which is not necessarily due to the light response.

EMI answers

1. Theme: History

1. B   The symptoms described are characteristic of retinal detachment with short-sightedness being a risk factor for the development of a spontaneous 'rhegmatogenous' detachment. Cataract and glaucoma tend to affect older patients and are of gradual onset, not characteristically causing symptoms of flashing lights.

2. A   As both eyes are affected the pathology is likely to be postchiasmal. The past medical history of hypertension and hypercholesterolaemia raises the risk of a cerebrovascular accident, which if affecting the visual pathway on the left side of the brain would lead to the symptoms on the contralateral side.

3. H   Complete uniocular, sudden onset loss of vision suggests optic nerve pathology. In an elderly woman with an associated temporal headache, giant cell arteritis is a possible diagnosis and must be excluded.

2. Theme: History

1. E   The symptoms described are consistent with closed-angle glaucoma. The history of similar previous episodes which resolved suggests she has a chronic, intermittent form of the condition. Long-sightedness is a risk factor for the development of closed-angle glaucoma.

2. J   Recurrent red itchy eyes, particularly if seasonal and seen in an atopic individual, are highly suggestive of allergy.

3. D   The symptoms are consistent with anterior uveitis, which is often unilateral and idiopathic but may be associated with ankylosing spondylitis and inflammatory bowel disease. The condition is usually recurrent requiring to be managed by an ophthalmologist and only settling with topical steroids.

CRQ answers

CRQ 1

a. The answers to the following questions aid in suggesting the site and type of pathology. Whether the visual disturbance:

- affects one or both eyes
- causes reduced acuity or visual field loss or both
- causes other symptoms such as flashing lights and floaters.
- is intermittent or constant
- is associated with other symptoms, such as headache
- was of acute or chronic onset.

b. Past ocular and medical history, drug history, family history and social history.

c. Visual acuity, external eye, pupil responses, ocular motility, visual fields and ophthalmoscopy.

d. Visual acuity, pupil responses, visual fields and ophthalmoscopy are most relevant to a presenting complaint of visual disturbance.

e. Observe for signs that may suggest the presence of a field defect.

Grossly assess a binocular field using palms of hands as targets.

Perform a more elaborate uniocular technique using counting fingers as a target.

Test the right eye then left, ensuring the targets are presented in the middle of each quadrant and at an equal distance between the patient and examiner.

CRQ 2

a. The nature of the onset of the symptoms. If the symptoms were of acute onset with severe headache then an aneurysm applying pressure to the third cranial nerve might be responsible, but if the symptoms have been gradually getting worse and tend to be more prominent toward the end of the day then myasthenia gravis may be responsible. The most common cause of double vision in this age group is a microvascular event of the cranial nerve, which usually presents acutely but with no pain. The nature of the double vision. If the double vision is purely horizontal then a sixth cranial nerve palsy is more likely than a third or fourth, which would present with vertical or torsional double vision.

b. Information on the patient's past medical and current drug history may reveal relevant conditions such as hypertension and diabetes, which are risk factors for a microvascular aetiology. Exploring the patient's past ocular history can reveal previous episodes and the associated cause.

c. Perform a cover test and then extraocular movements.

d. Associated clinical signs which may suggest an aetiology include: ptosis, a down-and-out pointing eye and a dilated pupil suggest a third nerve palsy. Prominent globes with swollen, red periorbital tissues suggest thyroid eye disease.

OSCE answers

OSCE 1

a. A: Eye piece
B: Dial to alter power of lens within the eye piece
C: Collar to turn the light source on and vary its brightness.

b. Cornea, anterior chamber, iris, lens and red reflex, vitreous, optic disc, arcade blood vessels, peripheral retina and macula.

c. The student is standing too far from the patient and is therefore forced to lean forward, which is both uncomfortable and tiring. To avoid this the student should instead initially place their feet adjacent to the patient. The view of the fundus is likely to be small and frequently obscured because the student is holding the ophthalmoscope too far from the patient's eye. The student's hand is placed too far down the handle of the ophthalmoscope out of reach of the dial that alters the power of the eye-piece lens. The student will be unable to alter the power of the eye-piece lens without repositioning their hand during the examination.

OSCE 2

a. Chiasmal bi-temporal hemianopias and post-chiasmal hemi- and quadrantanopias are the types of field defect most reliably identified using a 'counting fingers' technique to confrontation. Prechiasmal optic nerve and retinal diseases are difficult to confidently assess without using visual field plotting machines.

b. 'To confrontation' means the examiner is comparing their visual field with the patient's.

c. It is important to initially observe the patient for any clinical signs that might suggest the type of visual field defect present, then confirm that the patient understands the test and that their visual acuity is good enough to see the targets that are to be presented. Before performing a uniocular 'counting fingers' test, assess the binocular field grossly using the palms of the hands as a target.

d. The student is not presenting the target at an equal distance between himself and the patient and their eyes are not at the same level. As a consequence, a point much wider and higher in the patient's field is being tested than the student's. The technique is therefore not 'to confrontation'.

Viva answers

1. Initially set the ophthalmoscope to zero to examine the red reflex then change the lens to a +10 for the anterior segment structures. Place your feet adjacent to the patient to avoid leaning forward during the examination. Hold the ophthalmoscope relatively high up the handle so as you can alter the lens dial during the examination without repositioning your hand. Hold the eye-piece close to your own eye and when examining the fundus ensure the

ophthalmoscope is very close to the patient's eye, almost touching their lashes. Rack down through the lenses until the optic disc is seen, then examine in order the optic disc, arcade vessels, peripheral retina and macula commenting on abnormal and relevant negative findings.

2. Using a bright light and magnification examine in order the

- skin around the eyes
- eyelids
- 'white' of the eye, which includes the conjunctiva and sclera
- cornea
- anterior chamber.

Always remember to evert the eyelids to examine for inflammatory papillae in allergic eye disease and foreign bodies in trauma.
Use of fluorescein drops aid in highlighting abnormalities of the corneal epithelium such as dendritic ulcers or abrasions.

16 The eyelids and lacrimal system

Chapter overview

The eyelids and surrounding orbicularis oculi muscle protect the eye from blunt trauma and foreign bodies. The blinking actions of the lids ensure that the tears are distributed evenly over the cornea maintaining a smooth, comfortable and optically clear surface.

Common and important lid problems include:

- infection and inflammation
- abnormalities of position
- tumours.

Conditions of the lacrimal system discussed here include:

- kerato-conjunctivitis sicca (dry eyes)
- lacrimal outflow obstruction (watery eyes)
- dacryocystitis.

16.1 Infection and inflammation

Learning objectives

You should:

- be able to distinguish the differences between the different forms of eyelid inflammation
- be able to suggest appropriate management for the different conditions.

The eyelashes and eyelid meibomian glands are common sites of staphylococcal infection.

Hordeolum (stye)

This is a common cause of acute painful swelling of the eyelid and is often due to staphylococcal infection of an eyelash follicle.

Clinical features
There is an acute, red, tender swelling of the lid margin which 'points' at the lash line.

Management
Topical broad-spectrum antibiotics and steam bathing will help during the acute infection. Systemic antibiotics are of unproven benefit unless a preseptal cellulitis is developing. 'Styes' usually discharge spontaneously and resolve within 1 to 2 months.

Chalazion

If the opening of a meibomian gland on the lid margin becomes blocked, the gland will swell creating a chalazion. Meibomian glands open just posteriorly to the lashes with the body of the gland running perpendicularly to the lid margin within the tarsal plate. There are 15 to 30 glands within each tarsal plate.

Clinical features
A red, localised, occasionally tender swelling occurs within the lid. Chalazia are often associated with blepharitis (see below).

Management
The majority of acute chalazia will settle spontaneously over a 1–3-month period, often leaving a small residual firm, painless nodule. Any associated blepharitis should be treated with lid hygiene as outlined below. If a large or painful chalazion persists, incision and drainage will often hasten resolution. Topical antibiotics are often prescribed although their therapeutic benefit is unproven.

Blepharitis

Blepharitis is chronic inflammation of the lid margins and associated meibomian glands. It is a common cause

197

of irritable red eyes. It may develop spontaneously for no obvious reason or be associated with acne rosacea, eczema or psoriasis.

Clinical features

The lid margins are red and swollen. There may be crusting around the lashes in severe disease. This is a chronic disease in which the eyes are persistently gritty and sore. Patients are more likely to develop chalazia, an abnormal tear film, secondary conjunctivitis and marginal keratitis.

Management

The lids should be cleaned using cotton buds dipped in a dilute solution of sodium bicarbonate or baby shampoo. This removes crusts and clears meibomian gland orifices. Topical antibiotic ointment should be rubbed into the lid margins. If local measures are ineffective, and in those with acne rosacea, systemic tetracycline is recommended. Artificial tear supplements may be required. Any secondary infection or associated skin condition should be treated appropriately.

16.2 Lid position abnormalities

Learning objectives

You should:

● be able to diagnose correctly the three main eyelid position abnormalities: ptosis, entropion and ectropion

● appreciate the different causes of ptosis and investigate and manage appropriately

● be able to assess entropion and ectropion competently and refer appropriately if surgical correction is required.

Ptosis

Drooping of the upper eyelid is known as ptosis and may be congenital or acquired. Causes include:

● neurogenic
— third cranial nerve palsy
— Horner's syndrome (see Fig. 140)
● myogenic causes
— weakness of the levator muscle (e.g. 'senile ptosis')
● neuromyogenic
— myasthenia gravis
● mechanical causes
— cysts or swelling of the upper lid

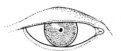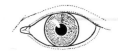

Fig. 140 Right Horner's syndrome.

Clinical features

The upper lid usually overlies the cornea by 1 mm; in ptosis, this position is lower than normal. The diagnosis is made clinically by measuring the marginal reflex distance (MRD) in each eye. The MRD is the distance in mm between the corneal light reflex and the upper lid (see Fig. 131, Chapter 15). The normal MRD is 4–5 mm. If this distance is reduced then a ptosis is present.

Management

If an underlying cause such as myasthenia gravis is identified this should be treated appropriately. Surgery for acquired ptosis consists of reattaching the levator complex and/or shortening it to raise the height of the lid away from the visual axis to a more cosmetically acceptable symmetrical height. In congenital ptosis, surgical correction is required promptly if the visual axis is occluded to prevent the development of amblyopia. The indication for surgery is otherwise cosmetic and is deferred until the child is due to go to school. As ptosis may induce astigmatism, all affected children should be referred to an ophthalmologist for visual acuity assessment and refraction. Surgery usually consists of attaching the upper lid to the brow muscles using a subcutaneous sling.

Lower lid entropion

In entropion the eyelid turns in and the lashes abrade the cornea. The most common cause is senile laxity of the lower lid tissues although acquired cases can also develop due to scarring forms of conjunctivitis. The most common worldwide form of scarring conjunctivitis is trachoma, which can lead to corneal ulcers and scarring leading to blindness. Congenital cases (epiblepheron) are usually self limiting.

Clinical features

This is usually a condition of the elderly. The lashes rub on the cornea and conjunctiva causing redness, pain and the feeling that there is something in the eye. Instillation of fluorescein will often reveal small corneal abrasions. If the entropion is not obvious, it may be necessary to ask the patient to forcibly close the eyes and then open them again to induce the entropion.

Management

Treatment is surgical by shortening the horizontal length of the lid or by placing everting sutures. Prior to surgery if the patient is unfit or unable to cooperate with local anaesthetic surgery then symptomatic relief can often be obtained by applying traction with sticky tape to the lower lids creating a more comfortable everted position.

Complications

- bacterial conjunctivitis
- corneal abrasion
- corneal ulcer and scarring
- blindness.

Lower lid ectropion

In ectropion, the lower lid turns out and the exposed tarsal conjunctiva becomes red and thickened (Fig. 141). This is usually a result of senile laxity of the orbicularis oculi muscle and the other normally supporting lid tissues.

Clinical features
The eye is uncomfortable because of exposure of the lower aspect of the cornea. If fluorescein dye is instilled small punctate epithelial erosions (PEE) may be seen on the corneal surface representing dried areas of corneal epithelium. The eye may water because tears cannot drain into the everted lower lacrimal punctum.

Management
The symptoms of grittiness and exposure may improve with the use of artificial tears. If symptoms persist then surgical treatment is required by an ophthalmologist. Objectives of surgery include repositioning of the punctum and reduction of lid laxity.

Complications

- bacterial conjunctivitis
- exposure keratitis
- corneal ulcer and scarring
- rarely blindness.

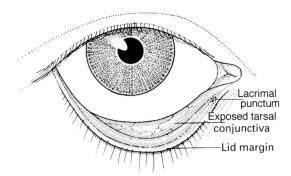

Fig. 141 Lower lid ectropion.

16.3 Tumours

Basal cell carcinoma

Basal cell carcinomas (BCC) account for 95% of eyelid tumours. The remaining 5% comprise squamous cell carcinoma, sebaceous gland carcinoma and malignant melanoma. These three uncommon lid tumours are more serious than BCCs as they can metastasise. They require thorough investigation, wide local excision and careful follow up. The clinical features and management of these rarer tumours is beyond the scope of this text.

Clinical features
BCCs are usually raised painless lesions with a pearly telangiectatic margin and an ulcerated centre. They are commonly found on the lower lid margin.

Management
Diagnosis can usually be made by characteristic clinical appearances. Treatment is by surgical excision or radiotherapy. Both methods have similar success rates, however, local excision is usually preferred since complete surgical clearance can be confirmed histologically.

Complications
Nasally placed tumours tend to be locally invasive and can penetrate deep into the orbit. BCCs characteristically rarely metastasise.

16.4 Abnormal lacrimal flow

- be able to treat dry eye symptomatically and consider the occasional systemic associations
- be able to refer dry eye for further management and investigation when appropriate.

Lacrimal outflow obstruction (watery eyes)

Tears drain from the conjunctival sac through the lacrimal puncta and canaliculi into the lacrimal sac in the medial wall of the orbit. From there they drain down the nasolacrimal duct to its opening in the nose beneath the inferior turbinate (Fig. 142). Obstruction at any point along this pathway results in epiphora (watering of the eye). This may be congenital or acquired.

Congenital nasolacrimal duct obstruction

Membranous obstruction of the lower end of the nasolacrimal duct may be present if incomplete canalisation occurs.

Clinical features
The eyes water from birth (congenital epiphora). The condition may be bilateral although usually asymmetrical. The eyes may be intermittently sticky but rarely red or inflamed. In the vast majority of children (> 90%), the membranous obstruction opens spontaneously during the first year of life and the symptoms resolve completely.

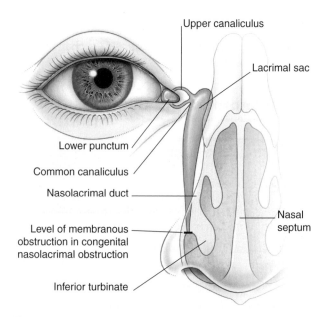

Upper canaliculus

Lacrimal sac

Lower punctum

Common canaliculus

Nasolacrimal duct

Level of membranous obstruction in congenital nasolacrimal obstruction

Inferior turbinate

Nasal septum

Fig. 142 The lacrimal drainage system.

Fluorescein disappearance test (FDT)
This test is useful in the assessment of watering eye in a young child. A drop of 1% fluorescein is placed into each eye. The drainage of fluorescein-stained tears are then observed. If after 5 minutes, fluorescein-stained tears are still seen then nasolacrimal duct obstruction is likely.

Management
The affected infant's mother should be reassured that this is a self-limiting condition and be advised to clean the eye regularly and to massage the lacrimal sac to express any stagnant contents. Routine probing of the ducts for either investigative or therapeutic reasons is not recommended during the first 12 months of life; this may damage the ducts and reduce the chances of the lumen spontaneously clearing. Since there is such a high rate of spontaneous resolution, investigation and surgery is only considered if epiphora persists beyond 12 to 18 months. Surgery consists of a probe being passed down the nasolacrimal duct to open the obstruction.

Infective conjunctivitis is rare. Antibiotics should only be prescribed if the eye becomes red and sticky.

Acquired lacrimal outflow obstruction

The causes of acquired obstruction of the lacrimal outflow system include:

- involutional stenosis
- infection (bacterial, viral, fungal)
- trauma.

Clinical features
There is painless watering of the eye, which may be worse in cold winds. The eyelids should appear healthy with no eyelid position abnormality and a normal tear film. Other causes of epiphora include ectropion, entropion and a dry eye. These should be excluded and nasolacrimal obstruction confirmed before referral for surgery.

Management
If the patient is very symptomatic, fit enough and suitably motivated to undergo a general anaesthetic procedure and other causes of epiphora have been excluded then referral to ophthalmology for surgical correction is appropriate. The obstruction is bypassed by creating a direct communication between the lacrimal sac and the nasal mucosa. This is known as a dacryocystorhinostomy (DCR). Performing DCRs using a nasal endoscope is becoming more commonplace. This technique is less invasive and can be performed under local anaesthetic.

Complications
The stagnant fluid which collects in the blind-ended lacrimal sac may give rise to infection. In its most mild

form this may appear as a conjunctivitis but may also lead to acute or chronic dacryocystitis (lacrimal sac infection, see below). Dacryocystitis can lead to preseptal or orbital cellulitis.

Dacryocystitis

Dacryocystitis is an infection of the lacrimal sac, often secondary to nasolacrimal duct obstruction.

Clinical features

Acute dacryocystitis. This is an extremely painful, tender, red swelling at the medial canthus. Pus builds up in the lacrimal sac and without treatment may discharge through the skin.

Chronic dacryocystitis. Chronic infection causes a painless swelling of the sac. Mucopurulent material accumulates in the sac and can be expressed through the lacrimal puncta by pressure on the swelling.

Management

Acute dacryocystitis requires systemic antibiotics. Once the infection has settled, an operation is necessary to avoid recurrent attacks. The operation aims to recreate the communication between the lacrimal sac and the nose and is known as a dacryocystorhinostomy (DCR).

Chronic dacryocystitis, if prone to acute painful exacerbations, will often also require a DCR. By allowing the tears to flow normally again, epiphora will improve and recurrent episodes of acute dacryocystitis will cease.

Complications

Lacrimal sac infections can lead to episodes of preseptal and orbital cellulitis. Orbital cellulitis can cause irreversible visual loss and very rarely intracerebral infection.

Keratoconjunctivitis sicca (dry eyes)

The tears lubricate the ocular surface and contain antibacterial substances that protect against infection. Keratoconjunctivitis sicca is an extremely common cause of ocular discomfort, especially in the elderly.

The underlying pathology is atrophy and fibrosis of the lacrimal gland caused by:

- senile changes in the lacrimal gland
- connective tissue diseases, e.g. Sjogren's syndrome, which is characterised by keratoconjunctivitis sicca, dry mouth and autoimmune diseases such as rheumatoid arthritis.

Clinical features

The patient complains of dry, gritty eyes. The symptoms may be worse towards the end of the day and in dry warm atmospheres. Paradoxically, the eyes may water from reflex secretion because of the surface irritation. By placing small strips of filter paper into the lower fornix, an assessment of tear production can be made. This is known as Schirmer's test. An assessment of the quality and quantity of the tear film can also be made by observing the height of the tear meniscus at the lid margin (see Fig. 131, chapter 15), the tear film break-up time and for the presence of punctate epithelial erosions (PEE) on the corneal surface.

Management

Artificial tear drops and lubricating ointments may provide symptomatic relief. There is no other recognised means to increase tear production but the rate of drainage can be reduced by blocking the lacrimal puntal openings on the eyelid margins. This can be performed reversibly by the use of plugs or definitively and irreversibly by cautery.

Self-assessment: questions

Multiple choice questions

1. Lower lid entropion:
   a. is associated with facial nerve paralysis
   b. is usually treated surgically
   c. is common in the elderly
   d. may be treated by applying traction with sticky tape to evert the lids
   e. is a cause of corneal abrasion

2. Congenital epiphora:
   a. is caused by infection
   b. has a high spontaneous resolution rate
   c. should be treated urgently by probing the nasolacrimal duct
   d. is present from birth
   e. is associated with amblyopia

Extended matching items questions (EMIs)

1.

A entropion	G keratoconjunctivitis sicca
B ectropion	H ptosis secondary to a
C senile ptosis	third nerve palsy
D Horner's syndrome	I ptosis secondary to
E blepharitis	myasthenia gravis
F Sjogren's syndrome	J congenital ptosis

For the symptoms and signs listed below select the most appropriate diagnosis from the above:

1. An out-turning eyelid causing drying to the surface of the eye.
2. An in-turning eyelid causing abrasions to the corneal surface from abrading eyelashes.
3. A droopy upper lid, noted since birth.

2.

A malignant melanoma	F Sjogren's syndrome
B hordeolum	G dacryocystitis
C basal cell carcinoma	H squamous cell carcinoma
D chalazion	I lacrimal gland swelling
E blepharitis	J Horner's syndrome

For the symptoms and signs listed below select the most appropriate diagnosis from the above:

1. Painless, pink, raised, pearly edged telangiectatic lump on the medial aspect of the lower eyelid with a central ulcerated area.

2. A very tender, red, hot, raised lump on the skin just nasal to the medial canthus associated with a watering eye.
3. Red swollen lid margins with blocked meibomian orifices, associated with a poor tear film and acne rosacea.

Constructed response question (CRQs)

CRQ 1

> A 65-year-old female has had a watering eye for some years. Over the last 3 days, she has developed a painful tender swelling at the medial aspect of the orbit. The swelling is red and was very tender to touch until there was a discharge of green pus though the skin this morning.

a. What is the likely diagnosis?
b. What are the potential complications of this condition?
c. Will the symptoms of watering eye ever resolve?
d. What is the management?

CRQ 2

> A 50-year-old man attends his GP complaining of several years of red swollen eyelids and red gritty 'burning' eyes. His skin appeared red with several sebaceous pustules.

a. What is the most likely diagnosis?
b. What management would you recommend?
c. Name two common complications of this condition.

Objective structured clinical examination questions (OSCEs)

OSCE 1

A mother takes her 9-month-old son to her GP. She says the child's right eye has watered since he was born and every couple of months becomes sticky. The left eye is never affected. She has seen most of the other doctors in the practice and has been prescribed topical antibiotic drops that usually clear the stickiness within a few days but not the constant watering. Today the child has a watering right eye with a watery discharge.

a. What is the most likely diagnosis?

b. What examination would help to make a diagnosis?
c. What treatment and advice would you offer?
d. If the problem persisted, at what age would you consider referral for an ophthalmology opinion?
e. What treatment should generally be avoided in these children?

OSCE 2

A 48-year-old woman attends her GP complaining that the appearance of her eyes has changed over the past month.

a. Describe the appearance of her eyes in Fig. 143.
b. List some causes of ptosis.

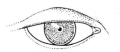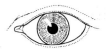

Fig. 143

c. In your opinion what is the most likely aetiology of this patient's ptosis.
d. What are the indications for surgical correction of a ptosis?

Viva questions

1. Discuss basal cell carcinoma.

2. Discuss dry eyes.

Self-assessment: answers

Multiple choice answers

1. a. **False.** Facial nerve paralysis is often a cause of ectropion, not entropion.
   b. **True.** Surgery everts the lid to its normal position.
   c. **True.** As a result of senile laxity of the lower lid tissues.
   d. **True.**
   e. **True.**

2. a. **False.** It results from incomplete canalisation of the nasolacrimal duct.
   b. **True.**
   c. **False.** Because of the high spontaneous resolution, probing is not indicated in the first year.
   d. **True.** By definition.
   e. **False.** There is no known association with amblyopia.

EMI answers

1.

1. B   An ectropion is where the lower eyelid turns out leading to corneal exposure and drying. The patient often complains of a gritty eye.
2. A   An entropion is where the lower eyelid turns in causing abrasions to the surface of the eye.
3. J   A ptosis is of the lower-positioned upper lid. If it is noted from birth it is by definition a congenital ptosis.

2.

1. C   This is the classical appearance and description given to this common non-metastasising but locally invasive skin tumour.
2. G   If the nasolacrimal duct becomes blocked, stagnant fluid collects within the sac. During an episode of dacryocystitis, the stagnant fluid becomes infected. As the sac is found just nasal to the medial canthus this area becomes red, swollen and tender. Because the nasolacrimal duct is blocked, the eye is always watery.
3. E   This is the classical appearance and description given to this common condition of the lid margins.

CRQ answers

CRQ 1

a. The diagnosis is acute dacryocystitis which has discharged anteriorly through the skin.
b. Chronic discharging sinus from the sac to the skin and a pre-septal or orbital cellulitis.
c. No, the passage of tears from the eye to the nose is irreversibly blocked.
d. Treatment is initially with systemic antibiotics. Once the infection has resolved a dacryocystorhinostomy may be required if the eye continues to water or if chronic recurrent infection occurs.

CRQ 2

a. Blepharitis associated with acne rosacea.
b. Blepharitis management includes lid hygiene, topical antibiotics and artificial tears. Acne rosacea often improves with systemic tetracycline.
c. Chalazia develop because the meibomian gland orifices are blocked predisposing to swelling and chronic inflammation within the gland. Marginal keratitis often also occurs in patients with blepharitis. Poor tear film with dry eyes.

OSCE answers

OSCE 1

a. Congenital nasolacrimal obstruction.
b. Fluorescin disappearance test (FDT).
c. Recommend regular cleaning and gentle massage of the lacrimal sac to remove stagnant pooling tears.
d. 12 to 18 months of age.
e. Try to avoid topical antibiotics unless the eye becomes red and sticky. Consider surgical probing only after 12-16 months of age.

OSCE 2

a. Right ptosis and miosis.
b. Aetiology of ptosis:

- Neurogenic: third cranial nerve palsy or Horner's syndrome
- Myogenic: congenital dystrophic levator muscle or age-related levator disinsertion
- Neuromyogenic: myasthenia gravis
- Mechanical: cysts or tumours of the upper lid.

c. The patient has sudden onset mild ptosis with associated miosis. Clinically this appears to be a right-sided oculo-facial sympathetic palsy or Horner's syndrome.

d. Surgery is indicated if:

- the appearance is cosmetically unacceptable
- the eyelid is interfering with vision, especially in young children as this may induce amblyopia.

Viva answers

1. Basal cell carcinoma is the most common eyelid tumour. The most important aetiological factor is exposure to sunlight. Basal cell carcinoma commonly arises on the lower lid or medial canthal region. The tumour is usually raised with a pearly margin and an ulcerated centre. The tumour is locally invasive and must be completely removed. Treatment is with radiotherapy or surgical excision.

2. Keratoconjunctivitis sicca (dry eyes) is a very common problem, especially in the elderly. It is caused by reduced tear production because of atrophy of the lacrimal gland. The eyes feel dry and gritty. The most common causes are ageing atrophy of the lacrimal gland and Sjogren's syndrome. Sjogren's syndrome is an autoimmune condition characterised by dry eyes and mouth commonly associated with rheumatoid arthritis. Treatment is with artificial tear drops and lubricating ointments. If the symptoms persist, blocking the punctual openings on the lid margins with plugs to reduce tear drainage may improve symptoms.

17 The conjunctiva, cornea and sclera

Chapter overview

In this chapter the common conditions which affect the conjunctiva, cornea and sclera are discussed.

These conditions represent the common causes of red eyes. An understanding of the surface anatomy of the eye and eyelids is necessary to appreciate the different red eye conditions and their associated symptoms and signs.

Emphasis is placed on taking a history as this is important in suggesting a likely aetiology for the common red eye conditions before an examination is commenced.

The appropriate investigations and treatments for the various conditions are discussed. Attention is drawn to drugs that are contraindicated in certain eye conditions and in specific patients with coexistent disease.

17.1 The conjunctiva

Learning objectives

You should:

- appreciate the common conditions that affect the conjunctiva
- differentiate the conditions by history and examination
- recommend appropriate management.

The conjunctiva is a clear mucous membrane which covers the globe and the inner surface of the eyelids. The most common conditions of the conjuctiva include infective and allergic conjunctivitis.

Infection

Acute conjunctivitis caused by bacteria, viruses or chlamydia is usually a bilateral condition characterised by red eyes, grittiness and discharge.

Bacterial conjunctivitis

Bacteria often cause a purulent discharge. The most common pathogens are staphylococci, streptococci and *Haemophilus influenzae*.

Clinical features
Patients may give a history of acute onset, red, gritty eyes with a purulent discharge that characteristically causes the eyelids to be stuck together on wakening. The redness is diffuse and most prominent deep in the conjunctival fornices rather than around the cornea. The vision is usually unaffected.

Diagnosis
The diagnosis is usually made on clinical grounds, although pathogenic organisms may be identified by culture of conjunctival swabs.

Management
Treatment is with a broad-spectrum topical antibiotic drop or ointment, such as chloramphenicol.

Adenoviral conjunctivitis

Adenovirus is a common cause of acute conjunctivitis with keratitis (inflammation of the cornea). Other viral causes of conjunctivitis include herpes simplex and molluscum contagiosum.

Clinical features
Although bilateral, this infection is often asymmetrical. The eyes are red with a watery discharge. The redness is diffuse but most prominent deep in the fornices rather than around the cornea. There are superficial punctate corneal lesions, which can often be seen particularly if

stained with fluorescein. These lesions are largely responsible for the symptoms of grittiness and photophobia. Occasionally they can reduce visual acuity. The preauricular lymph nodes are also often enlarged and tender.

Diagnosis

The diagnosis is based on clinical findings. Viral swabs may be used to confirm the diagnosis.

Management

Antiviral agents are ineffective and consequently treatment is symptomatic. The condition is highly contagious and the patient should be advised on hygiene techniques to reduce spreading the infection, e.g. not sharing a face towel with another family member.

Complications

The keratitis can become chronic. If this occurs mild topical steroid drops can help resolve the corneal lesions, improving symptoms.

Chlamydia conjunctivitis

Conjunctivitis caused by *Chlamydia trachomatis* can be divided into two distinct groups: endemic trachoma and sexually transmitted conjunctivitis.

- Endemic Trachoma — this infection is common in developing countries in areas of poor sanitation. It affects several million people worldwide and is one of the leading causes of preventable blindness.
- Sexually transmitted conjunctivitis — this condition tends to affect young adults. A bilateral conjunctivitis develops approximately 2 weeks after sexual exposure. The eyes become red with follicular changes in the fornices and palpebral conjunctiva. The discharge tends to be mucopurulent and stringy with non-tender enlargement of the preauricular lymph nodes. This is not sight threatening.

Diagnosis

Current tests include taking scrapings from the conjunctival sac for PCR, ELISA or immunofluorescence.

Management

If the diagnosis is suspected clinically then topical chlortetracycline is initially prescribed and appropriate swabs taken. Once the diagnosis is confirmed, referral to genito-urinary medicine (GUM) is necessary to perform further investigations to confirm the GU infection. Treatment with systemic doxycycline or azithromycin is recommended as well as initiation of contact tracing.

Complications

Endemic chlamydial conjunctivitis (trachoma) as it occurs in developing countries can lead to scarring of the tarsal plates with 'in-turning' of the eyelid margins (entropion) leading to corneal abrasions, infection and scarring of the cornea from the abrading eyelashes (trichiasis). This can lead to loss of vision. Trachoma is the second most common cause of blindness in the world after cataract.

Neonatal conjunctivitis (ophthalmia neonatorum)

This is a conjunctivitis occurring in the first month of life. It is a notifiable disease. The usual source of infection is the mother's genital tract or the environment, and the most common causative organisms are chlamydia and staphylococci. Gonococcal infections are very rare but may cause severe conjunctivitis with keratitis. Herpes simplex can also cause neonatal conjunctivitis with keratitis.

Clinical features

The clinical features are dependent on the aetiology. Chlamydia may cause a mucopurulent discharge up to several weeks after birth. It is important to recognise, investigate and treat early as this organism may spread causing a pneumonitis. Gonococcus tends to present earlier with a more purulent discharge.

Diagnosis and management

Appropriate microbiological investigations should be performed promptly. Treatment should be started before results of tests are available based on the likely aetiology suggested by the history and clinical examination.

Bacterial infections resolve quickly with topical broadspectrum antibiotics. Chlamydial infection should be treated with systemic erythromycin rather than a tetracycline as this binds to calcium, thus staining growing teeth. If a sexually transmitted disease is confirmed then the mother should be referred to genito-urinary medicine.

Complications

Chlamydial neonatal conjunctivitis may rarely lead to pneumonitis while gonococcal infection can cause corneal ulceration with perforation.

Allergic conjunctivitis

The hallmark of allergy is itch. The most common manifestations are hay fever conjunctivitis and vernal conjunctivitis.

Hay fever conjunctivitis

Hay fever conjunctivitis is a very common self-limiting acute conjunctivitis caused by a type 1 immediate hypersensitivity reaction to pollens.

Clinical features

The eyes become red and itchy with a watery discharge. There may be marked oedema and swelling of the conjunctiva (chemosis). The condition tends to be seasonal and patients often have a history of asthma or eczema (atopy).

Diagnosis

The diagnosis is clinical. Patch testing may be useful in identifying a precipitating antigen.

Management

Avoiding the precipitating antigen may reduce episodes. Topical antihistamine drops may be used prophylactically as well as during an attack to improve symptoms. Under ophthalmological supervision topical steroids may be prescribed.

Vernal keratoconjunctivitis (spring catarrh)

Vernal keratoconjunctivitis (VKC) is an allergic condition normally only seen in children. It is caused by the release of inflammatory mediators from conjunctival mast cells and basophils in response to environmental antigens. This leads to bilateral ocular inflammation particularly affecting the palpebral conjunctiva.

Clinical features

The most prominent symptoms include itch and photophobia. Reduced visual acuity is often noted due to corneal abnormalities and associated poor tear film. There tends to be a mucopurulent discharge with exacerbations occurring in the spring. Boys are more commonly affected than girls. There is a tendency to spontaneous remission in adolescence, but this is not always the case. There is an association with atopy.

Management

The most important element of management is antigen avoidance. The most common antigenic precipitant is the house-dust mite. Measures to reduce exposure include: vacuum cleaning and dusting the child's bedroom and consideration of a wooden rather than carpeted floor, the use of 'sealed' pillowcases and duvet covers and placing soft toys in the freezer to kill the mite. Combining reduction of antigen load with anti-inflammatory medication is more likely to achieve symptomatic improvement.

A hierarchal treatment regimen is employed in VKC. Initially topical mast cell stabilizers, antihistamines and steroids are prescribed. If symptoms are not relieved then systemic antihistamines, steroids and newer immunosuppressant steroid-sparing agents such as cyclosporin can be used.

Complications

Corneal scarring is the most common sight-threatening complication.

Glaucoma and cataract may develop secondary to steroid treatment.

Non-ocular systemic complications may occur if oral steroids and other steroid-sparing anti-inflammatory drugs are used.

17.2 The cornea

Learning objectives

You should:

- understand the anatomy of the cornea
- appreciate the common conditions which affect the cornea
- be able to make a diagnosis by taking a history and performing an examination
- be able to suggest appropriate management for the different conditions.

The cornea is the major refracting structure of the eye and its clarity is essential for good vision. The cornea is made up of three structural layers:

1. The surface of the cornea is a combination of the tear film and a multilayered epithelial membrane continuous with the conjunctiva at the limbus.
2. The middle layer of the cornea is the stroma, which consists of collagen fibres combined in such a way that they allow the passage of light. The stroma is continuous with the sclera.
3. Lining the inner aspect of the stroma is a layer of endothelium. The endothelium actively pumps water out of the stroma maintaining the overall clarity of the cornea.

Keratitis and corneal ulceration

Keratitis is any inflammatory or infective process affecting the cornea.

Marginal keratitis

This is a common inflammatory condition affecting the cornea. It is caused by hypersensitivity to staphylococcal antigens and is often seen in patients with blepharitis.

Clinical features

The patient complains of a gritty red eye with photophobia. The redness tends to be sectorial, localised around an opacified area of the peripheral cornea with irregular overlying epithelium that faintly stains with fluorescein. This is termed a marginal ulcer and is often seen in association with blepharitis and acne rosacea.

Management
The condition is usually self-limiting but may resolve more quickly by instilling a mild topical steroid and a broad-spectrum antibiotic. Treating any associated blepharitis with lid hygiene or acne rosacea with systemic antibiotics will reduce the chance of recurrence.

Bacterial keratitis

The combination of normal lid anatomy, healthy tear film, intact corneal epithelium and a normal immune system protects the cornea from infection. If corneal infection develops it is usually associated with a predisposing factor such as:

- lid abnormalities (entropion, ectropion, lid retraction)
- keratoconjunctivitis sicca
- trauma (corneal abrasion)
- contact lens wear
- corneal paraesthesia
- immunocompromised host
- keratitis
- corneal ulceration.

Clinical features
The clinical features vary with the pathogen. The condition is usually unilateral. The patient presents with a red eye associated with a discharge. There is intense pain and photophobia with reduced vision particularly if the ulcer is in the centre of the cornea. An opacified area of the cornea represents the stromal focus of infection. An overlying corneal epithelial defect may be easily seen if stained with fluorescein. Often there is a secondary anterior uveitis with inflammatory cells circulating in the anterior chamber. These cells may settle in the inferior aspect of the anterior chamber creating a white fluid level known as a 'hypopyon'.

Diagnosis
The causative organism is identified by microscopy and culture of conjunctival swabs and scrapings from the corneal ulcer.

Management
The patient is usually admitted for round-the-clock intensive topical antibiotic treatment. 'Blind' treatment is started before results of microbiology investigations are known. The antibiotics may be altered once the organism is identified and antibiotic sensitivities are

known. Any predisposing abnormalities should be reversed such as augmenting the tear film with copious artificial tears or surgically correcting an entropion.

Complications
- corneal perforation
- corneal scarring
- loss of the eye.

Herpes simplex (dendritic ulcer)

Exposure to herpes simplex virus is very common, with 90% of the adult population showing antibodies to the virus. The virus remains latent in the trigeminal ganglion and may become reactivated, causing a corneal dendritic ulcer.

Clinical features
The condition is classically unilateral with recurrences always occurring on the same side. Photophobia, pain and blurred vision are common symptoms. The eye appears diffusely red, with a watery discharge. The virus characteristically produces a branching, dendritic epithelial defect (Fig. 144) that stains with fluorescein. With successive attacks scarring of the cornea can occur.

Diagnosis
The diagnosis is clinical although the virus can be cultured from swabs.

Management
Topical acyclovir will normally help ulcers to heal within 1 to 2 weeks. Topical steroids must *not* be prescribed. The steroid will reduce the local effect of the immune system making the eye more comfortable but stopping the ulcer healing. This often results in the ulcer becoming larger and deeper leading to an overall longer duration of infection and possibly more scarring with

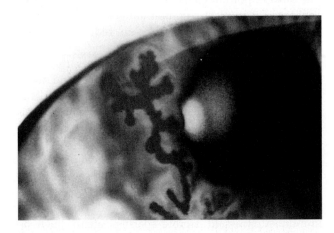

Fig. 144 Dendritic ulcer.

loss of vision. Because of this risk, patients with an acute red eye *must* not be given topical steroids except under the supervision of an ophthalmologist.

Complications

- corneal scarring and loss of vision
- corneal paraesthesia with secondary bacterial ulceration.

Keratoconus

Keratoconus is a structural abnormality of the cornea in which the normal collagen of the stroma is weakened and prone to thinning and bowing forward. The cornea thus gradually becomes more conical in shape losing its ability to focus light accurately onto the retina.

The condition may occasionally run in families. It is more commonly seen in atopic individuals and may be associated with eye rubbing. Individuals with Down's syndrome are also more prone to developing keratoconus.

Clinical features

Patients usually present around puberty or early adult life because of blurring of vision in one or both eyes. This is caused by the development of irregular astigmatism, which increases as the cornea becomes more conical.

Management

Initially the visual acuity may be improved with spectacles, but usually contact lenses are required to correct the high degree of astigmatism. Corneal grafting may be required later if contact lenses can no longer be fitted or the cornea becomes scarred.

Complications

If the inner membrane of the cornea (Descemet's membrane) suddenly ruptures, acute localised corneal oedema at the tip of the cornea can develop. This causes immediate profound loss of vision. As the oedema resolves marked scarring often develops.

17.3 The sclera and episclera

Learning objectives

You should:

- appreciate the common conditions which affect the sclera and episclera
- be able to differentiate the conditions by history and examination
- appreciate the possible systemic conditions associated with scleritis
- recommend appropriate management of the different conditions.

The sclera is the tough white collagenous wall of the eye. It is continuous with the cornea at the limbus. The episclera is an overlying layer of blood vessels, nerves and connective tissue.

Episcleritis

Episcleritis is a self-limiting inflammatory condition of the episcleral tissues. The condition is more common in females. The cause is unknown.

Clinical features

The patient complains of mild irritation, usually in one eye. The affected eye displays sectorial injection in the interpalpebral area. Two forms exist: nodular and diffuse episcleritis. In the nodular type, there is a raised yellow nodule on the episclera with surrounding hyperaemia. In the diffuse type, there is no nodule but diffuse hyperaemia occurs.

Management

The condition usually resolves spontaneously within a few weeks. Resolution may be hastened by instilling a mild topical steroid or non-steroidal anti-inflammatory under ophthalmic supervision.

Scleritis

Pathologically scleritis represents a form of immune complex deposition. Most cases are idiopathic. Systemic associations include any type III hypersensitivity

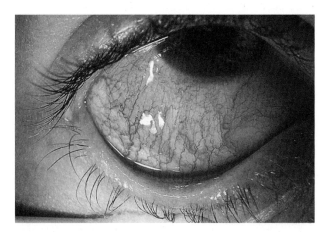

Fig. 145 Scleritis.

vasculitic disease. Rheumatoid arthritis is the most common systemic association.

Clinical features
The most characteristic feature is severe ocular pain, which serves to differentiate scleritis from episcleritis. The globe is exquisitely tender and appears either diffusely red or injected in a sectorial fashion (Fig. 145).

Management
Investigations for an underlying connective tissue disease are performed. The mainstay of treatment is the use of topical and systemic steroids although other immunosuppressive drugs are sometimes used.

Complications
If scleritis affects the posterior globe then swelling of the retina can occur resulting in loss of vision. Rarely the sclera can become dramatically thin: this is known as 'scleromalacia perforans'. The contents of the eye can be seen through the thinned sclera, which bulges because of the intraocular pressure. Despite its name it rarely actually perforates.

Self-assessment: questions

Multiple choice questions

1. Vernal conjunctivitis:
   a. Is rarely sight threatening
   b. is characterised by a purulent discharge
   c. Is more common in males
   d. Is characterised by intense ocular itch
   e. Can require systemic immunosuppression

2. Herpes simplex keratitis:
   a. Is usually treated with topical steroids in the acute phase
   b. Is associated with a purulent discharge
   c. Is characterised by a dendritic corneal ulcer
   d. Is a recurrent disease
   e. Can cause corneal paraesthesia

Extended matching items questions (EMIs)

1.

A bacterial conjunctivitis	F herpes simplex keratitis
B adenoviral conjunctivitis	G marginal keratitis
	H trachoma
C scleritis	I allergic conjunctivitis
D uveitis	J episcleritis
E neonatal conjunctivitis	

For the symptoms and signs listed below select the most appropriate diagnosis from the above:

1. Unilateral photophobic red eye with a watery discharge. Central corneal dendritic-shaped epithelial defect.
2. Bilateral gritty, watering eyes with diffuse conjunctival injection and punctate corneal epithelial erosions and associated preauricular and submandibular lymphadenopathy. The patient also has a sore throat and flu-like illness.
3. Chronic bilateral sticky red eyes with a mucopurulent discharge. In-turning eyelashes and corneal scarring. This is the second most common cause of preventable and treatable visual loss in the world.

2.

A acyclovir	F tetracycline
B timoptol	G lid hygiene
C chloramphenicol	H artificial tears
D gentamicin	I steroid
E erythromycin	J fucithalmic

For the conditions below select the most appropriate treatment from the above:

1. Chlamydia conjunctivitis in an adult.
2. Scleritis.
3. Herpes simplex conjunctivitis and keratitis.

Constructed response questions (CRQs)

CRQ 1

> A young mother brings a 14-day-old girl to the clinic with a sticky red eye. The eyelids are swollen and closed.

a. What is the diagnosis?
b. What organisms may cause this infection?
c. How is the diagnosis confirmed?
d. How should the problem be managed?

CRQ 2

> A 30-year-old management executive has had an acute red eye for 4 days. The patient normally wears soft contact lenses and thinks he may have hurt the eye putting the lenses in. The lids are stuck together in the mornings because of a green discharge, and for the last 24 hours the pain has become severe and vision reduced. On examination, the eye is extremely red and there is a central corneal epithelial defect. There is a white opacity under the epithelial defect and a hypopyon.

a. What is the likely diagnosis?
b. What factors predispose to infection?
c. How should this patient be managed?
d. What complications may occur?

Objective structured clinical examination questions (OSCEs)

OSCE 1

> A 65-year-old woman presents with a painful red eye of 2 weeks' duration. She describes the pain as a 'deep ache'.

a. What important questions would you ask to help make a diagnosis?

The patient states that the eye is not itchy or sticky and that there is no discharge. She has rheumatoid arthritis.

b. What important ocular signs would you look for in this patient in considering a differential diagnosis of a red eye?
c. What is the likely diagnosis?

> The patient's visual acuity is 6/6 corrected in both eyes. The globe is very tender to touch. The eye is not sticky and there is no discharge.

d. What are the common treatments used in this condition?
e. List three conditions which may be precipitated or worsened by the use of high-dose oral steroid treatment.

OSCE 2

> A 21-year-old student returns from a holiday in Ibiza 2 weeks before important examinations. She complains of a photophobic red right eye for 1 week.

a. What questions would you ask in the history to help identify an aetiology?

> The patient complains that her vision is very blurred in the right eye. This is the fourth similar episode in the past 3 years. A watery discharge is present. She has had a cold sore on her lip for the past 10 days. The visual acuity in the right eye is reduced to 6/60. Figure 146 shows the appearance of the right cornea.

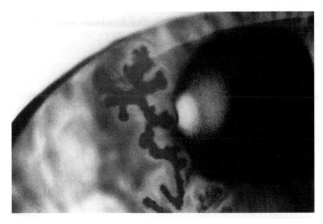

Fig. 146

b. What is the common stain used to highlight diseases of the surface of the cornea?
c. Describe the findings.
d. What is the likely diagnosis?
e. List three factors that increased the chances of this student developing a recurrent attack.
f. Describe the appropriate management for the problem.
g. What topical medication is contraindicated during an active infection?

Viva questions

1. Discuss viral conjunctivitis.

2. Discuss keratoconus.

Self-assessment: answers

Multiple choice answers

1. a. **False.** Vernal conjunctivitis may be complicated by keratitis, which is sight threatening.
   b. **False.** Purulent discharge is associated with infection, not allergy.
   c. **True.**
   d. **True.** This is the outstanding symptom.
   e. **True.** Topical steroids must only be used for short periods of time because of the risk of developing glaucoma and cataract, therefore systemic steroids and steroid-sparing agents may require to be used.

2. a. **False.** Topical steroids cause local suppression of the immune system, which leads to increased viral replication worsening the clinical appearance.
   b. **False.** Herpes simplex keratitis is associated with a watery discharge.
   c. **True.**
   d. **True.** Herpes simplex remains latent in the trigeminal ganglion where it may become reactivated.
   e. **True.** Herpes simplex infection can damage the local sensory nerve supply causing corneal surface paraesthesia.

EMI answers

1.

1. F   Herpes simplex virus characteristically causes a unilateral infection, unlike most other infective conjunctivitis conditions, which tend to be bilateral. Photophobia rather than itch is the predominant symptom and therefore infective keratitis is more likely than an allergic conjunctivitis. The characteristic corneal epithelial defect is dendritic shaped.
2. B   Adenoviral conjunctivitis and keratitis is characteristically bilateral. Local lymph nodes are often swollen and the patient may have a systemic illness with a sore throat and flu-like illness. Most other infective causes of a conjunctivitis do not cause a systemic illness.
3. H   Trachoma is a bilateral condition seen in children and adults in developing countries in areas of poor sanitation. The infective organism is *Chlamydia trachomatis*. It characteristically causes a bilateral conjunctivitis which with time

becomes scarring causing the eyelids to turn inwards. The rubbing of the eyelashes on the cornea leads to abrasions, infection and scarring of the cornea with associated loss of vision. This is second only to cataract in the world's leading causes of visual loss.

2.

1. F   Topical chlortetracycline is useful as an initial treatment in a conjunctivitis that is suspected of being the result of sexually transmitted chlamydia. Once the diagnosis is confirmed then referral to genito-urinary medicine (GUM) is required and systemic treatment is then required to treat any associated GU infection. Erythromycin is used systemically in neonatal chlamydia conjunctivitis as tetracycline stains growing teeth.
2. I   Scleritis is a type III mediated hypersensitivity response where immune complex deposition occurs. Topical and systemic steroids are often prescribed.
3. A   Acyclovir is the treatment of choice in active herpes simplex keratitis. Steroids are contraindicated as they prolong the episode and can cause local ocular side effects including raised intraocular pressure and the development of cataract.

CRQ answers

CRQ 1

a. The child is only 14 days old. Any conjunctivitis occurring within the first month of life is by definition a 'neonatal' conjunctivitis (ophthalmia neonatum).
b. The infection is usually caused by either infective agents from the mother's birth canal or from the environment. Infective agents include: chlamydia, gonococcus, herpes simplex and staphylococci.
c. Conjunctival swabs.
d. Appropriate topical antibiotics are prescribed based on the aetiology suggested by the history and clinical examination. Once the results of microbiology investigations are available, treatment can be altered and tailored to sensitivities of the causative organism. If chlamydia is confirmed systemic treatment with erythromycin is required and the child should be seen by a paediatrician because of the risk of pneumonitis. If chlamydia or

any other sexually transmitted organism is identified then the mother must be referred to the genito-urinary clinic for investigation, treatment and contact tracing.

CRQ 2

a. The likely diagnosis is bacterial keratitis because there is a purulent discharge, an epithelial defect with associated opacified cornea and a hypopyon.

b. The major predisposing factor is soft contact lens wear, which may cause a corneal abrasion and introduce infection. Other potentially predisposing factors include:

- lid abnormalities (entropion, ectropion, lid retraction)
- dry eye
- trauma (corneal abrasion)
- corneal paraesthesia
- immunocompromised host.

c. The patient should be admitted for intensive antibiotic drops. Conjunctival swabs and scrapings of the ulcer should be examined microscopically and cultured for organisms.

d. Corneal scarring with loss of vision and corneal perforation with endophthalmitis and loss of the eye.

OSCE answers

OSCE 1

a. Questions in taking a history from patients with a red eye revolve around:
1. discharge   – sticky; bacterial conjunctivitis (occasionally bacterial corneal ulcer)
   – watery or stringy; viral or allergic conjunctivitis
2. discomfort – gritty; bacterial or viral conjunctivitis
   – itchy; allergic conjunctivitis
3. pain or ache – uveitis, scleritis, acute angle closure glaucoma, corneal ulcers
4. vision   – normal conjunctivitis, decreased a little in uveitis and scleritis, very reduced in others
5. general and ocular previous medical history.

b. It is important to consider characteristic signs of certain red eye conditions such as (see Table 1, p. 236):
- unilateral/bilateral

- zone of infection – diffuse: conjunctivitis, scleritis, glaucoma
  – sectional: episcleritis, corneal ulcer
  – circumcorneal: uveitis
- pupil   – normal size and reactions
  – small
  – mid dilated
- measure vision – use pinhole if necessary.

c. Scleritis.

d. Topical and systemic steroids and other steroid-sparing immunosuppressive drugs.

e. Immunosuppression with increased risk of infection and reactivation of TB, hypertension, diabetes, osteoporosis, peptic ulceration, psychosis.

OSCE 2

a. Is the vision affected?
Is this the first episode?
Is there a discharge and what is the nature of the discharge?
Does she have any intercurrent illnesses?

b. Fluorescein drops help to identify any epithelial defects.

c. Dendritic-shaped epithelial defect in the centre of the cornea.

d. Herpes simplex keratitis.

e. Sunlight (from Ibiza), tiredness (from being up all night dancing or travelling), and stress (from travelling and imminent examinations).

f. Topical acyclovir ointment treats active herpes simplex infection.

g. Topical steroids are contraindicated during active herpes simplex infection as they prolong the course and have potentially serious ocular side effects of increasing intraocular pressure and the development of cataract.

Viva answers

1. Many different viruses can cause a conjunctivitis often also associated with a keratitis. Organisms include: adenovirus, herpes simplex and molluscum contagiosum. Adenoviral infection may be preceded by upper respiratory tract infection and fever, especially in children. Complications include keratitis and secondary bacterial conjunctivitis. The keratitis takes the form of punctate lesions over the entire cornea, which slowly resolve. Treatment is symptomatic.
Herpes simplex is characteristically unilateral and recurrent always in the same eye. An acute dendritic ulcer may form, which if untreated or poorly

managed by instilling steroids may become a larger confluent 'geographical' ulcer. Scarring can often occur as a chronic complication leading to visual loss. Topical acyclovir is the treatment of choice.

2. Keratoconus is characterised by a gradual thinning and bowing forward of the cornea leading to it developing a conical shape. The abnormal shape does not focus light on to the retina correctly and therefore the vision is reduced. Although the cause is unknown, it is more common in atopic patients and patients with Down's syndrome. Patients often present in late childhood and early adult life with blurring of vision that gradually worsens. Initially spectacles and contact lenses improve the vision, but as the astigmatism worsens and becomes more irregular, the vision cannot be corrected. Eventually a corneal graft may be necessary for visual rehabilitation, especially if the cornea has become scarred, but this is unusual.

18 The optics of the eye

Chapter overview

This chapter discusses the normal optical state of the eye as well as the common abnormal optical states including myopia, hypermetropia, astigmatism, presbyopia and cataract.

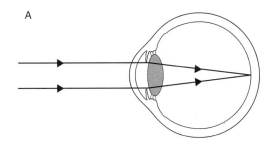

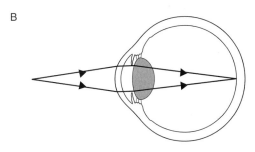

Fig. 147 A. Normal eye. Emmetropia. **B.** Accommodation. The lens becomes thicker and more curved to increase its power, which allows focus on a near object.

18.1 Physiology of the optics of the eye

The eye has two main focusing elements. The first and most powerful focusing surface is the static cornea. The second and less powerful focusing element is the dynamic lens. Although the lens is less powerful than the cornea it is importantly different as it can vary its focusing power to allow near as well as distant objects to be brought into focus on the retina. This process is known as accommodation (Fig. 147).

The lens is a biconvex structure situated immediately behind the iris. It consists of a central nucleus surrounded by a peripheral cortex contained within a transparent membrane, the lens capsule. The lens is held in place by the lens zonules. The lens zonules are attached to the encircling ciliary muscle. When the ciliary muscle contracts and shortens, the zonules become lax and the lens assumes a more rounded shape with a reduced diameter and increased thickness with higher focusing power. This is the situation when the eye is accommodating. When the ciliary

muscle is relaxed it has a larger diameter which pulls on the zonules stretching the lens to have a greater diameter, reduced thickness and a less curved overall shape with reduced focusing power. With age the power of the ciliary muscle and the intrinsic elasticity of the lens reduce so the power of accommodation lessens. This becomes clinically significant in most individuals by the fifth decade when spectacles are required to observe near objects. This is known as presbyopia.

If parallel light from a distant object on entering a 'relaxed' non-accommodating eye focuses directly onto the retina, the eye is considered to be physiologically normal or emmetropic. If the light comes to a focus short of the retina then the eye is considered short-sighted or myopic and if the light focuses behind the retina it is considered long-sighted or hypermetropic. Occasionally an eye can have different focusing powers at different axes of the eye. If this occurs then the light is focused to many different plains and the image is always perceived as a blur. This is known as astigmatism.

18.2 Disorders of refraction

Learning objectives

You should:

- appreciate the different types of refractive error

- understand the anatomical reasons for refractive errors

- know the ocular diseases associated with the different types of refractive error

- appreciate how refractive errors are corrected to improve visual acuity.

Myopia (short sight)

In myopia, the globe is bigger and therefore the eye is from front to back relatively longer than normal. As a consequence the image of a distant object is brought to focus in front of the retina and a blurred image is formed at the retina. Distance vision is therefore reduced but can be corrected by using a concave (diverging) spectacle lens. These individuals have good near vision, hence the term short sight (see Fig. 148). Because the globe is abnormally big compared with the normal-sized retina, tension is created at the periphery of the retina where it attaches to the globe. This area of the retina is prone to developing tears and holes, which may lead to retinal detachment. Individuals with myopia are consequently more prone to spontaneous and traumatic retinal detachment.

Hypermetropia (long sight)

In hypermetropia, the globe is smaller and the eye is relatively shorter than normal from front to back. As a consequence the image of a distant object is theoretically brought to a focus behind the plane of the retina and a blurred image is formed on the retina. A convex (converging) lens will correct this. If the degree of hypermetropia is not great, then this may be achieved by accommodation, so that most young people with mild hypermetropia have good distance vision, even without glasses (Fig. 149). Because the eye is smaller, the structures in the anterior part of the eye tend to be 'anatomically crowded', which increases the chance of developing closed-angle glaucoma especially if the pupil is dilated.

Astigmatism

Regular astigmatism

The refractive power of the cornea is dependent upon its curvature. In astigmatism, the corneal curvature is not uniform, making it impossible to bring an image into sharp focus on the retina. An astigmatic cornea can be considered to be more the shape of a rugby ball than a football (normal), being more curved in one axis than another. An astigmatic spectacle lens can neutralise the differences in corneal curvature bringing a single sharp image to be focused on the retina.

Irregular astigmatism

If the cornea has a very uneven surface because of corneal scarring or keratoconus then even an astigmatic lens cannot fully neutralise the astigmatism and form a

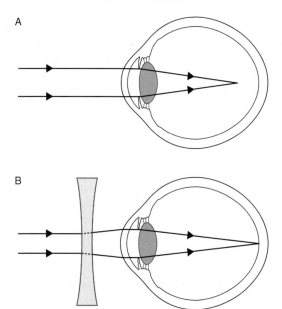

Fig. 148 A. Myopia. **B.** Corrective lens for myopia.

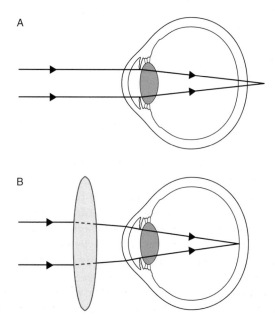

Fig. 149 A. Hypermetropia. **B.** Corrective lens for hypermetropia.

focused image on the retina. This is known as irregular astigmatism.

Presbyopia

Accommodation for near work is dependent upon the plasticity of the lens and the power of the ciliary muscle. With increasing age, the lens becomes more rigid and it cannot assume the more rounded and thicker shape associated with higher focusing power. The ciliary muscle also weakens and the combination of these effects leads to a reduced ability to increase the focusing power of the eye for near. By the fifth decade most individuals will begin to hold reading material progressively further away. This is a normal process termed presbyopia. Reading glasses are required in order to focus on a near object.

Neutralising refractive errors

A simple method of determining whether reduced vision is caused by a refractive error or not is to demonstrate that the acuity improves with the use of a pinhole. The patient observes a Snellen chart through a tiny aperture (the pin-hole) made in a piece of card. The pinhole only allows a narrow pencil of light to enter the eye. The narrow shaft of light is not altered by the refractive surfaces of the eye and consequently passes on through to the retina unaltered and in focus. If the visual acuity is better with the use of the pin-hole compared with the unaided vision then refractive error accounts for the difference. If the vision does not improve then the reduced vision is likely to be due to media opacities, retinal or optic nerve disease or central neurological disease such as stroke.

Formal testing for spectacles, or 'refraction', requires a more complex assessment and is carried out by an optometrist or ophthalmologist.

Treatment of refractive disorders
There are a number of methods used in treating refractive errors:

- spectacle correction is the traditional method of improving vision
- contact lenses are preferred by some patients; the previously popular hard lenses have been replaced with rigid lenses (gas permeable) or soft lenses
- refractive surgery: there are several methods available to alter the intrinsic refractive power of the eye. Some procedures are irreversible (EXCIMER laser surgery) while others are reversible (intrastromal rings). Refractive surgery is generally more suited to reducing the refractive power of the cornea and therefore in treating myopia rather than

hypermetropia. In cases of extreme myopia clear lens extraction can be combined with laser surgery.

18.3 Disorders of the lens

Learning objectives

You should:

- appreciate what a cataract is
- understand the causes of cataract
- know the common symptoms of a cataract
- understand the management of age-related and congenital cataracts
- appreciate the potential complications of cataract surgery.

Cataract

Cataract is the presence of opacity in the lens. It is only considered clinically relevant if the patient has symptoms from the opacity. This is the most common cause of treatable visual impairment worldwide. Opacification of the lens commonly forms in three distinct portions. An opacity in the central portion of the lens is termed nuclear sclerosis: this is the most common form of age-related lens opacity. Cataract in the periphery of the lens has a radial spoke-like pattern and is called cortical cataract. An opacity at the posterior aspect of the lens is called a posterior subcapsular cataract; this type of cataract can be particularly visually disabling causing early loss of reading vision and glare in bright lights.

Most cataracts are the consequence of ageing. There is some evidence that increased exposure to ultraviolet light, dehydration and low dietary antioxidant intake can increase the rate of cataract development. A minority of cataracts develop secondary to specific problems:

- ocular trauma
- ocular disease e.g. uveitis
- metabolic disorders: diabetes is the most common with galactosaemia and hypercalcaemia being very rare
- drugs: notably prolonged use of systemic steroids
- congenital and hereditary cataract.

Clinical features
Patients with cataract can have a variety of symptoms such as:

- no symptoms (an incidental finding), which is very common
- reduced visual acuity leading to difficulty with
  — reading the newspaper

— reading prices of items in shops
— watching the television
— recognising faces in the street
— mobility
— reading signs
● glare
— in daylight
— in low sunlight
— from car headlights
● monocular diplopia

The lens opacity can be noted on ophthalmoscopy as a disturbance of the red reflex. If the lens opacity is very advanced the pupil can appear white on macroscopic examination. This is known as 'leucocoria'.

Management
The only definitive means of dealing with cataract is surgical removal of the opacified lens. Surgery should be considered when the vision is reduced to the point where the patient is having problems with activities of daily living because of poor vision. This does not represent any consistent critical level of Snellen acuity and can be very different from patient to patient. The risks and benefits of surgery must be explained to the patient in language they understand. The patient must then decide for themselves whether to proceed. Most operations are performed under local anaesthetic by infiltrating anaesthetic around the globe. The pupil is widely dilated to allow access to the lens. Cataract extraction is the most common operation performed worldwide. Methods of cataract extraction include:

● intracapsular cataract extraction (ICCE)
● extracapsular cataract extraction (ECCE)
● phaco-emulsification (a modified type of ECCE).

Intracapsular extraction. The lens is removed intact, i.e. the lens capsule and its contents are extracted in entirety. Because the lens has been removed and not replaced, this leads to profound blurring of vision, which requires correction with very strong spectacle lenses. Because of their thickness, the strong spectacles are associated with many optical aberrations, which commonly results in spectacle intolerance. Contact lenses do not cause these optical problems but are inconvenient to use, particularly in the elderly. This technique is rarely employed in the UK today but is a rapid, inexpensive method and is commonly used to remove cataracts in developing countries.

Extracapsular extraction. This involves removal of the lens nucleus and cortex from within the capsule, leaving the capsule intact (except for a hole in the anterior surface that is used to remove the contents). This is less disrupting for the eye than ICCE. The major advantage of this technique is that the remaining capsule can

be used to hold a replacement, artificial, plastic intraocular lens, which is permanently implanted into the eye at the time of surgery (Figs 150 and 151). These lenses are available in different refractive powers, and the power of the implant is determined preoperatively to give the patient clear vision for distance. Spectacles are usually still required for reading and near work.

Phaco-emulsification. A small incision is made close to the limbus of the eye and a round tear in the anterior capsule of the lens is made. The lens is fragmented and sucked out of the eye by a sharp, oscillating, hollow tip known as a phaco-emulsification probe. A small, often foldable, lens is inserted via the incision and placed within the capsule bag upon the posterior capsule. The incision wound is normally self-sealing and does not require any sutures (Fig. 152). This technique allows rapid patient visual rehabilitation.

Postoperative care. Topical steroids and antibiotics are prescribed routinely for a short period after cataract surgery to prevent infection and reduce inflammation.

Complications of cataracts
A longstanding cataract can with time become white and swollen. This is known as a 'mature' cataract. The

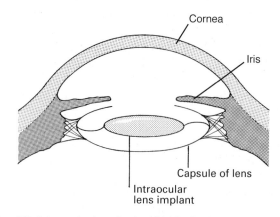

Fig. 150 Intraocular lens implant inside the lens capsule at the end of an operation.

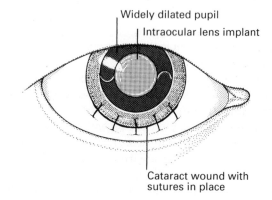

Fig. 151 Surgeon's view (upside down) of an extracapsular operation at the end of surgery.

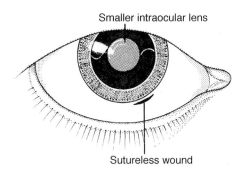

Smaller intraocular lens

Sutureless wound

Fig. 152 The surgeon's view (upside down) of phaco-emulsification at the end of surgery. Note the small wound and intraocular lens.

swollen cataract can lead to anterior uveitis and raised intraocular pressure. The only definitive treatment of these complications is to remove the cataract.

Complications of cataract surgery
Cataract extraction surgery is generally a successful procedure.
  Common complications include:

- astigmatism induced by the wound incision
- postoperative uveitis, which is usually mild and settles with topical steroids
- cystoid macular oedema: an accumulation of fluid within the retina, which can lead to reduced visual acuity. This normally settles spontaneously after a few months.
- opacification of the posterior capsule which holds the lens: this is more common in younger patients and can lead to blurred vision. It can be easily treated using a laser to disrupt and clear the opacified capsule.

  Rare complications:

- intraocular infection (endophthalmitis): the infection is usually acquired at the time of surgery. If diagnosed early and treated appropriately then useful vision may be maintained, but otherwise this is a devastating complication with poor visual outcome.
- retinal detachment: if this is diagnosed early and treated appropriately with laser or surgery then good vision can be preserved.
- corneal decompensation: if the number of endothelial cells which line the cornea become reduced they may no longer be capable of maintaining the clarity of the cornea. The cornea

becomes hazy and is considered to have decompensated. Definitive treatment is by surgically replacing the opacified cornea with clear donor material. This is called a penetrating keratoplasty.
- choroidal haemorrhage: this is a very rare intraoperative complication more common in elderly hypertensive patients. It can lead to devastating effects on vision. Small incision cataract surgery protects from some of the complications of this most feared of problems.

Congenital cataract

Congenital cataracts are a rare but important cause of visual impairment in childhood. They can cause highly variable effects on vision. They usually affect both eyes but may be very asymmetrical.
  Causes include:

- idiopathic (> 50% of patients)
- familial congenital cataract syndromes
- intrauterine rubella infection
- inborn errors of metabolism: galactosaemia is the most common
- chromosomal abnormalities such as Down's syndrome

Clinical features
All infants should be screened routinely at birth for the presence of lens opacities by observing the red reflex of each eye with a direct ophthalmoscope. Screening is important to start early treatment and reduce the chance of developing amblyopia. In a child with a dense lens opacity the diagnosis can be made more easily as the pupil appears white (leucocoria).

Management
The treatment of paediatric cataract is challenging. A balance is sought between conservative (optical aids) and surgical (cataract extraction) interventions while maximising the long-term potential vision of the eye. In practice a combination of both optical and surgical interventions are employed. All children with cataract must be referred to an ophthalmologist urgently.

If the cataract is very dense and clearly causing gross visual impairment and likely to induce a lazy eye (amblyopia) then surgical removal is indicated.

If the lens opacity is only partial then the management may include prescribing spectacles and monitoring the child's visual acuity.

Self-assessment: questions

Multiple choice questions

1. Cataracts:
   a. Are more common in diabetics
   b. May be treated by drugs
   c. Are a cause of ocular pain
   d. Cause sudden loss of vision
   e. That are drug induced are often caused by systemic steroids

2. Which of the following are complications of cataract surgery:
   a. Retinal detachment
   b. Retinal vein occlusion
   c. Infection
   d. Uveitis
   e. Astigmatism

Extended matching items questions (EMIs)

1. Theme: Treatments

A myopia
B dense congenital cataract with poor vision
C hypermetropia
D regular astigmatism
E mild congenital cataract with good vision
F age-related nuclear sclerotic cataract
G age-related posterior subcapsular cataract
H presbyopia
I irregular astigmatism
J keratoconus

For the treatments listed below select the most appropriate diagnosis from the above:

1. This condition can be corrected by prescribing a convex, converging 'plus' lens.
2. This condition can be corrected by prescribing a concave, diverging 'minus' lens.
3. This condition needs urgent surgery to avoid deprivational amblyopia.

2. Theme: Symptoms

A myopia
B dense congenital cataract with poor vision
C hypermetropia
D regular astigmatism
E mild congenital cataract with good vision
F age-related nuclear sclerotic cataract
G age-related posterior subcapsular cataract
H presbyopia
I irregular astigmatism
J keratoconus

For the symptoms listed below select the most appropriate diagnosis from the above:

1. This condition may present in childhood with blurred vision for near but clear for distance.
2. This condition causes vision to be clear for near but blurred for distance.
3. This condition commonly presents in the fifth decade of life with difficulty reading the newspaper.

Constructed response questions (CRQs)

CRQ 1

> A 67-year-old man is referred to the eye clinic because his optometrist has noted reduced visual acuities in both eyes of 6/12 uncorrected. The vision does not improve with a new prescription or a pin-hole.

a. What is the most likely diagnosis?
b. Discuss other possible diagnoses (information from other sections is required to answer this question).
c. What kind of symptoms is the patient likely to complain of?

After a full examination a diagnosis of cataracts in both eyes is made.

d. Briefly describe the operation of phaco-emulsification cataract extraction and lens implantation.

The patient does not complain of any significant visual symptoms despite the reduced visual acuities.

e. Should this man proceed with cataract extraction?

CRQ 2

> A 36-year-old woman complains of increasingly blurred vision when reading the newspaper. The television still appears clear and she has no problems reading street signs. Using a pin-hole she can read small print clearly. Her mother recently suffered an attack of closed-angle glaucoma.

a. What refractive problems might this patient be suffering from?
b. Is she likely to have relatively small or relatively large eyes?
c. What type of spectacle correction would improve her symptoms?
d. In 30 years' time what further problems might she complain of?

Objective structured clinical examination questions (OSCEs)

OSCE 1

> A 2-week-old boy is referred with an abnormal red reflex on ophthalmoscopy.

a. What is the most likely diagnosis?

> On examination there is a central dense opacity seen in both lenses (Fig. 153). The child does not seem to be able to 'fix and follow' on the mother's face.

b. What is the recommended management?

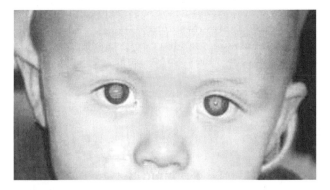

Fig. 153

> The child undergoes bilateral cataract extraction and is fitted with contact lenses postoperatively.

c. What is the ophthalmologist attempting to prevent developing in this child?

> The child reaches the age of 10 but has become intolerant of contact lens wear.

d. What are the management options now?
e. What are the ocular risks associated with cataract surgery?

OSCE 2

> A 69-year-old woman presents to Accident and Emergency complaining of a painful red right eye with profoundly reduced visual acuity. She had undergone uncomplicated cataract extraction in the symptomatic eye 5 days previously.

a. List some of the postoperative complications of cataract surgery.

> Figure 154 shows the appearance of the eye on presentation.

b. Describe the main abnormality seen in the anterior chamber.

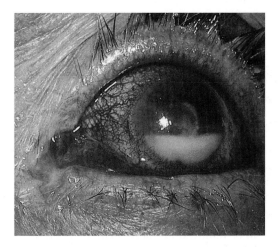

Fig. 154

> The red reflex is absent and the visual acuity is only perception of light.

c. In your opinion what complication has this patient developed?
d. How should her management proceed?

Viva questions

1. Regarding myopia describe the symptoms, cause and type of lenses that correct the vision. State the ocular conditions that are characteristically associated with myopia.

2. Regarding hypermetropia describe the symptoms, cause and type of lenses that correct the vision. State the ocular conditions that are characteristically associated with hypermetropia.

Self-assessment: answers

Multiple choice answers

1. a. **True.** Patients suffering from diabetes are prone to early cataract development.
   b. **False.** Surgery is the only effective method.
   c. **False.** Cataract does not cause pain in the eye.
   d. **False.** Cataract causes a gradual loss of vision.
   e. **True.** Prolonged use of systemic steroids can lead to early cataract development.

2. a. **True.** A rare complication.
   b. **False.** Cataract surgery does not normally cause retinal vein occlusion.
   c. **True.** A rare complication.
   d. **True.** This is usually mild.
   e. **True.** Astigmatism maybe induced by the wound incision.

EMI answers

1. Theme: Treatments

1. C   Hypermetropic eyes are relatively small. Light focuses posterior to the retinal plane. A converging, convex, 'plus' lens is required.
2. A   Myopic eyes are relatively large. Light focuses anterior to the retinal plane. A diverging, concave, 'minus' lens is required.
3. B   Visually impairing congenital cataract requires to be removed promptly to avoid deprivational amblyopia. If the child sees well despite the congenital cataract it does not require to be removed for its own sake.

2. Theme: Symptoms

1. C   These are the symptoms of hypermetropia also known as long sight.
2. A   These are the symptoms of myopia also known as short sight.
3. H   As ageing changes occur in the lens and the accommodative apparatus, the ability to focus for near reduces until commonly in the fifth decade near vision becomes blurred. This is known as presbyopia.

CRQ answers

CRQ 1

a. The most common cause of gradual deterioration of vision in this age group is cataract.

b. Other possible causes for these symptoms in a gentleman of this age include age-related macular degeneration and primary open-angle glaucoma that has advanced to a late stage.
c. He may complain of difficulty reading the newspaper and price tags in shops, watching television, navigating in the home and outside, recognising faces, and glare in bright lights.
d. The pupil is fully dilated. Local anaesthetic is infiltrated around the globe. A small incision is made close to the limbus of the eye and a round tear in the anterior capsule of the eye lens is made. The lens is fragmented and sucked out of the eye by a phaco-emulsification probe. A new lens is placed within the capsule bag upon the posterior capsule. The incision wound is normally self-sealing and does not require any sutures.
e. If the patient does not have any visually impairing symptoms then the cataract extraction is not necessary. The cataract itself will not harm the eye and does not need removal for its own sake with the associated risks of surgical intervention.

CRQ 2

a. Hypermetropia and early presbyopia. She is having difficulty seeing at short distance but can see clearly at long distance: she is therefore long-sighted (hypermetropic). She may have presented at this age because she is losing the ability to accommodate (presbyopia), which is 'unmasking' her hypermetropia. She also appears to have a family history of hypermetropia.
b. Hypermetropia is associated with relatively small eyes with anatomically crowded anterior segment structures.
c. Spectacles with convex (plus lenses) to converge the light to focus on the back of her eye.
d. Theoretically she has an increased risk of developing acute closed-angle glaucoma as hypermetropia is a risk factor for this condition. She may also develop any of the other common visually impairing age-related eye conditions such as cataract or age-related macular degeneration.

OSCE answers

OSCE 1

a. Congenital cataract.

b. Cataract extraction without intraocular lens implantation and contact lens placement postoperatively.

c. Deprivational amblyopia.

d. Spectacles or further surgery with placement of an intraocular lens.

e. Astigmatism, cystoid macular oedema, uveitis, posterior capsule opacification, endophthalmitis, retinal detachment, choroidal haemorrhage and corneal decompensation.

OSCE 2

a. Anterior uveitis, intraocular infection (endophthalmitis), cystoid macular oedema, opacification of the posterior capsule, retinal detachment, corneal decompensation.

b. A pale fluid level is seen in the anterior chamber. This represents a collection of inflammatory cells known as a hypopyon.

c. An intraocular infection known as endophthalmitis.

d. She should be referred as an emergency to the ophthalmology team.

Viva answers

1. Myopia means difficulty in seeing clearly for distance. Because the individual has a large eye, the light focuses short of the retina. A diverging (concave or minus) lens will focus the light on to the retina. Myopic eyes are prone to retinal detachment and an early form of macular degeneration.

2. Hypermetropia is defined as difficulty seeing clearly for near. Because the individual has a small eye, the light focuses behind plain of retina. A converging (convex or plus) lens will focus the light onto the retina. Hypermetropic eyes are prone to convergent squints and acute closed-angle glaucoma.

19 The uveal tract

Chapter overview

This chapter outlines the anatomy and function of the uveal tract as well as the common conditions that may affect it.

The most common disorder of the uveal tract is uveitis. The anatomical classification of uveitis and the associated symptoms and signs will be discussed.

The investigation and management plans for the different uveitis entities are explained.

Choroidal tumours are briefly discussed with emphasis on the diagnosis and management of choroidal malignant melanoma.

19.1 Uveitis

Learning objectives

You should:

- understand the anatomy of the uveal tract

- be able to classify the different uveitis entities

- appreciate the symptoms and signs of the different uveitis entities with special emphasis on anterior uveitis

- differentiate uveitis from the other causes of red eye by taking a history and performing an examination

- be able to manage anterior uveitis appropriately

- appreciate the complications of uveitis.

The uveal tract: structure and function

The uveal tract consists of three components from anterior to posterior.

- iris
- ciliary body
- choroid.

The iris is a diaphragm that contains a central opening (the pupil) which controls the amount of light entering the eye.

The ciliary body secretes aqueous humour and contains the ciliary muscle, which controls the focusing power of the lens.

The choroid is the highly vascular and deeply pigmented middle layer of the eye sandwiched between the inner retina and outer sclera.

Classification of uveitis

Inflammatory conditions of the uveal tract are referred to as 'uveitis'. Depending on the component of the uveal tract predominantly involved this can be classified into four main groups:

- *Anterior uveitis.* The iris is predominantly involved, commonly known as 'iritis'
- *Intermediate uveitis.* The ciliary body is predominantly involved
- *Posterior uveitis.* The choroid is predominantly involved, commonly known as 'choroiditis'
- *Pan-uveitis.* The whole uveal tract is inflamed.

Anterior uveitis (iritis)

Anterior uveitis is the most common of the four manifestations of uveitis. The other forms are fortunately rare as they can often have severe effects on visual function.

Clinical features
Anterior uveitis is usually unilateral. The patient has a photophobic, painful, watering, red eye with moderately reduced visual acuity. The presence of a sticky discharge or symptoms of itch and grittiness are not characteristic and instead would suggest a conjunctivitis.

Examination of the eye reveals diffuse redness that is most prominent around the limbus (junction of the

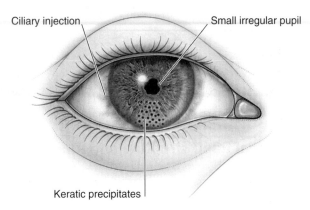

Ciliary injection   Small irregular pupil

Keratic precipitates

Fig. 155 Anterior uveitis.

cornea and sclera). This is also known as ciliary or circumcorneal injection. The pupil is usually small but may also be irregular because of adhesions between the anterior lens surface and the pupil margin (posterior synechia) (Fig. 155).

Slit lamp examination is helpful in making the diagnosis as this reveals flare (proteinaceous exudates) and cells (immune cells) in the anterior chamber which have leaked from the dilated swollen iris blood vessels.

A complete, detailed examination of the eye including the posterior segment is necessary to reveal any associated ocular cause for the condition.

Diagnosis and investigation

The diagnosis is clinical, based on identifying characteristic eye signs.

A structured history aimed at identifying the known systemic disease associations or ocular causes is most useful. If an underlying systemic association is suggested by the history then investigations can be tailored to this and an appropriate specialist referral made. An underlying systemic association is more commonly found if the condition is bilateral, chronic or both.

Systemic associations include:

- ankylosing spondylitis
- inflammatory bowel disease (both Crohn's and ulcerative colitis)
- sarcoidosis
- Reiter's syndrome
- Behçet's syndrome
- psoriatic arthropathy
- juvenile idiopathic arthritis
- tuberculosis
- syphilis

Ocular associations include:

- postoperative uveitis (e.g. following cataract surgery)
- blunt trauma to the eye
- retinal detachment
- corneal ulcer

In the majority of cases of unilateral acute anterior uveitis no cause can be identified and they are therefore considered idiopathic.

Management

Intensive topical steroid drops reduce the inflammation. Most patients require a 4–8-week reducing regimen. Cycloplegic drops such as cyclopentolate and atropine aid in relieving the prominent symptom of photophobia. Dilating the pupil also breaks pre-existing posterior synechiae and reduces the formation of new adhesions. Analgesia and dark glasses may help symptomatically.

If the condition becomes chronic and is resistant to topical treatment then local depot injection of steroids can be used as well as systemic steroid treatment.

Complications

Acute unilateral anterior uveitis is generally an uncomplicated condition compared with the other forms of uveitis. Complications, if they do occur, can be due to the condition itself or to the side effects of the treatment prescribed and are more common if the condition becomes chronic.

Complications include:

- Raised intraocular pressure
  The rise in pressure can also be due to the uveitis itself causing compromise to the drainage angle. Approximately one-third of the general population may respond to topical and systemic steroids by raising intraocular pressure. The pressure usually returns to the normal range when the inflammation settles and steroids are discontinued.
- Cataract formation
  Chronic steroid use, given either systemically or topically, can lead to early lens opacity formation.
- Cystoid macular oedema
  Fluid collection within the macular area can lead to central loss of vision.
- Corneal band keratopathy
  Chronic ocular inflammation can lead to the development of calcium deposition on the cornea.

Posterior uveitis (choroiditis)

This condition is rare, but can cause significant visual impairment. Choroiditis can manifest itself in a variety of ways owing to the broad spectrum of possible aetiologies. A thorough discussion of this subject is beyond the scope of this book; however a brief outline follows.

Clinical features

The patient usually presents with visual impairment. This can be acute or chronic. The symptoms can vary from mild peripheral flashing lights and floaters to dense central loss of vision. The eye can appear white and comfortable or be painful, photophobic and red.

Choroiditis can overlap with the other uveitis entities and can often involve the retina and overlying blood vessels as well. The vitreous may demonstrate inflammatory cells and dense 'floaters'. The fundus may show areas of focal or diffuse white infiltrates. The view of the fundus may be poor due to the inflammatory cells in the vitreous.

Diagnosis and investigation

The causes of choroiditis fall into two main groups:

- Infective
  — toxoplasma
  — tuberculosis
  — syphilis
  — toxocara
- Inflammatory
  — sarcoidosis
  — Behçet's syndrome
  — Wegner's granulomatosis
  — systemic lupus erythematosus
  — multiple sclerosis
  — juvenile idiopathic arthritis
  — specific ocular inflammatory syndromes

Core investigations include:

- full blood count and plasma viscosity
- chest X-ray
- urinalysis
- syphilis serology

Other more specific investigations should be dictated by the history, and ocular and systemic clinical findings. Despite investigation, in approximately half of cases a cause will still not be identified.

Management

Management is dependent on the assumed cause and whether the condition appears to be sight threatening or not. Generally non-sight-threatening disease is simply observed. Treatment is only instigated if it worsens and becomes sight threatening. If an infective cause is identified then appropriate antimicrobials should be commenced. If the aetiology appears to be immune then immunosuppressive agents are prescribed. Anti-inflammatory treatment can range from local depot injections of steroid to systemic steroid and steroid-sparing agents such as cyclosporin. Immunosuppressive drugs have side effects such as hypertension and renal toxicity. These effects should be monitored carefully during therapy.

Complications

Complications are the same as for anterior uveitis, but also include:

- profound irreversible loss of vision
- systemic side effects from treatment
- systemic effects of underlying disease.

Intermediate uveitis

Intermediate uveitis represents a uveitis syndrome where inflammation of the ciliary body is predominant. The patients are often in their 3rd or 4th decade of life and present with floaters and visual disturbance. The peripheral fundus appears inflamed with characteristic 'snow banking' of inflammatory cells inferiorly.

The systemic associations are similar to the list of posterior uveitis inflammatory aetiologies but with multiple sclerosis being more common.

The investigation and management is also similar. Visual loss can occur due to macular oedema.

Pan-uveitis

Pan-uveitis is a rare condition with a poor visual outcome where the whole uveal tract is chronically inflammed. The classic pan-uveitis syndrome is sympathetic ophthalmia. This is a condition precipitated by a penetrating injury to one eye that incites a uveitis in the other healthy or 'sympathising' eye. Sympathetic ophthalmia can present at any time after an injury and requires similar management to inflammatory posterior uveitis.

19.2 Choroidal tumours

Learning objectives

You should:

- appreciate that different types of tumours can affect the choroid

- know how choroidal tumours might present

- understand how a diagnosis is made

- be able to describe in broad terms the management of a malignant melanoma

- appreciate the significance of the diagnosis for the patient.

Choroidal malignant melanoma

This is the most common primary intraocular tumour. Secondaries from breast and lung tumours commonly metastasise to the choroid, but these frequently remain undiagnosed as they are usually asymptomatic occurring in the later terminal stages of the disease.

Choroidal malignant melanoma may occur in any age group but becomes more common with increasing age. These tumours often remain quiescent for long periods but may suddenly undergo a period of rapid growth. They arise from the melanocytes of the choroid.

Clinical features

The patient may present with visual disturbance due to the melanoma itself, or an associated retinal detachment or vitreous haemorrhage. Often however the patient is asymptomatic and the lesion is noted during a routine optometry consultation.

On fundal examination a round or oval, smooth-bordered mass can be seen. The colour can be highly variable, sometimes appearing dark brown but can be pale and 'amelanotic'. An associated retinal detachment may be present.

Diagnosis

A diagnosis can usually be made on the basis of clinical examination and the characteristic findings on ocular ultrasound.

Management

Management depends upon

- the size of the lesion
- the position within the fundus
- any evidence of extension beyond the globe
- the health of the fellow eye
- the age of the patient.

Treatment options range from observation with regular follow up including serial clinical photographs and ultrasound measurements in small tumours to removal of the eye in larger tumours. Many treatment modalities are in use to preserve the globe and useful vision. These include local resection, cryotherapy, laser treatment, radiotherapy and systemic chemotherapy. The choice of treatment must be fully discussed with the patient to allow him or her to take part in the decision-making process.

Complications

- loss of the eye
- metastatic disease, especially to the liver and lungs.

Self-assessment: questions

Multiple choice questions

1. Choroidal malignant melanoma:
   a. on fundoscopy often appears clinically as a raised pigmented lesion
   b. may present as visual disturbance
   c. tends to metastasise to the liver
   d. can be diagnosied with the aid of an ultrasound examination
   e. always requires extensive surgical excision

2. Anterior uveitis:
   a. usually has a well-defined aetiology
   b. is usually painful
   c. commonly affects one eye
   d. is associated with systemic toxoplasmosis
   e. affects children with juvenile idiopathic arthritis

Extended matching items questions (EMIs)

1. Theme: The uvea

A photophobic, watering, red eye with limbal injection and mildly reduced visual acuity
B sectorial injection of one eye with a deep 'aching' pain
C sticky, gritty red eye with purulent discharge
D painful complete uniocular loss of vision with associated nausea
E A gritty red eye with localised peripheral corneal opacification
F asymptomatic
G floaters and reduced visual acuity with vitreous inflammation and multiple pale retinal patches
H itchy red eye with swollen lids
I painless uniocular sectorial injection of the conjunctiva with no visual disturbance
J painless loss of vision with diffuse flame-shaped retinal haemorrhages and tortuous veins

From the symptoms and signs listed above choose the most appropriate diagnosis from below:

1. Choroidal malignant melanoma.
2. Anterior uveitis.
3. Posterior uveitis.

2. Theme: The uvea

A herpes simplex conjunctivitis
B non-infective, idiopathic, sight-threatening posterior uveitis

C active but non-sight-threatening toxoplasmosis
D anterior uveitis
E adenoviral conjunctivitis
F subconjunctival haemorrhage
G episcleritis
H choroidal malignant melanoma
I Fuch's heterochromic cyclitis
J bacterial conjunctivitis

From the diagnoses listed above select the most appropriate management from below:

1. Topical steroids, dilating drops (such as cyclopentolate), analgesia and dark glasses.
2. Systemic immunosuppression.
3. Radiotherapy.

Constructed response questions (CRQs)

CRQ 1

A 35-year-old male presents with a red right eye. He complains of the vision being reduced with associated photophobia for the last 24 hours. There is no history of trauma and no stickiness or discharge. He has a past medical history of ankylosing spondylitis. Examination reveals a red eye with ciliary injection. The pupil is miosed. There is no corneal staining with fluorescein.

a. What is the most likely diagnosis?
b. What is the treatment?
c. Discuss the differential diagnosis (information from other sections is required to answer this question).

CRQ 2

A 76-year-old female is referred to the eye department by her optometrist because a large 'grey' raised mass was noted on a routine fundal examination. Her vision is unaffected. She has had a poor appetite recently and has lost 2 stone in weight over the past 6 months.

a. What is the differential diagnosis?
b. How might a lesion like this normally present?
c. What might explain this woman's poor appetite and weight loss?

Objective structured clinical examination questions (OSCEs)

OSCE 1

An 82-year-old woman presented to the eye department complaining of visual disturbance. She was aware of a 'shadow' in her temporal field. Figure 156 is a photograph of the retina of her symptomatic left eye.

a. Describe the findings seen in this photograph.
b. Describe an appropriate differential diagnosis.
c. What test would help to make a diagnosis?

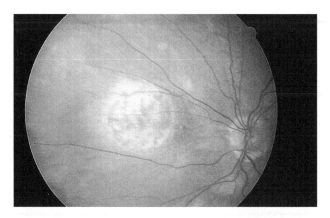

Fig. 156

OSCE 2

A 23-year-old man presented with a 2-day history of a red photophobic right eye. There was a watery discharge. The vision was 6/12. Figure 157 shows his symptomatic eye.

a. Describe the findings seen in the photograph.
b. What is the likely diagnosis?
c. What are the common systemic associations of this condition?
d. Describe the appropriate management of this condition.

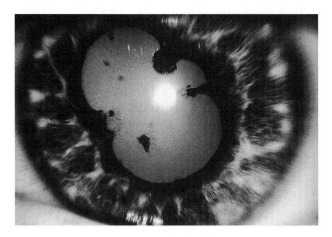

Fig. 157

Viva questions

1. Discuss the aetiology and investigation of posterior uveitis.

2. Describe the classification of uveitis and the structure that is predominantly inflamed in each group.

Self-assessment: answers

Multiple choice answers

1. a. **True.** Melanomas are usually raised pigmented lesions but can often also appear pale and amelanotic.
   b. **True.** They are often asymptomatic, however, and only referred after being noted during fundoscopy by an optometrist.
   c. **True.** Metastastic disease tends to be to the liver and lungs.
   d. **True.** Melanomas have characteristic appearances on ultrasound examination.
   e. **False.** Management depends upon the size, site, state of fellow eye, general health of the patient and the patient's management preferences.

2. a. **False.** The underlying aetiology is rarely identified.
   b. **True.** Pain and photophobia are characteristic and predominant symptoms.
   c. **True.** Acute anterior uveitis is usually unilateral. If bilateral then an underlying systemic association is likely to be found.
   d. **False.** Toxoplasmosis is one of the many causes of posterior uveitis or choroiditis.
   e. **True.** Children with juvenile idiopathic arthritis should be screened regularly for anterior segment inflammation.

EMI answers

1. Theme: The uvea

1. F   Most choroidal malignant melanomas are 'picked up' as incidental findings during fundoscopy and are asymptomatic. The eye would rarely be red.
2. A   Limbal injection is characteristic of anterior uveitis (iritis). Photophobia is usually a prominent symptom. There is never a purulent discharge, which would be more characteristic of an infective conjunctivitis. The vision is often reduced but rarely as profoundly as in closed-angle glaucoma or retinal vessel occlusion.
3. G   Posterior uveitis may present with a variety of symptoms and signs. This stem represents a common presentation.

2. Theme: The uvea

1. D   This describes standard management of anterior uveitis. Patients often require a 4–8-week course.

2. B   Sight threatening non-infective posterior uveitis requires systemic immunosuppression. Usually steroids are initially prescribed. If the uveitis persists then a steroid sparing agent such as cyclosporin is usually started to replace the steroid. This helps to reduce the well-recognised side effects of systemic steroids.
3. H   Choroidal malignant melanomas can be treated by a number of means. Radiotherapy is a commonly used modality.

CRQ answers

CRQ 1

a. The symptoms of photophobia with reduced visual acuity, in the absence of itch or a discharge, are highly suggestive of an anterior uveitis (iritis). Identifying a well-recognised systemic association such as ankylosing spondylitis raises the suspicion of this being anterior uveitis.
b. Topical steroids, cycloplegics, analgesia and dark glasses.
c. The differential diagnosis of a red eye is: conjunctivitis (infective or allergic), corneal abrasion/foreign body, subconjunctival haemorrhage, episcleritis, scleritis, corneal ulceration (infective or inflammatory), uveitis, and acute-angle closure glaucoma.

Table 1 lists the principal differences in these diagnoses.

CRQ 2

a. Choroidal malignant melanoma, choroidal naevus, metastasis.
b. Asymptomatic (incidental finding on ophthalmoscopy) or visual disturbance due to:

   - the mass itself obscuring the visual axis
   - an associated retinal detachment
   - vitreous haemorrhage.

c. She may have metastatic disease from a primary choroidal melanoma. Characteristically malignant melanoma metastasises to the liver and lungs. Alternatively if the lesion is a metastasis then she must have a primary elsewhere and probable other metastatic disease leading to anorexia and weight loss.

Table 1 Differential diagnosis of the red eye.

	Vision	Pain	Discharge	Area	Fluorescein staining	Pupil	Laterality
Conjunctivitis	Normal	Gritty	Sticky	Generalised	No	Normal	Both
Subconjunctival haemorrhage	Normal	No	No	Diffuse	No	Normal	One
Episcleritis	Normal	No	No	Interpalpebral	No	Normal	One
Corneal ulcer	Reduced	Yes	Yes/No	Limbal	Yes	Normal	One
Scleritis	Reduced	Yes	No	Variable	No	Normal	One/both
Uveitis	Reduced	Yes	No	Limbal	No	Small	One
Acute-angle closure glaucoma	Reduced	Yes	No	Diffuse	No	Mid-dilated	One (Second eye at risk)

OSCE answers

OSCE 1

a. An oval-shaped lesion is seen nasal to the optic disc. It has poorly demarcated borders. The horizontal diameter is approximately three disc diameters and the vertical two and half discs. There is no associated haemorrhage or obvious retinal detachment.
b. Choroidal malignant melanoma, choroidal naevus, metastasis.
c. Ocular ultrasound.

OSCE 2

a. This is a photograph of the anterior segment of an eye. It demonstrates an abnormality of the iris. Adhesions are seen between the iris and the lens. These are known as posterior synechiae. They are likely to be associated with inflammatory cells and flare in the anterior chamber.
b. Anterior uveitis.
c. Among many others: ankylosing spondylitis, inflamatory bowel disease (both Crohn's and ulcerative colitis), sarcoidosis, Reiter's syndrome, Behçet's syndrome, psoriatic arthropathy, juvenile idiopathic arthritis, tuberculosis, syphilis
d. Topical steroids, dilating drops (cyclopentolate or atropine), analgesia, dark glasses.

Viva answers

1. The aetiology of posterior uveitis falls into two main groups: inflammatory, such as sarcoidosis or Behçet's syndrome, or infective such as toxoplasma or tuberculosis. In 50% of cases no cause will be identified.
   The standard core investigations include a full blood count and plasma viscosity, chest X-ray, urinalysis and syphilis serology. Other investigations are dictated by the history and clinical findings.

2. The anatomical site that is predominantly inflamed classifies uveitis. Four main groups are described:

   - *Anterior uveitis.* The iris is predominantly involved, commonly known as 'iritis'
   - *Intermediate uveitis.* The ciliary body is predominantly involved
   - *Posterior uveitis.* The choroid is predominantly involved, commonly known as 'choroiditis'
   - *Pan-uveitis.* The whole uveal tract is inflamed.

20 The retina

Chapter overview

This chapter deals with the two of the most common causes of visual impairment in developed countries: diabetic retinopathy and age-related macular degeneration (ARMD). Diabetic retinopathy is the most common cause of blindness in the working population while age-related macular degeneration (ARMD) is the most common in the elderly population.

The classification of diabetic retinopathy is described, based on the characteristic signs seen on fundoscopy. The other less common retinal vascular diseases are discussed with emphasis on assessing for systemic cerebrovascular risk factors.

The characteristic symptoms of retinal detachment are discussed along with the risk factors for developing the condition.

Investigation of retinal disease

Fluorescein angiography

This test involves the patient receiving an injection of fluorescein dye into a vein of the arm. From the arm the dye passes to the right side of the heart, then through the lungs and back to the left side of the heart. From there it enters the aortic arch, internal carotid artery, ophthalmic artery and then the eye. The fundus is observed during the test and serial photographs of the dye travelling through the circulation of the eye are taken with a blue light to induce fluorescence of the dye. The dye normally remains within the lumen of retinal blood vessels but leaks out of choroidal blood vessels. Figure 158 shows a normal angiogram. If there is disease of the choroidal or retinal tissues then the dye behaves differently and may demonstrate leakage or occlusion of blood vessels. Using the results of the angiogram combined with the clinical appearance, certain diagnoses can be made more confidently.

There is a small risk of anaphylactic shock and collapse during fluorescein angiography and a resuscitation trolley must therefore be available when performing this test.

20.1 The retina: structure and function

Tiny light-sensitive cells (photoreceptors) at the back of the eye collect information about the visual world. There are two types of photoreceptors:

Rod photoreceptors are very sensitive to dim light but cannot assess the colour (frequency) of the light.

Cone photoreceptors are sensitive to bright light and because there are three different types of cones they are capable of assessing the frequency of light.

Each light photoreceptor transmits its information down nerves to the brain. The optic nerve is a collection of all these nerves. All the photoreceptors together make up a thin light-sensitive layer at the back of the eye known as the retina. The retina is divided into three separate anatomical and functional areas:

1. The peripheral retina is the area beyond the temporal arcade blood vessels. This area is dominated by rod photoreceptors. Functionally it has low visual acuity (as the photoreceptors are relatively widely spaced) and poor colour vision but it functions well in dim light and is very sensitive to movement. This part of the retina serves the peripheral visual field.
2. The macula is the area of the retina within the temporal arcade blood vessels. This part of the retina is functionally dominated by the cone photoreceptors and therefore has good colour vision. The photoreceptors are more tightly packed

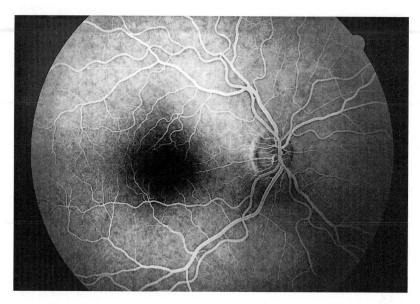

Fig. 158 Normal fluorescein angiography with background choroidal fluorescence and the arteries and veins showing up with no area of leakage.

together and consequently this area has better visual acuity than the periphery. The posterior pole serves the central 20 to 30° of vision.

3. The fovea is the central part of the macula. Cone photoreceptors are very densely packed in this area functionally providing sharp central visual acuity for fixating and identifying fine-detailed objects.

It is important to emphasise that the eye is only a means of collecting information about the visual world: it itself does not 'see'. 'Seeing' is a complex conscious and subconscious processing property of the brain based on information provided by the eye.

20.2 Retinal detachment

Learning objectives

You should:

- recognise the symptoms of retinal detachment

- be able to identify the individuals at risk of developing the condition

- be able to outline appropriate primary care management

- understand the techniques of surgical repair.

The retina can detach from the back of the eye by several mechanisms, two of which are:

- Fluid accessing the subretinal space from the vitreous by flowing through a retinal hole or tear.

This is known as a 'rhegmatogenous' detachment and is the most common mechanism (Fig. 159).

- Severe proliferative diabetic retinopathy may lead to contracting scar tissue pulling the retina off the back of the eye causing a 'tractional' detachment (see section on diabetic retinopathy).

Predisposing factors for 'rhegmatogenous' detachment include:

- myopia
- cataract surgery

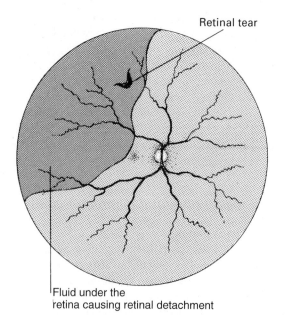

Retinal tear

Fluid under the retina causing retinal detachment

Fig. 159 Retinal detachment.

- blunt trauma
- YAG laser posterior capsulotomy
- inherited peripheral retinal degeneration
- posterior vitreous detachment.

Posterior vitreous detachment

The vitreous is a gel that fills the posterior segment of the globe. In young people the vitreous is attached to the retina but with age it peels away leading to a 'posterior vitreous detachment'. Patients often complain of floaters and peripheral flashing lights during the vitreous detachment. These symptoms normally settle after a few months. In the process of detaching, the vitreous can occasionally pull a small hole or tear in the retina, which may progress to a retinal detachment.

Clinical features of rhegmatogenous retinal detachment

Most patients present complaining of peripheral flashing lights and 'floaters'. As these symptoms are commonly caused by a posterior vitreous detachment, an associated retinal detachment is more likely if the floaters are accompanied by the awareness of 'a bit of the vision missing'. The missing bit is characteristically in the peripheral inferonasal field, as retinal tears most commonly develop in the superotemporal retina, although they can be anywhere. The patient often describes this as a 'black curtain' or 'shadow'. Fluid flows from the vitreous via a hole into the subretinal space causing the retina to detach with loss of function.

On examination the patient may already have reduced visual acuity that varies as the detached retina moves with eye movement and head position. A field defect may be noted. On ophthalmoscopy an anteriorly placed, slightly pale area of retina may be seen ballooning forwards.

Management

The subretinal fluid is usually drained. The globe is then pressed onto the retina by an external plastic buckle. Alternatively the vitreous can be removed to reduce traction on the retina, and gas or oil placed inside the eye, which presses the retina onto the choroid. The goal is to achieve a flat retina and seal the hole with either laser or cryotherapy.

20.3 Age-related macular degeneration

Learning objectives

You should:

- know the symptoms of age-related macular degeneration (ARMD)

- appreciate the different clinical appearances of ARMD

- recognise the individuals at risk of developing the condition

- appreciate the classification of the condition and the significance for visual outcome

- appreciate that in developed countries it is the most common cause of visual impairment in the elderly population

- appreciate that there is currently no satisfactory treatment that halts the disease process

- appreciate that the mainstay of management is based on offering practical support including low visual aids and occupational therapy assessment.

Age-related macular degeneration (ARMD)

This degenerative change of the macula is the commonest cause of reduced vision in the elderly. ARMD can be classified into two types: 'dry' (Fig. 160) and 'wet' (or disciform) degeneration (Fig. 161).

'Dry' ARMD

Clinical features

The patient usually complains of a gradual deterioration in vision. Ophthalmoscopy demonstrates pigmentary mottling at the macular region around areas of pale atrophic-looking retina. Well-demarcated yellow deposits known as hard drusen may be seen in association with these changes (see Fig. 160). The condition is bilateral although it may be asymmetrical.

Management

There is no treatment available that either improves or halts the degenerative changes. With the use of good lighting, magnifiers and bigger print, the patient can maximise their functional reading vision. The patient may be eligible for partial sight or blind registration. The advantage of such registration is that the patient may receive financial, practical, social and educational bene-

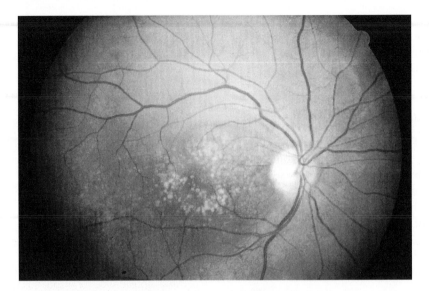

Fig. 160 Dry ARMD. There is evidence of drusen and pigmentary disturbance at the macula.

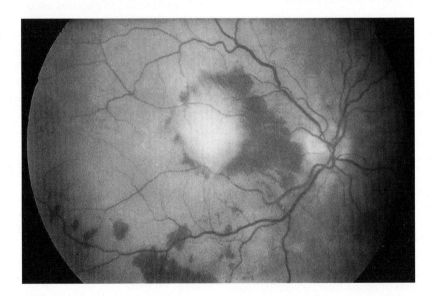

Fig. 161 Disciform ARMD. There is evidence of a pale raised lesion in the macular area with haemorrhage around the lesion. Some of this haemorrhage has spread inferiorly.

fits from local social services and visual impairment societies. The current definition of 'blind' in the UK is 'a person who is so blind that they are unable to perform work for which vision is required'. This generally equates to vision of equal to or less than 3/60 or a patient with a significant visual field defect such as a hemianopia or grossly constricted fields from glaucoma.

'Wet' ARMD

This condition characteristically causes more profound and rapid loss of vision than 'dry' ARMD. Because of degenerative changes in the interface between the retina and choroid, blood vessels from the choroid can grow under the retina. These new fragile vessels can leak fluid or bleed causing catastrophic loss of macular function.

Clinical features

Patients may initially complain of distortion of vision. They may state that door frames have a 'bend' in them when they know them to be straight. This is known as 'metamorphopsia'. As the condition progresses sudden profound loss of central vision may occur.

The fundal appearance of ARMD is dependent on its stage of evolution. If the patient is complaining of metamorphopsia then often only a slightly raised, faint grey lesion is discernible near to the fovea. This would represent a patch of subretinal blood vessels. If the blood vessels leak fluid then a larger pale raised area may often be seen associated with more peripheral yellow exudative deposits. If the blood vessels bleed then dark subretinal blood may be seen (Fig. 161). By this stage in the disease the patient will usually have suffered profound loss of central vision. The condition is normally bilateral although there is usually a period of time between the eyes being affected (which can be months to years).

Management

If the condition is diagnosed early certain patients may benefit from laser treatment. A new treatment called photodynamic therapy is currently undergoing trials. This treatment may help in slowing the growth of new patches of blood vessels thus reducing the long-term visual morbidity. Every effort should be made to improve visual function with optical aids and larger reading material (see 'dry' ARMD).

20.4 Retinal artery occlusion

Learning objectives

You should:

- recognise the symptoms and clinical appearance of central retinal artery occlusion (CRAO)

- be able to describe the immediate emergency management of the condition

- understand the poor prognosis for vision

- appreciate that CRAO is very often the symptom of a more significant underlying arterial disease

- appreciate that the patient is at risk of further serious ocular and systemic disease such as stroke

- know what the associated underlying diseases are and be able to perform appropriate investigations

- know how to treat the more common underlying diseases to reduce the risk of further cardiovascular morbidity.

Arterial occlusion causes sudden profound uniocular visual loss (usually to counting fingers or less).

Risk factors for an arterial occlusion include:

- carotid artery disease
- smoking
- hypertension
- diabetes (this is a risk factor for *all* arterial disease; it is treatable and must be excluded in all cases of CRAO)

- hypercholesterolaemia
- cardiac arrhythmia
- heart valve disease
- giant cell arteritis

The commonest cause is an embolus from an atheromatous plaque in the internal carotid artery. If the visual disturbance lasts for less than 24 hours then this is known as 'amaurosis fugax'. An embolus is assumed to have passed through the retinal circulation with no irreversible consequences. This is the eye equivalent of a cerebral transient ischaemic attack.

Clinical features

Central retinal artery occlusion causes complete painless uniocular loss of vision. A branch arterial occlusion leads to loss of function in one part of the retina usually resulting in an 'altitudinal' field defect in which the upper or lower half of the visual field is lost. The patient will complain of visual field loss corresponding to that area of the retina.

Visual acuity is normally profoundly reduced to counting fingers or less. A dense relative afferent pupillary defect is present. Fundoscopy reveals a swollen pale retina characteristically with a 'cherry-red spot' at the centre of the macula. An embolus may be seen lying within an arteriole.

Diagnosis

A clinical diagnosis can be made based on the history, visual acuity, pupil reflexes and characteristic fundal appearances.

Management

If the patient presents within 6–12 hours of onset of the visual disturbance then efforts should be made to dislodge the embolus. Techniques include massage of the globe, lowering of intraocular pressure with intravenous diamox and 'rebreathing' into a paper bag to precipitate vascular dilation (by increasing systemic carbon dioxide levels).

A standard systemic examination and investigation protocol should be performed to exclude an underlying reversible cause of emboli. Systemic examination should specifically exclude an irregular pulse, hypertension, a carotid bruit and any heart murmurs. Hyperviscosity states should be excluded and the cholesterol level checked. A carotid ultrasound examination is recommended to exclude significant stenosis.

Medical or surgical management should be instigated to reduce future cardiovascular morbidity. Interventions include low-dose aspirin, lipid-lowering agents, hypertension treatment and, in cases with significant carotid stenosis, carotid endarterectomy is considered. Patients should stop smoking.

20.5 Retinal vein occlusion

Learning objectives

You should:

- recognise the symptoms and clinical appearance of a central retinal vein occlusion (CRVO)

- understand the potential ocular complications and the prognosis for vision

- appreciate that laser treatment can reduce the risk of developing ocular complications

- appreciate that CRVO may be the symptom of a more significant underlying disease

- be able to name the associated underlying disease and perform appropriate investigations

- be able to describe how to treat the more common underlying diseases.

Visual loss in retinal vein occlusions is not usually as profound as in retinal artery occlusions. Branch retinal vein occlusions are more common than central vein occlusions.

Risk factors for a vein occlusion include:

- increasing age
- hypertension
- diabetes
- hyperviscosity syndromes

Clinical features

In a central retinal vein occlusion (Fig. 162) the patient complains of a sudden generalised loss of vision. This will affect only part of the visual field in those with branch vein occlusion.

The characteristic fundal appearance of vein occlusions include:

- flame-shaped haemorrhages
- dilated tortuous veins
- cotton-wool spots
- macular oedema
- iris new vessel growth

Management

It is important to consider the problem on two levels. First any systemic risk factors that may have precipitated the vein occlusion need to be identified and treated. Second the ocular consequences have to be considered. The two main causes of loss of vision are macular oedema and the development of a painful red eye with raised intraocular pressure (rubeotic glaucoma). Laser treatment is sometimes helpful.

20.6 Diabetic retinopathy

Learning objectives

You should:

- be able to classify diabetic retinopathy based on the clinical signs

- appreciate the different causes of visual loss in diabetic retinopathy

- appreciate that in developed countries it is the most common cause of visual impairment in the working population

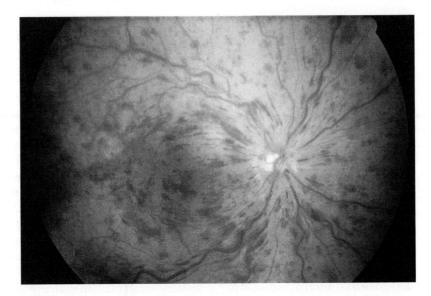

Fig. 162 Central retinal vein occlusion. Note the flame-shaped retinal haemorrhages and the dilated tortuous veins.

- appreciate that good glycaemic control will reduce the chance of developing long-term visual loss

- appreciate that controlling associated cardiovascular risk factors can reduce the chance of developing long-term visual loss

- advise that smoking will worsen diabetic retinopathy and exercise will help

- appreciate that appropriate laser treatment will reduce the chance of developing long-term visual loss

- understand how laser treatment works

Diabetic retinopathy is the most common cause of blindness in the working population. Individuals with diabetes must have annual systemic examinations and ophthalmoscopy in order that medical treatment is optimised and laser treatment performed early to prevent visual loss.

Classification
Diabetic retinopathy is usually categorised as:

- background retinopathy
- preproliferative retinopathy
- proliferative retinopathy
- maculopathy

Pathophysiology
The loss of normal glycaemic control leads to damage to the cells that line blood vessels. This leads to:

- dilating local blood vessels, which leak protein and lipid-rich fluid causing hard exudate deposition, and retinal oedema, which define diabetic maculopathy

- the release of angiogenic growth factors that lead to new vessel growth, defining proliferative diabetic retinopathy.

The retinal changes can be assessed on ophthalmoscopy by identifying specific clinical signs. These signs help classify the stages of diabetic retinopathy. A form of classification with the defining clinical features is outlined below.

Clinical box
Clinical features and diagnostic classification of retinopathy

Background retinopathy
- dot and blot haemorrhages
- microaneurysms
- fine yellow exudates (called hard exudates)
- normal vision

Preproliferative retinopathy
- cotton-wool spots
- irregular dilatation of the retinal veins (venous beading)
- intraretinal microvascular abnormalities (IRMA)
- normal vision

Proliferative retinopathy
- new vessel growth on retina
- normal vision unless becomes complicated by maculopathy
- hard exudates in macular area
- oedema at macula
- vision may be normal but becomes reduced

Proliferative retinopathy

The hallmark of proliferative disease is new vessels growing on the retina (Fig. 163). These may be complicated by:

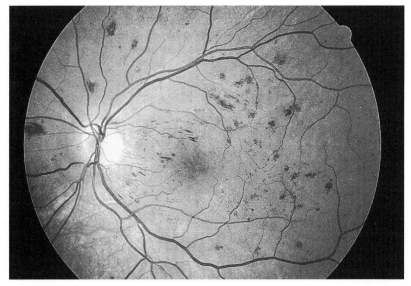

Fig. 163 Background diabetic retinopathy.

- vitreous haemorrhage, as a result of bleeding from fragile new vessels. This presents as acute painless profound loss of vision. On ophthalmoscopy the red reflex is absent. The haemorrhage normally clears spontaneously over 2 to 3 months. If the haemorrhage persists then surgical intervention is required to remove the blood.
- tractional retinal detachment, because of contraction of the supporting connective tissue
- rubeotic glaucoma, caused by growth of new vessels at other sites within the eye, such as the drainage angle.

If vitreous haemorrhage, tractional retinal detachment or rubeotic glaucoma develop then the acuity is reduced (new vessels alone are usually associated with normal vision).

Maculopathy

- oedema of the macula
- hard exudates
- usually reduced visual acuity

Management
Background and preproliferative retinopathy do not require laser treatment; however, patients still require regular fundal examination and systemic examination for cardiovascular risk factors such as hypertension and hypercholesterolaemia. Control of associated cardiovascular risk factors will reduce the chance of retinopathy progression and visual loss. The patient should be strongly discouraged from smoking. It should be emphasised that exercise is protective. The more advanced the retinopathy the more regular the examinations should be.

Once the retinopathy progresses to the proliferative stage, argon laser ablation of the peripheral retina is indicated. Laser treatment reduces the amount of ischaemic tissue present and therefore reduces the overall oxygen demand.

Oedematous maculopathy requires direct but gentle laser treatment. Ischaemic maculopathy, where the retinal capillary bed has become occluded, does not respond to laser treatment. It is occasionally necessary to perform fluorescein angiography to differentiate the two conditions.

Vitrectomy involves removal of the vitreous. This is useful for cases of vitreous haemorrhage or traction retinal detachment.

Complications of diabetic retinopathy
Visual loss can occur by four mechanisms:

- maculopathy
- vitreous haemorrhage
- tractional retinal detachment
- rubeotic glaucoma.

Self assessment: questions

Multiple choice questions

1. Features of non-proliferative diabetic retinopathy include:
   a. dot and blot haemorrhages
   b. new vessel formation at the optic disc
   c. venous beading
   d. cotton-wool spots and retinal new vessel growth
   e. intraretinal microvascular abnormalities (IRMAs)

2. Vein occlusions of the retina:
   a. are associated with carotid bruits
   b. may lead to a painful red eye with raised intraocular pressure known as rubeotic glaucoma
   c. may cause painless uniocular loss of vision
   d. can be associated with an underlying systemic condition, such as hypertension
   e. are often seen in healthy, young individuals

Extended matching items questions (EMIs)

1. Theme: Retina (1)

A widespread retinal pallor and thickening with a central macular red spot
B widespread flame-shaped intraretinal haemorrhages, tortuous veins, multiple cotton-wool spots and iris new vessel growth
C a bright yellow deposit is seen within a vessel at the apex of pale thickened quadrant of retina
D widespread dot and blot haemorrhages, multiple cotton-wool spots, venous beading, intraretinal microvascular abnormalities and new vessels at the disc
E widespread flame-shaped intraretinal haemorrhages and tortuous veins
F widespread dot and blot haemorrhages and microaneurysms
G pigmentary changes at the macula
H pale area of retina seen ballooning forwards
I retinal thickening at the macula with a ring of yellow exudate
J a quadrant of flame-shaped haemorrhages, one cotton-wool spot and an associated tortuous vein

Match the signs above with the most appropriate diagnosis from below:

1. Branch retinal artery occlusion.
2. Preproliferative diabetic retinopathy.
3. Central retinal vein occlusion.

2. Theme: Retina (2)

A dry age-related macular degeneration
B 2-day-old central retinal artery occlusion
C longstanding branch retinal artery occlusion
D background diabetic retinopathy
E central retinal vein occlusion with iris new vessel growth
F preproliferative diabetic retinopathy
G diabetic maculopathy with reduced visual acuity
H 4-hour-old central retinal artery occlusion
I large retinal detachment, with the macula still attached
J 3-month-old branch retinal artery occlusion

Match the condition above with the most appropriate investigation and management from the list below:

1. Attempt to dislodge the occluding embolus by performing ocular massage, reducing intraocular pressure and 'rebreathing'. In addition perform a cardiovascular disease risk assessment examination with particular emphasis on the identification of reversible embolic risk factors. Treat any reversible risk factors and prescribe long-term low-dose aspirin.
2. Refer urgently to an ophthalmologist for surgical repair.
3. Perform a cardiovascular disease risk assessment examination. Treat any condition identified. Make an urgent referral for laser pan-retinal photocoagulation.

Constructed response questions (CRQs)

CRQ 1

An 80-year-old woman attended as an emergency in the afternoon with loss of vision in her right eye. She had woken that morning with reduced vision measuring on examination hand movements (HM) in the affected eye. The left eye could see 6/9. The eyes were comfortable. She has a past medical history of ischaemic heart disease, but is otherwise well.

a. What is the differential diagnosis?
b. Describe how each possible diagnosis can be confirmed and treated.

CRQ 2

A 29-year-old insulin-dependent diabetic patient presents with sudden, painless complete loss of vision in her right eye. She has never been seen in the eye department before.

a. What are the possible causes of the visual loss?
b. What are the important clinical signs to look for on examination?
c. What treatment is she likely to need?

Objective structured clinical examination questions (OSCEs)

OSCE 1

A 42-year-old woman presented with sudden painless loss of vision in one eye.

a. Describe the clinical findings in Figure 164.

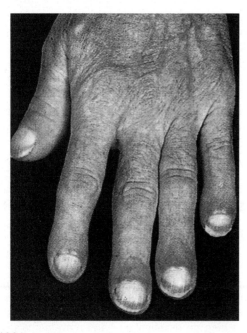

Fig. 164

b. What are the recognised systemic associations of this finding?
c. How might these systemic associations have led to her presentation?
d. Describe some investigations which would help in identifying an underlying cause.

OSCE 2

A 92-year-old man presented to his GP complaining of difficulty watching television and recognising faces in the street. His visual acuities measured 3/60 in both eyes corrected.

a. Describe the fundal appearances of the patient's left eye as seen in Figure 165.
b. What is the differential diagnosis?
c. State the legal definition of 'blind' in the UK.
d. What can be done to help this patient?

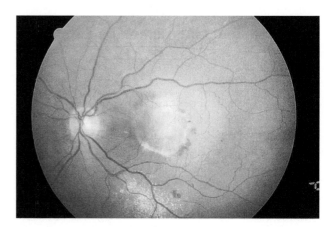

Fig. 165

Viva questions

1. Describe the risk factors for retinal detachment and the common presenting symptoms.

2. Describe the potential causes of visual loss due to diabetic retinopathy.

Self-assessment: answers

Multiple choice answers

1. a. **True.** Dot and blot haemorrhages as well as microaneurysms are the first signs of diabetic retinopathy and are characteristic of 'background' retinopathy.
   b. **False.** New vessel formation defines proliferative retinopathy.
   c. **True.** Irregular retinal veins, also known as venous beading, are evidence of increasing fundal ischaemia but alone in the absence of new vessel formation are characteristic of preproliferative retinopathy.
   d. **False.** Cotton-wool spots represent infarcts of the nerve-fibre layer. They are signs of progressive ischaemia and are commonly seen in preproliferative and proliferative diabetic retinopathy. If seen in combination with new vessel growth then by definition this must be proliferative diabetic retinopathy.
   e. **True.** IRMAs are a sign of progressive ischaemia. They represent the opening up of collateral channels between the venous and arterial sides of the retinal blood supply. They are commonly seen in preproliferative and proliferative diabetic retinopathy. In the absence of new vessel growth then by definition this is a sign of non-proliferative diabetic retinopathy.

2. a. **False.** Retinal arteriole occlusions are characteristically associated with carotid stenosis.
   b. **True.** Retinal vein occlusions may create an ischaemic fundus. The ischaemic tissue releases angiogenic factors, which causes new vessel growth. The new vessels often grow on the iris and into the drainage angle causing raised intraocular pressure and a painful red eye.
   c. **True.** Venous occlusions commonly present with painless loss of vision. Arterial occlusions are similarly painless but often cause more profound visual loss. Retinal detachments may cause painless unilateral visual loss but often with the symptoms of flashing lights and floaters. Optic neuritis can cause a progressive unilateral loss of vision but characteristically the eye is painful on extraocular movement. Temporal arteritis may cause unilateral visual loss but often with an associated headache and systemic symptoms. Any postchiasmal pathology characteristically causes bilateral visual disturbance.
   d. **True.** Retinal vein occlusions are common in patients with hypertension, diabetes and hyperviscosity syndromes.
   e. **False.** Young, healthy individuals rarely present with retinal vein occlusions. The condition is more common in individuals over the age of 70 years.

EMI answers

1. Theme: Retina (1)

1. C   Retinal arteriole occlusions appear as pale, oedematous areas of retina. Emboli are the most common cause of occlusions. Occasionally the embolus can be seen within the lumen of the 'feeding' arteriole. In a branch occlusion only a sector of the retina is affected rather than the whole retina.
2. D   Preproliferative disease is seen clinically as flame-shaped haemorrhages, cotton-wool spots, IRMAs, and venous beading, but no new vessel growth.
3. B   Central retinal vein occlusions are characterised by poor visual acuity with an associated relative afferent pupil defect. The fundus is generally very haemorrhagic and cotton-wool spots may be present. Because of the release of angiogenic factors from the ischaemic tissue, iris new vessel growth may occur, and this usually leads to painful rubeotic glaucoma.

1. Theme: Retina (2)

1. H   If the patient presents within 12 hours of onset efforts should be made to dislodge the occluding arteriole embolus. The visual disturbance may be reversed if the blood supply is restored. Beyond 12 hours there is little evidence that the visual outcome will be improved. A source for the embolus should be sought and treated to reduce the risk of cerebrovascular disease.
2. I   Retinal detachment requires urgent surgical repair to prevent further visual disturbance. If the patient postures appropriately the progression of the detachment can be slowed.
3. E   Patients who develop central retinal vein occlusions are at higher risk of developing cerebrovascular disease. A systemic examination to exclude hypertension, hypercholesterolaemia and diabetes is required. Any previously unrecognised conditions should be treated.

CRQ answers

CRQ 1

a. An elderly woman with sudden loss of vision in one eye is most likely to have had an event affecting the vascular supply to the retina or optic nerve, i.e. central retinal vein occlusion, central retinal artery occlusion (or amaurosis fugax, if the loss of vision had been for less than 24 hours) or anterior ischaemic optic neuropathy. Other possibilities include wet age-related macular degeneration, vitreous haemorrhage or retinal detachment. Another possibility is that the woman has had a longstanding loss of vision in her right eye that she has just noticed because the vision in her left eye is normal. This may happen when the patient covers their better eye.

b. Examination of the retina will provide most of the information in order to make a diagnosis. Central retinal vein occlusion will be recognised by the presence of diffuse flame-shaped haemorrhages over the retina, whereas the retina in a central retinal artery occlusion is pale with a cherry-red spot at the macula and an embolus may be seen within the retinal arterial tree. The optic disc in anterior ischaemic optic neuropathy is swollen with haemorrhages around the nerve head. The macula in wet age-related degeneration is pale and raised, often with surrounding haemorrhage. Retinal details are obscured by blood in cases of vitreous haemorrhage and folds of detached retina may be apparent in those with retinal detachment. Optic neuritis usually has no abnormal clinical findings except reduced vision and an afferent pupillary defect. It is important to ensure that this patient has no underlying treatable condition that has contributed to her loss of vision.

CRQ 2

a. Vitreous haemorrhage is the most likely cause, as it tends to be an acute loss with no pain. Maculopathy and tractional retinal detachment both tend to cause a more slowly progressive visual disturbance. Rubeotic glaucoma is characteristically painful.

b. Visual acuity reduction, abnormal pupil reflexes, corneal clarity, new vessel growth on the iris, intraocular pressure, the red reflex and fundoscopy. A vitreous haemorrhage will often have very poor vision such as hand movements and an absent red reflex.

c. Vitrectomy and argon laser pan-retinal photocoagulation.

OSCE answers

OSCE 1

a. Finger clubbing.

b. Neoplasia, chronic obstructive airways disease, bronchiecstasis, chronic hypoxia, endocarditis (among many).

c. Neoplasia: metastasis to the choroid
Endocarditis: retinal arteriole embolus from a heart-valve vegetation.

d. Full blood count, plasma viscosity/ESR/CRP, chest X-ray, carotid ultrasound scan, blood gases, blood culture, echocardiogram.

OSCE 2

a. The central part of the macula appears pale with well-demarcated but irregular borders. There is no associated haemorrhage or exudate.

b. The appearances are in keeping with age-related macular degeneration.

c. The patient should be added to the blind register if they are so blind that they are unable to do work for which vision is essential. In most circumstances this equates to visual acuity of worse than 3/60 corrected in the better eye, a visual field less than 10° or a hemianopia. If a patient has a hemianopia it is at the discretion of the examining consultant ophthalmologist as to whether the patient should be added to the blind register, often based on the level of visual acuity.

d. Ensure he is wearing his best spectacle correction. Issue low visual aids for near and distance. Add to blind register to allow access to social services and help from the local visual impairment society, if he fulfils the criteria for registration.

Viva answers

1. Risk factors for retinal detachment include myopia, ocular surgery, trauma, peripheral retinal degenerations, posterior vitreous detachment and YAG laser posterior capsulotomy. Common presenting symptoms include flashing lights and floaters with peripheral visual disturbance like a shadow, which can progress and affect central vision.

2. Maculopathy: Fluid from leaky blood vessels collects in the layers of the retina causing the clinical appearance of retinal thickening with consequent loss of function.
Vitreous haemorrhage: The new vessels which define proliferative diabetic retinopathy are fragile and prone to bleeding. If this occurs the vitreous

fills with blood causing painless uniocular loss of vision.

Tractional retinal detachment: In severe longstanding proliferative diabetic retinopathy, the retina can become progressively detached by contracting fibrovascular complexes leading to loss of vision.

Rubeotic glaucoma: In severe proliferative diabetic retinopathy, new vessel growth can occur on the iris and the drainage angle obstructing the trabecular meshwork. The intraocular pressure becomes raised leading to a painful, red eye, with corneal haze and loss of vision.

21 Strabismus

Chapter overview

This chapter describes the causes and classification of squint (ocular misalignment). The conditions that cause the different types of squint are described, with emphasis placed upon the characteristic clinical symptoms and signs that help to make a diagnosis. The management of each condition is then described.

Each eye has six extraocular muscles (the medial, lateral, inferior and superior rectus muscles, and the inferior and superior obliques). The movements of each eye are finely coordinated with those of the opposite eye, so that both eyes normally function as one unit when fixating an object of interest in different fields of gaze. When the eyes become misaligned so that the visual axis of one eye is not directed to the same fixation point as the other, then a squint, or strabismus, is present.

Classification of squints:

- **Concomitant**
  - convergent (esotropia) (Fig. 166A)
  - divergent (exotropia) (Fig. 166B)
  - vertical (hyper/hypotropia) (Fig. 166C)
- **Incomitant**
  - cranial nerve palsies
  - dysthyroid eye disease
  - myasthenia gravis
  - trauma

A concomitant squint is one that stays the same size no matter in which direction the patient looks and the patient has a full range of eye movements, whereas an incomitant one varies in size depending on the direction of gaze and there is evidence of weakness or tightness of one or more of the extraocular muscles. This distinction

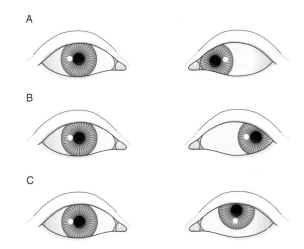

Fig. 166 Squints. **A.** Left esotropia. **B.** Left exotropia. **C.** Left hypertropia.

is important as it has implications regarding underlying aetiology, which is important in terms of investigation and management.

21.1 Concomitant squints

Learning objectives

You should:

- understand the classification of squints
- recognise a squint in a child
- be able to perform a cover test
- be able to refer patients appropriately
- understand the basis of the management of childhood squint
- appreciate the importance of preventing amblyopia.

Concomitant squints are common, and up to 5% of all children have them, the majority of which are convergent. Virtually all squints presenting in childhood are concomitant. They are caused by an anomaly of the developing ocular motility system with no underlying organic disease. It is important to be able to identify squints in children, as if left untreated, they may result in poor vision in one eye (amblyopia).

Convergent squint (esotropia)

There is a strong association between hypermetropia (long-sightedness) and childhood esotropia.

This type of squint usually becomes evident at the age of about 18 months to 3 years, when the child's near reflex (i.e. the ability to converge and focus on a near object) is developing, so that the eyes tend to over-converge when trying to focus on a near object.

Clinical features
One eye turns inwards (Fig. 166A), which is confirmed by the cover test. This eye commonly becomes amblyopic without treatment. The eye movements are full.

The squint may start as intermittent but becomes constant with time. There are usually no symptoms (such as double vision) as the patient develops suppression of the squinting eye.

Management
In this age group, any child with a squint should be tested for glasses (refracted), and any correction given to see if this improves or alters the angle of squint. If there is any amblyopia (see below) this should be treated by patching the better eye. In patients whose vision is not corrected with spectacles, surgery is usually required.

Complications
The main complication of childhood squint is the development of amblyopia. Strabismic amblyopia is a condition in which there is a reduction in vision in one eye because it squints. Treatment of amblyopia consists of patching, or covering, the other non-amblyopic eye for several hours each day to visually stimulate the amblyopic eye and, therefore, to assist its normal visual development. Any spectacle correction should be worn when patching is being carried out. Patching is only effective during the period of visual maturation (i.e. up to 8 years of age).

Pseudo-esotropia

Infants and small children often appear to have convergent squints when, in fact, their eyes are straight. This is because children's faces have wide nasal bridges and prominent epicanthal folds, which make their eyes appear convergent. The cover test is used to confirm that there is no squint.

Divergent squint (exotropia)

Divergent squints are much rarer in children than convergent ones. The age of onset of this type of squint is from the very young infant to 5–6 years of age. The aetiology is unknown.

Clinical features
One eye tends to turn outwards (Fig. 166B), especially when looking in the distance. It often commences as an intermittent squint, but this becomes constant with time. The child tends to close one eye when looking in the distance. There is a full range of extraocular movements with no refractive error and no double vision.

Management
Surgery consists of weakening the lateral rectus muscle and/or strengthening the medial rectus to move the eye into a more central position.

21.2 Incomitant squints

Learning objectives

You should:

- understand the classification of squints
- appreciate the different causes of incomitant squint
- be able to diagnose by history and examination the different causes of incomitant squint
- be able to perform a cover test
- understand the management of the different conditions
- know how to refer appropriately.

This type of squint is usually caused by pathology of the nerve supply to the extraocular muscles or of the muscles themselves.

Incomitant squints may appear in children or adults. All children with squints should be examined with care to ensure that they do not have an incomitant squint. The features of incomitant squint depend on which muscles or nerves are affected. The presentation is usually of acute double vision.

Motor nerve palsies

The motor nerves to the extraocular muscles may be affected by a variety of disease processes such as:

- microvascular disease (in association with hypertension, diabetes or atherosclerosis)
- demyelination
- intracranial aneurysms
- infection (e.g. herpes zoster, meningitis)
- trauma
- intracranial neoplasms.

Clinical features
The features depend on the affected nerve.

Third nerve palsy. All muscles except the lateral rectus and superior oblique are innervated by the third (oculomotor) nerve. Features of a third nerve palsy include:

- divergent, hypotropic eye
- dilated, unreactive pupil
- ptosis (droopy upper lid).

In many patients, the condition is partial, either by sparing the pupil or lid or by leaving some movements partially or fully intact. A painful third nerve palsy must be considered as a neurosurgical emergency as this may be caused by enlargement of a posterior communicating artery aneurysm, which may be at risk of bleeding with catastrophic consequences.

Fourth nerve palsy. The fourth, or trochlear, nerve innervates the superior oblique muscle. The affected eye cannot look downwards fully while adducted (turned inwards). Patients notice diplopia in which the images are on top of each other (vertical diplopia) and tilted at an angle to each other (torsional diplopia). To compensate for this the patients commonly tilt their heads away from the affected side (Fig. 167).

Sixth nerve palsy. Sixth (abducent) nerve palsy is the most common cranial nerve palsy. It causes an isolated lateral rectus weakness, which presents as double vision in which the images are side by side. The diplopia is maximal (i.e. the images are most widely separated) on looking towards the affected side and when looking in the distance (Fig. 168).

Management

The majority of nerve palsies improve spontaneously over a few months. An orthoptist can monitor the improvement of a palsy by examining the patient and recording the movements. During this time, the patient should be treated symptomatically to relieve any diplopia. This is done by patching one eye to occlude the second image or by sticking a plastic prism on to the glasses in front of one eye to allow the eyes to function together.

In the long term, those that do not improve require definitive treatment to improve ocular alignment. In the majority of patients, this involves surgery to the affected muscles. In some patients botulinum toxin injections may be used to weaken antagonist muscles. Toxin may be used in isolation or as a supplement to surgery.

Dysthyroid eye disease

Thyroid gland dysfunction can be associated with a disturbance of eye movements.

Clinical features

Patients often present with vertical or horizontal diplopia. In addition they usually have other features of dysthyroid eye disease, such as ocular discomfort and redness, lid retraction, lid lag and proptosis (Fig. 169). The abnormality of muscle function is not a weakness but a restriction caused by contraction of the affected muscles.

Patients with characteristic eye findings who have not previously been diagnosed as dysthyroid should have their thyroid function tested (thyroxine, triiodothyronine and thyroid-stimulating hormone). CT or MRI scanning demonstrates thickened rectus muscles.

Management

The underlying thyroid disorder should be treated. This, however, probably does not influence the clinical course of the eye disease. The condition runs an active course during which there may be continuing changes in the eye position, and during this time the patient should be kept comfortable with prisms or patches. After some months or years, this eventually stabilises and at this point the resultant ocular motility defects can be treated definitively, by operating to weaken (or recess) the restricted extraocular muscles.

Complications

- chronic diplopia
- exposure keratitis
- irreversible loss of vision.

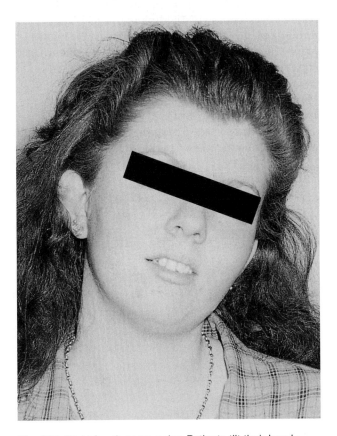

Fig. 167 Right fourth nerve palsy. Patients tilt their head away from the affected side.

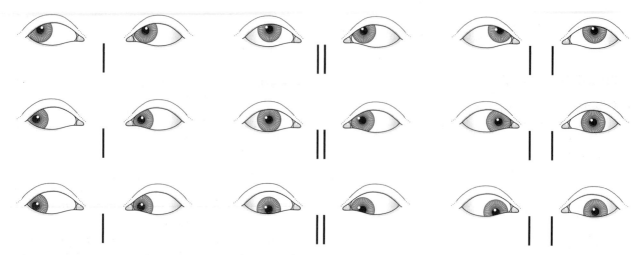

Fig. 168 Left sixth nerve palsy. A single image is seen on looking to the right, and the double images become progressively further apart when looking left.

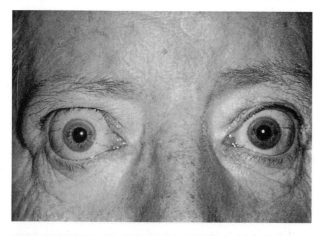

Fig. 169 Dysthyroid opthalmoscopy. Both upper and lower lids are retracted. Both eyes show proptosis.

Myasthenia gravis

Myasthenia gravis is an autoimmune condition in which neuromuscular transmission is affected by antibodies to the acetylcholine receptors.

Clinical features
The most common ocular sign is ptosis, although the patient may complain of diplopia, which may vary throughout the day and is characteristically worse at night. There is no pattern to the motility disturbance and it may simulate any nerve palsy.

Management
Treatment is with pyridostigmine.

Patients suspected of having myasthenia should have a therapeutic trial of pyridostigmine.

Self-assessment: questions

Multiple choice questions

1. Features of a sixth nerve palsy include:
   a. reduced abduction of the affected eye
   b. reduced vision in the affected eye
   c. oblique double vision
   d. horizontal double vision
   e. maximum double vision on looking away from the affected side
2. Regarding thyroid eye disease:
   a. it may be associated with thyroid gland dysfunction
   b. it may cause visual loss
   c. it often presents as red and gritty eyes
   d. extraocular muscle surgery may be required
   e. thickened rectus muscles often show on CT or MRI scanning

Extended matching items questions (EMIs)

1. Theme: Strabismus

A   An 84-year-old man who is blind in one eye complains of constant double vision from his only good eye.

B   A 42-year-old female presents with intermittent double vision, worse towards the end of the day, associated with variable bilateral ptosis.

C   An 81-year-old female presents with painless sudden-onset horizontal double vision.

D   A 47-year-old male presents complaining of blurred vision for near with occasional double vision. He does not wear reading glasses.

E   A 25-year-old woman presents with a manifest divergent squint with no double vision. She has a history of a convergent squint as a child.

F   A 12-month-old child presents with intermittent convergent squint with a full range of eye movements.

G   A 53-year-old male with a history of hyperthyroidism presents with painful eye movements and blurred vision. Both eyes appear red and protruding. There is bilateral upper and lower lid retraction.

H   A 93-year-old female presents with gradually reduced vision in both eyes

I   A 27-year-old female presents with sudden onset severe headache, photophobia, nausea, vertical double vision and ptosis.

J   A 5-year-old boy presents with an intermittent manifest convergent squint which is worse for near. He does not complain of double vision.

Match the diagnoses below with the most appropriate clinical description above:

1. Subarachnoid haemorrhage from an aneurysm causing a third nerve palsy.
2. Severe thyroid eye disease.
3. Myasthenia gravis.

2. Theme: Strabismus

A   Weakness of down gaze in adduction of the right eye with a head tilt to the left. The patient complains of double vision with 'tilting' of the images.

B   Intermittent double vision worse towards the end of the day associated with variable bilateral ptosis.

C   Vertical double vision associated with a right ptosis and a 'down and out' eye position on the same side.

D   Weakness of all eye movements of the left eye except abduction and depression.

E   A manifest convergent squint with weakness of right abduction.

F   Weakness of all eye movements of the right eye except abduction and depression.

G   Constant double vision with marked restriction of up gaze. The eyes appear prominent. There is bilateral lower lid retraction.

H   Weakness of down gaze in adduction of the left eye with a head tilt to the right. The patient complains of double vision with tilting of the images.

I   Vertical double vision associated with a left ptosis and a 'down and out' eye position on the same side.

J   A manifest convergent squint with weakness of left abduction.

Match the diagnoses below with the most appropriate clinical descriptions from above:

1. Myasthenia gravis.
2. Right fourth cranial nerve palsy.
3. Right sixth nerve palsy.

Constructed response questions (CRQs)

CRQ 1

A 27-year-old man presents to Accident and Emergency with severe sudden-onset headache. He is also complaining of vertical double vision associated with a slight droop of his left upper lid.

a. What diagnosis needs to be excluded in this patient?
b. What signs might you look for when examining his eyes?
c. What further questions would you like to ask him?
d. What investigations will help in managing the patient?

CRQ 2

> A 68-year-old woman presents to her GP complaining of horizontal double vision. The double vision is worse for distance and on looking to the left but does not bother her for near. She is otherwise asymptomatic. She has a past medical history of obesity and a family history of cerebrovascular accidents.

a. What cranial nerve palsy is most likely to be responsible for this patient's double vision?
b. What are the possible aetiologies of the cranial nerve palsy?
c. What investigations would be appropriate to perform in the surgery?

> The patient is referred to the eye department for further management.

d. What important signs must the ophthalmologist examine for in order to clinically exclude a space-occupying lesion?
e. What are the management options for improving the symptoms of double vision?

Objective structured clinical examination questions (OSCEs)

OSCE 1

> A 54-year-old woman is referred to the eye clinic. She has a past medical history of hyperthyroidism and thyroid eye disease.

a. Describe the clinical signs seen in Figures 170 and 171

> Her eyes are currently comfortable with no redness or symptoms of grittiness and burning.

b. What problems may this patient complain of?
c. Outline the general management of thyroid eye disease.

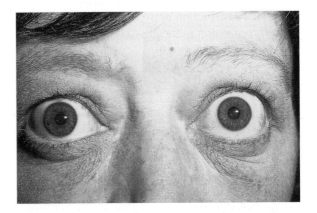

Fig. 170

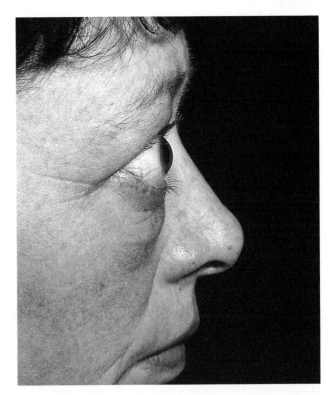

Fig. 171

OSCE 2

A young girl was referred to the eye clinic because her parents noticed that her eyes appeared to 'squint' when she held objects close to her eyes.

a. Describe the findings in Figure 172.

The girl was refracted and the glasses were pre-scribed.

b. What type of spectacles are seen in Figure 173 and what type of refractive error do they correct?
c. What effect do the spectacles have upon her squint as seen in Figure 174?
d. What symptoms is the girl likely to complain of?
e. Outline the general management of squints in childhood.
f. Why is it important to treat squints?

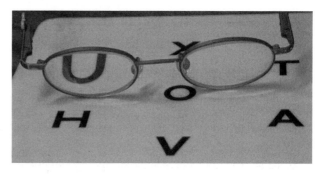

Fig. 173

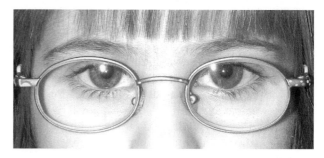

Fig. 174

Viva questions

1. What is a pseudo-esotropia?

2. What is the difference between a concomitant and an incomitant squint?

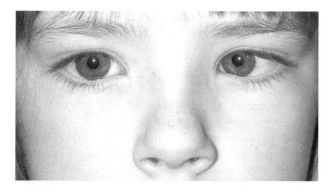

Fig. 172

Self-assessment: answers

Multiple choice answers

1. a. **True.** The lateral rectus muscle abducts the eye. The sixth cranial nerve (abducens) supplies the lateral rectus and therefore the characteristic finding is a weakness of abduction.
   b. **False.** The optic nerve is the second cranial nerve.
   c. **False.** The extraocular muscles which serve vertical eye movements are not affected in a sixth nerve palsy and therefore oblique or vertical double vision are unlikely to occur.
   d. **True.** Weakness of the lateral rectus muscle results in purely horizontal double vision.
   e. **False.** In looking away from the side with the abduction weakness, the affected eye will move into adduction, where there is no limitation of movement and therefore the vision will become single. By looking toward the side with the abduction weakness, the double vision will become worse.

2. a. **True.** It is often associated with hyperthyroidism.
   b. **True.** If the optic nerve is compressed from swollen orbital tissues, a 'compressive' optic neuropathy can develop, which can lead to visual loss.
   c. **True.** A common presentation of thyroid eye disease is bilateral red, gritty eyes.
   d. **True.** Although double vision may be improved by prisms surgery to the extraocular muscles is often performed.
   e. **True.** The thickened muscles are responsible for the diplopia and proptosis.

EMI answers

1. Theme: Strabismus

1. I   The clinical description is consistent with a subarachnoid haemorrhage and a third nerve palsy. Urgent investigations are necessary.
2. G   The clinical description is suggestive of severe thyroid eye disease with probable early compressive optic neuropathy. A specialised MRI scan which suppresses the signal from fat and thus highlights the extraocular muscles will help confirm the diagnosis. Urgent steps must be taken to decompress the orbit by medical, radiotherapy and surgical means.
3. B   The clinical description is consistent with myasthenia gravis. Many clinicians will

investigate this condition with a 'tensilon' test or systemic therapeutic trial of an appropriate acetylcholinesterase inhibitor such as pyridostigmine. If the symptoms improve then a diagnosis is confirmed.

2. Theme: Strabismus

1. B   The presentation of myasthenia can be highly variable. The signs characteristically worsen towards the end of the day because of fatigue. Ptosis is a characteristic finding.
2. A   The superior oblique muscle is supplied by the fourth cranial nerve. Weakness of this muscle causes torsional (tilting) double vision and a head tilt away from the side of the lesion.
3. E   The lateral rectus muscle is supplied by the sixth cranial nerve. Weakness of this muscle may present as a convergent squint and weakness of abduction of the affected eye.

CRQ answers

CRQ 1

a. Subarachnoid haemorrhage. The patient may have an associated left third nerve palsy as suggested by the symptoms and signs of vertical double vision and drooping upper lid. An aneurysm of the left posterior communicating artery may be the source of the bleed as this is closely associated with the course of the third cranial nerve.

b. The characteristic signs of a third nerve palsy include:

- ocular misalignment with the affected eye pointing 'down and out' due to the unopposed action of the lateral rectus and superior oblique muscles supplied by the still functional sixth and fourth cranial nerves respectively.
- ptosis because of weakness of the levator muscle of the upper lid supplied by the third nerve.
- dilated pupil due to loss of the parasympathetic supply to the sphincter muscle of the iris and consequent unopposed overaction of the sympathetic driven dilator muscle. The parasympathetic nerve fibres are thought to run in the more superficial layers of the third nerve and therefore may be more susceptible to a compressive insult such as an expanding aneurysm. Some authors believe that a dilated pupil may be an early and more prominent sign

of a third nerve palsy secondary to an expanding aneurysm and therefore more in need of urgent investigations. Clinical suspicion would also be increased in a painful palsy in a younger patient.

c. Identify the nature of the onset of the headache and any associated symptoms since onset: characteristically the onset of a subarachnoid haemorrhage is like being hit over the head by a bat and continues as 'the worst headache I've ever had'. Meningitic symptoms may develop such as photophobia and a stiff neck.

d. Imaging of the head to identify an aneurysm or subarachnoid blood and/or lumbar puncture to confirm the presence of blood in the cerebrospinal fluid and exclude other diagnoses.

CRQ 2

a. A left sixth nerve palsy with consequent abducting weakness of the left eye. This characteristically causes horizontal double vision which worsens when the affected eye moves into the direction of action of the weakened muscle. The abducting weakness does not affect the patient when converging for near work.

b. In order of likelihood:

- microvascular ischaemia of the nerve secondary to risk factors associated with cardiovascular morbidity
- space-occupying lesion
- raised intracranial pressure causing a 'false localising sign'
- mid-brain stroke
- demyelination
- vasculitis.

c. Investigations aimed at identifying cardiovascular disease risk factors:

- blood pressure
- urinalysis to exclude glycosuria and haematuria
- cholesterol level
- fasting blood glucose
- plasma viscosity to exclude a vasculitis such as giant cell arteritis.

d. Associated cranial nerve palsies and swollen optic discs suggesting a space-occupying lesion and raised intracranial pressure.

e. Occluding the vision from one eye either by patching or fogging a lens in the patient's spectacles. Alternatively, if the angle of squint is not too large, a prism may be applied to a spectacle lens, which will maintain binocularity.

OSCE answers

OSCE 1

a. Bilateral proptosis and lid retraction with the right eye appearing worse than the left.

b. Problems may include: corneal exposure leading to gritty uncomfortable eyes with mild blurring of vision, restrictive myopathy leading to double vision and tender eye movements, proptosis and 'puffy' periorbital tissues leading to concerns regarding cosmesis.

c. If an underlying thyroid gland dysfunction is present then this should be treated. Most patients can be managed conservatively with symptomatic treatment. Sometimes if double vision occurs prisms or extraocular surgery are required.

OSCE 2

a. Left convergent squint or esotropia.

b. Convex plus lenses to correct hypermetropia.

c. Wearing the glasses appears to straighten the eyes.

d. Probably none as the brain suppresses the image from the squinting eye and therefore double vision is not perceived.

e. Ensure the child is wearing an appropriate spectacle correction. If a 'lazy' or amblyopic eye is found then patching of the good eye will force the amblyopic eye to be used, usually improving the vision acuity. If a manifest squint persists despite appropriate spectacles and patching, perform surgery on the extraocular muscles to straighten the eyes.

f. To avoid amblyopia and cosmetically unacceptable squints.

Viva answers

1. Pseudo-esotropia is a condition in which a child appears to have a convergent squint because of the shape of their face, with the broad nose and epicanthal folds of childhood. The diagnosis can be made by confirming the eyes are straight on the basis of a normal cover test.

2. In a concomitant squint, the patient has a full range of extraocular movements with the angle of the deviation remaining the same in all directions of gaze. There is no weakness or limitation of eye movements. no matter in which direction the patient looks. In incomitant squints the angle of deviation varies depending upon which direction the patient looks. The variation in angle of squint is caused by muscle weakness or restriction of movement.

22 Glaucoma

Chapter overview

This chapter introduces the glaucomas, emphasising the common elements of all the glaucomas and the differences that define the various glaucoma syndromes.

The symptoms, pathophysiology, diagnosis and management are discussed with special emphasis on primary open-angle glaucoma (POAG), acute closed-angle glaucoma (ACAG) and congenital glaucoma.

22.1 The glaucomas

Learning objectives

You should:

- understand the classifications of glaucoma
- be able to describe the methods of diagnosing and assessing glaucoma
- recognise the symptoms of glaucoma
- be able to outline the management of the different types of glaucoma.

Introduction

The glaucomas are a group of conditions with the common pathological end point of optic nerve neuropathy commonly associated with raised intraocular pressure. The optic neuropathy can be observed clinically as optic disc cupping. The neuropathy leads to peripheral visual field loss and if untreated to blindness.

The exact pathophysiology of glaucomatous optic nerve neuropathy is unclear. It is, however, recognised that increasing age, family history of glaucoma, and raised intraocular pressure are risk factors for the development of the condition.

Intraocular pressure is dependent on the balance between the rate of production and drainage of aqueous humour (outflow). Aqueous fluid is produced by the ciliary body. It flows from the posterior chamber into the anterior chamber via the narrow gap between the lens and the iris (see Fig. 175). The fluid then drains mainly through the trabecular meshwork situated in the angle between the iris and the cornea, into the canal of Schlemm and subconjunctival venous circulation. Intraocular pressure within the normal population is less than 21 mmHg.

Raised intraocular pressure occurs when aqueous humour drainage becomes compromised. The 'build up' of aqueous humour leads to a rise in intraocular pressure. Raised intraocular pressure is not due to over-production of aqueous humour.

Reduction of the intraocular pressure in most patients can slow down and even halt the optic neuropathy and associated visual field loss. Both medical and surgical treatments are available to reduce pressure.

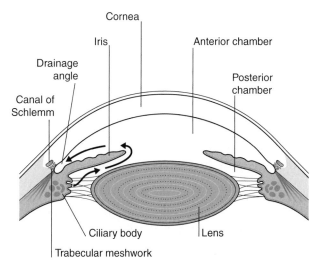

Fig. 175 Aqueous production, flow and drainage.

22.2 Primary open-angle glaucoma (POAG)

Learning objectives

You should:

- understand the anatomy of aqueous humour production and drainage
- understand the pathophysiology of POAG
- identify who is at risk of developing POAG
- recognise that POAG is initially asymptomatic but can lead to irreversible blindness
- understand that it is a condition suitable for screening in the community
- recognise which clinical signs are useful for screening
- appreciate that POAG requires lifetime treatment and follow up
- appreciate that some topical treatments may have serious systemic side effects.

Primary open-angle glaucoma is a bilateral condition usually seen in those over 40 years of age. It has a familial tendency with 10% of first-degree relatives developing the condition.

Clinical features

The onset is insidious and the patient is asymptomatic until very late in the disease. The condition is characterised by:

- raised intraocular pressure (>21 mmHg)
- optic disc cupping (see Fig. 176)
- characteristic visual field loss
- open drainage angle.

Patients with POAG may be identified at the asymptomatic stage by finding raised IOP (>21 mm Hg) and optic disc cupping with associated visual field defects. The visual field loss characteristically occurs initially as an arcuate pattern (see Fig. 177). The condition is therefore suitable for screening in the community. All patients attending an optometrist with a family history of POAG or over the age of 40 have these tests performed.

Management

Most referrals to the eye clinic come from optometrists. At the initial consultation the IOP is rechecked, the appearance of the optic disc recorded, the drainage angle observed and confirmed as 'open' and the visual fields assessed. An automated perimetry machine is

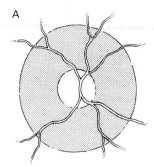
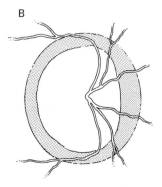
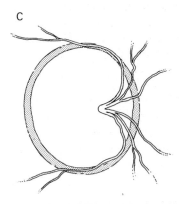

Fig. 176 Optic disc. **A.** Normal optic disc with small central cup. **B.** Early glaucomatous cupping with extension of the cup vertically. **C.** Advanced glaucomatous cupping.

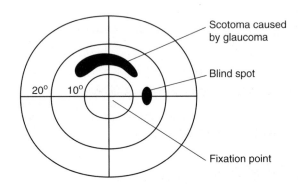

Fig. 177 Pattern of field loss in early open-angle glaucoma, in arcuate scotoma (or nerve fibre bundle defect).

commonly used to assess the visual fields and a print-out of the result added to the notes for future comparison. As previously discussed, reduction in IOP is the only treatment and can be achieved either medically or surgically.

Medical management

Medical management is normally first line and takes the form of a variety of topically applied intraocular pressure-lowering drops. One, two or even three drops may be prescribed at the same time depending on the control of the condition judged by optic disc cupping and visual field loss.

- beta-blockers (e.g. timolol) are the most common first-line treatment of POAG. They reduce aqueous production at the ciliary body. Beta-blockers should not be prescribed, even topically, to patients with reversible airways disease, heart block or heart failure as they are absorbed systemically and may aggravate these conditions
- sympathomimetics (e.g. brimonidine) reduce aqueous production
- prostaglandin analogues (e.g. latanoprost) increase aqueous drainage. They only need to be administered once per day. Common side effects include increased pigmentation of the iris and lengthening of the eyelashes.
- para-sympathomimetics (e.g. pilocarpine) reduce aqueous production and increase outflow via the trabecular meshwork. They cause miosis and often induce 'brow ache'. The miosis may lead to reduced visual acuity in patients with cataract. The drops need to be administered up to four times per day, which may reduce compliance in some patients.
- carbonic anhydrase inhibitors (e.g. dorzolamide drops topically and acetazolamide systemically) act at the ciliary body to reduce aqueous production.

Surgical treatment

A surgical trabeculectomy is an operation that creates a fistula between the anterior chamber and the sub-conjunctival venous plexus, bypassing the trabecular meshwork. This creates a new channel for aqueous drainage, which leads to reduced intraocular pressure. Trabeculectomy has a high success rate but may be complicated by intraocular infection, intraocular haemorrhage and premature cataract formation.

Ocular hypertension (OHT)

In some patients the IOP is greater than 21 mmHg but there is no evidence of optic disc cupping or typical visual field loss. This is termed 'ocular hypertension'. The patient does not require any treatment, although they should be reviewed regularly as they are at increased risk of developing glaucoma.

Low tension glaucoma (LTG)

A group of patients show evidence of optic disc cupping and typical visual field loss, despite consistently normal intraocular pressures (<21 mmHg). After an intracranial cause of visual field loss has been excluded, a diagnosis of 'low tension' glaucoma is made. This condition is very common and accounts for approximately 40% of patients suffering from glaucoma.

22.3 Acute closed-angle glaucoma (ACAG)

Learning objectives

You should:

- understand the anatomy of aqueous fluid/humour production and drainage
- understand the mechanism of the development of a closed angle
- appreciate who may be at risk of developing ACAG
- be able to make a diagnosis by taking a history and performing an examination
- be able to recommend appropriate management for a patient suffering from an acute attack.

Pathophysiology

ACAG develops when the normal flow of aqueous fluid between the lens and the iris at the pupil meets resistance. The resistance is known as 'pupil block' and is maximal when the pupil is mid-dilated. The aqueous fluid becomes trapped in the posterior chamber causing the iris to bow anteriorly (see Fig. 178). The peripheral iris obscures the trabecular meshwork in the drainage angle causing an acute, marked reduction in aqueous outflow. The IOP rises rapidly leading to pain and loss of vision. ACAG is more common in people with relatively small eyes with anatomically crowded anterior segment structures. Most patients with relatively small eyes are hypermetropic. The condition is also more common in elderly females, ocurring in the evening and winter months when the pupil is more likely to be mid-dilated. The instillation of dilating drops may also precipitate an attack.

Clinical features

The patient presents with an extremely painful red eye, which may be associated with nausea and vomiting.

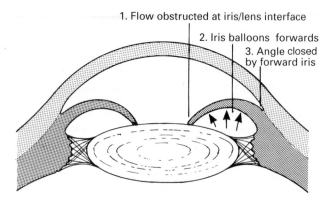

1. Flow obstructed at iris/lens interface
2. Iris balloons forwards
3. Angle closed by forward iris

Fig. 178 Sequence of events in acute closed-angle glaucoma.

The eye is diffusely red, there is no discharge, the cornea is cloudy and the pupil is mid-dilated and fixed. There is usually profound visual loss.

Prior to the acute episode, the patient may give a history of intermittent episodes of ocular pain and seeing haloes round lights, especially in the evenings.

The diagnosis is made on the basis of a typical history, in association with a shallow anterior chamber, extremely high IOP and a pupil that is mid-dilated and fixed. Digital pressure (i.e. simply pressing on the eye) reveals a brick-hard eye.

Management

The immediate aim is to make the patient feel more comfortable by prescribing analgesia and antiemetics as necessary. The IOP should then be lowered as quickly as possible using intravenous carbonic anhydrase inhibitors and topical hypotensive agents (see medical management of POAG). Intensive topical pilocarpine will miose the pupil, breaking the pupil block and opening the drainage angle to increase aqueous outflow.

After the acute attack has been reversed a laser peripheral iridotomy should be performed to prevent a further episode of ACAG. Because the fellow eye is similarly anatomically predisposed to an attack of ACAG, both eyes should be treated. A peripheral iridotomy is a small hole in the peripheral iris that allows aqueous fluid to flow directly from the posterior chamber into the anterior chamber, bypassing the pupil and any asso-

ciated 'pupil block'. This creates equal pressure in the posterior and anterior chambers reducing iris bowing and thus preventing a further episode of angle closure. Pressure control is not always achieved and medical treatment or tubeculectomy may be required (see POAG).

22.4 Congenital glaucoma

Learning objectives

You should:

- understand the anatomy of aqueous production and drainage

- be able to recognise the presentation features of congenital glaucoma.

- appreciate its implications for the child and parents

- appreciate that management is often surgical and follow up is lifelong.

Congenital glaucoma

Primary congenital glaucoma is an extremely rare condition which is usually bilateral and is due to abnormal development of the anterior chamber drainage angle. Most cases are sporadic; however, some have a familial background.

Clinical features

In the early stages, the cornea becomes oedematous, which causes photophobia and watering of the eye. Affected infants commonly rub their eyes. In untreated or poorly controlled disease, the eye becomes enlarged and may go blind.

Management

The drainage angle may be opened surgically (goniotomy) to increase outflow. Although treatment is usually surgical, drops may be employed to augment it.

Self-assessment: questions

Multiple choice questions

1. Primary open-angle glaucoma:
   a. causes severe pain
   b. is associated with a normal visual field
   c. has a familial tendency
   d. is associated with disc cupping
   e. may be treated by peripheral iridotomy

2. The following are characteristic of acute closed-angle glaucoma:
   a. myopic refractive error
   b. severe ocular pain
   c. mid-dilated fixed pupil
   d. normal vision
   e. nausea and vomiting

Extended matching items questions (EMIs)

1. Theme: Glaucoma

A the optic nerve
B trabecular meshwork
C Descemet's membrane
D corneal endothelium
E ciliary body
F iris–lens interface
G capsule of the lens
H Schwalbe's line
I vitreous cavity
J iris

Match the function from below with the correct structure from above:

1. The main site of aqueous humour drainage from the eye.
2. The site of 'pupil block'.
3. The main site of aqueous humour production in the eye.

2. Theme: Glaucoma

A timolol maleate
B dorzolamide
C brimonidine tartrate
D latanoprost
E adrenaline
F benoxinate
G cyclopentolate
H tropicamide
I pilocarpine
J acetazolamide

Match the description below with the correct drug from above:

1. This topical medication acts at the ciliary body and reduces aqueous humour production. It is contraindicated in patients with asthma and heart block.
2. This systemic medication acts at the ciliary body and reduces aqueous humour production.

3. This topical medication causes miosis and reduces intraocular pressure. It is helpful in breaking 'pupil block' in acute closed-angle glaucoma.

Constructed response questions (CRQs)

CRQ 1

A 78-year-old woman is referred to the eye clinic by her optometrist because at a recent routine appointment raised intraocular pressure (>21 mmHg), optic disc cupping and visual field loss were found. She is asymptomatic.

a. What condition is most likely to be responsible for the findings above?
b. Is it surprising that she is asymptomatic?
c. List some risk factors for developing this condition.
d. What initial management is she likely to be prescribed?

CRQ 2

A 56-year-old male was found by his optometrist to have raised intraocular pressures of 32 mmHg in both eyes. He also had optic disc cupping in both eyes with associated advanced visual field loss. After examination at the local eye clinic the drainage angle was confirmed as 'open' and a diagnosis of primary open-angle glaucoma (POAG) was made.

a. State the site at which aqueous humour is produced.
b. State the site of aqueous humour drainage.
c. What is the reason for raised intraocular pressure in POAG?

The patient was prescribed topical beta-blockers by the eye clinic.

d. State how topical beta-blockers reduce intraocular pressure.

The patient's intraocular pressure does not reduce on topical medical treatments and the visual field loss and optic disc cupping advance.

e. Explain how surgical trabeculectomy reduces intraocular pressure.

Objective structured clinical examinations questions (OSCEs)

OSCE 1

> A 69-year-old woman presented to her GP complaining of intermittent pain around her right eye. The episodes are associated with blurred vision characterised by the perception of haloes around bright lights. The episodes tend to develop in the evening but settle once she falls asleep. Over the past 24 hours, however, her right eye has been constantly painful and she has felt nauseated, vomiting twice.

a. What is the most likely cause of her symptoms? Figure 179 shows her spectacles.
b. State the type of lens in the spectacles.
c. What type of refractive error would these spectacles correct?
d. Is this patient's refractive error relevant to her presentation? Justify your answer.
e. Describe some of the common eye signs that you would expect to see in this patient's right eye on presentation.

> Her family doctor organises immediate referral to the local eye department.

f. What might the GP prescribe in the surgery to offer symptomatic relief until she is seen in the eye department?

OSCE 2

> A 71-year-old man who suffers from asthma is referred to the eye clinic because at a recent routine optometrist appointment an 'abnormal' optic disc was noticed in the right eye. The patient is asymptomatic.

a. Describe the abnormalities seen in Figure 180 of the patient's right optic disc.
b. What condition might the patient have?

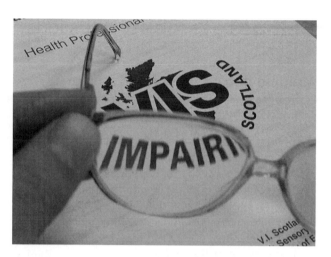

Fig. 179

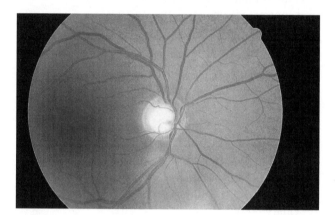

Fig. 180

c. What other tests might the optometrist perform to help make a diagnosis?
d. What field defect might the patient display?
e. What group of intraocular-pressure-lowering drugs are contraindicated in this man?
f. Name two other classes of topical intraocular-pressure-lowering drugs that would be suitable alternatives.

Viva questions

1. What is ocular hypertension (OHT)?

2. Discuss the treatment of primary open-angle glaucoma (POAG)?

Self-assessment: answers

Multiple choice answers

1. a. **False.** Pain is characteristic of acute closed-angle glaucoma.
   b. **False.** The diagnosis of glaucoma is dependent on the finding of optic disc cupping and associated consistent visual field defect.
   c. **True.** 10% of first-degree relatives of open-angle glaucoma sufferers will develop the condition.
   d. **True.** The diagnosis of glaucoma is dependent on the finding of optic disc cupping and associated consistent visual field defect.
   e. **False.** A peripheral iridectomy equalises the pressure between the posterior and anterior chambers, overcoming 'pupil block' and flattening the iris plane. This is an important procedure in the prophylaxis and treatment of angle-closure glaucoma; however, in open-angle glaucoma this will have no effect on the overall intraocular pressure. If medical treatment has failed or the patient is intolerant of topical medication then surgical trabeculectomy is indicated to reduce intraocular pressure.

2. a. **False.** Closed-angle glaucoma is more common in small, hypermetropic eyes with anatomically crowded drainage angles. Myopic eyes are larger and are very unlikely to develop closed-angle glaucoma.
   b. **True.** Patients presenting with closed-angle glaucoma characteristically complain of a painful red eye with reduced visual acuity.
   c. **True.** One of the most important features of acute closed-angle glaucoma, which differentiates it from other causes of a red painful eye, is the presence of a mid-dilated, unreactive pupil sometimes difficult to discern because of associated corneal haze.
   d. **False.** The endothelial cells which line the cornea constantly remove fluid from the corneal stroma maintaining its clarity. A significant and acute rise in intraocular pressure compromises the function of these endothelial cells. Loss of corneal clarity therefore occurs during an attack of acute closed-angle glaucoma leading to reduced visual acuity.
   e. **True.** Nausea and vomiting during an attack of acute closed-angle glaucoma is common.

EMI answers

1. Theme: Glaucoma

1. B The trabecular meshwork in the drainage angle is the main site of aqueous fluid/humour drainage.
2. F The flow of aqueous fluid/humour from the posterior chamber into the anterior chamber may slow and become 'blocked' at the narrow lens–iris interface. This can lead to 'bowing' forward of the iris and may lead to angle-closure glaucoma.
3. E The ciliary body is the single site of aqueous humour production.

2. Theme: Glaucoma

1. A Timolol is a beta-blocker. It is absorbed into the systemic blood stream and therefore caution is required in patients with asthma, heart block, bradycardia or heart failure. It may interact with verapamil and precipitate heart block.
2. J The only effective oral ocular hypotensive drug is acetazolamide. It is a diuretic and if used chronically may lead to a hypokalaemic metabolic acidosis. It is a sulfonamide derivative and may precipitate Stevens–Johnson syndrome.
3. I Pilocarpine is a parasympathetic agonist. It causes miosis. It reduces intraocular pressure and is used in breaking pupil block in acute closed-angle glaucoma.

CRQ answers

CRQ 1

a. Primary open-angle glaucoma (POAG).
b. No. This condition is characteristically asymptomatic until advanced disease occurs.
c. Increasing age, family history and raised intraocular pressure.
d. Medical: topical beta-blockers.

CRQ 2

a. Ciliary body.
b. The main drainage site is the trabecular meshwork.
c. The main reason for raised intraocular pressure is a reduction in aqueous humour drainage. A 'build-up' therefore occurs and intraocular pressure becomes raised. Increased production of aqueous humour is not a cause of raised intraocular pressure.

d. Beta-blockers act at the ciliary body by reducing aqueous humour production.

e. A surgical trabeculectomy is a fistualising procedure that connects the anterior chamber to the subconjunctival venous plexus. This creates a new channel for aqueous humour drainage, which leads to reduced intraocular pressure.

OSCE answers

OSCE 1

a. Acute closed-angle glaucoma, almost certainly preceded by chronic intermittent closed-angle glaucoma.

b. Convex, plus lens which converges light and so magnifies the image.

c. Hypermetropia.

d. Yes: hypermetropia is associated with smaller eyes. Smaller eyes tend to have anatomically crowded anterior segments, which are more prone to angle closure.

e. A red eye with reduced visual acuity, hazy cornea and a fixed, mid-dilated pupil. Digital palpation through closed eyelids would reveal a 'firm' eye compared with the fellow eye owing to the raised intraocular pressure.

f. Antiemetics and analgesia. There is no indication for patching or any other treatment until the patient is seen in the eye clinic.

OSCE 2

a. Optic disc cupping with an uneven neuroretinal rim.

b. The signs above are characteristic of glaucomatous optic nerve neuropathy. The patient may have primary open-angle glaucoma. As the patient is asymptomatic with no pain or redness, an 'open-angle' form is most likely.

c. Visual field examination using automated perimetry: by confirming visual field loss consistent with the optic disc appearance then the presence of glaucoma is more likely.

Intraocular pressure check, if the intraocular pressure is raised (>21 mmHg) then again glaucoma is more likely. Even if the pressure is within the normal range, 'low tension' glaucoma (LTG) may still be present.

d. Arcuate visual field defects.

e. Beta-blockers.

f. Suitable second-line agents include:

- carbonic anhydrase inhibitors (dorzolamide)
- parasympathomimetics (pilocarpine)
- sympathomimetics (brimonidine)
- prostaglandin analogues (latanoprost).

Viva answers

1. Ocular hypertension is a condition where the intraocular pressure is elevated beyond the normal range of 21 mmHg, but where there is no evidence of any optic disc cupping and the fields of vision are full. The patient should be observed and no treatment is required.

2. Medical and surgical treatment may be employed in the management of glaucoma. Medical treatment involves the use of a variety of classes of drugs which include, topically and systemically:

- beta-blockers
- sympathomimetics
- prostaglandin analogues
- para sympathomimetics
- carbonic anhydrase inhibitors.

All the drugs act to reduce intraocular pressure. One, two or even three drops may be prescribed at the same time depending on the control of the condition judged by optic disc cupping and visual field loss.

A surgical trabeculectomy is a fistualising procedure that connects the anterior chamber to the subconjunctival venous plexus. This creates a new channel for aqueous drainage, which leads to reduced intraocular pressure.

23 Ocular injuries

Chapter overview

This chapter describes the causes, effects and management of ocular trauma. Most trauma occurs in young males and is preventable by altering risky behaviour and wearing appropriate eye protection. While most trauma is trivial a significant minority of injuries lead to profound irreversible loss of vision despite surgical intervention. Emphasis is placed upon the history and clinical signs which suggest a serious eye injury requiring immediate intervention and referral to an ophthalmologist.

Introduction

Injuries to the eye are an important cause of ocular morbidity and visual impairment. The majority occur in young men. Most are superficial, with less than 30% being considered sight threatening. The common causes are sport and leisure activities, accidents in the workplace or home, assaults and road traffic accidents.

Prevention of injuries

The treatment of eye injuries is expensive and in many cases disappointing. The best method of reducing this burden is prevention. Although effective protective eyewear is available for most high-risk activities, such as sports and work, it is unfortunately infrequently worn properly.

23.1 Blunt injuries

Learning objectives

You should:

- appreciate the causes of blunt trauma
- appreciate that causes of blunt trauma are preventable
- understand the mechanical effects of blunt trauma upon the eye and orbit
- recognise the clinical signs of blunt trauma
- be able to recommend appropriate management and investigations
- appreciate the potential short- and long-term complications.

Blunt injuries are the most common type of eye injury. They are caused by a direct blow to the eye and surrounding tissues by an object such as a fist or a ball. Rapidly moving objects are more damaging than those moving at a lower velocity, even if they are larger and heavier.

If the eye is struck, the globe flattens antero-posteriorly and becomes stretched equatorially (Fig. 181); thus intra-ocular structures are damaged by a combination of contusional and tearing forces. No penetration takes place, although in severe cases rupture of the periorbital skin or eyeball may occur.

Clinical features

Common features of blunt ocular trauma include:

- periorbital haematoma (black eye)
- blow-out fracture (or orbital floor fracture). Significant blunt trauma leads to a rapid rise in intraorbital pressure. The contents of the orbit decompress into the sinuses surrounding the orbit causing a fracture of the floor of the orbit in which the orbital rim remains intact (Fig. 182). This often leads to double vision and the appearance of a sunken orbit (enophthalmos). It is often also associated with infraorbital paraesthesia
- subconjunctival haemorrhage (diffuse bleeding under the conjunctiva)

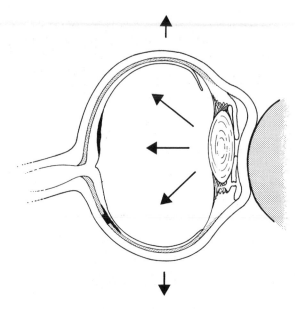

Fig. 181 When the eye is struck, it is deformed and intraocular structures are damaged.

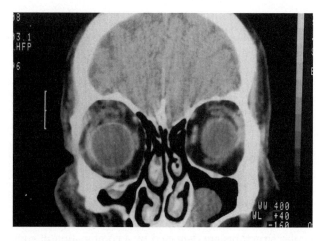

Fig. 182 A 'blow-out' fracture of the right orbit, shown on CT scan. The orbit is expanded and there is evidence of a prolapse of tissue into the maxillary antrum through the orbital floor (the tear-drop sign).

* corneal abrasion: an acutely painful injury that can be detected by instilling fluorescein drops into the conjunctival sac. The abraded area will stain bright green when viewed with a blue light
* hyphaema (blood in the anterior chamber; see Fig. 183). This indicates that the eye has suffered a significant injury with damage to the intraocular structures. The eye is usually acutely painful, especially if the intraocular pressure is elevated, which is a common effect of blood in the eye
* sight-threatening complications include retinal holes, choroidal tears and rupture of the globe.

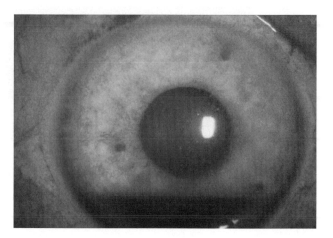

Fig. 183 Hyphaema.

Management

Black eyes and subconjunctival haemorrhages settle spontaneously over a few days without any treatment. Corneal abrasions are treated with antibiotic ointment and firm padding. Blow-out fractures only require surgical intervention if double vision persists or the appearance is cosmetically unacceptable. In cases of intraocular damage, full examination of the eye may not be possible until bleeding has settled and the eye is comfortable, which may be 3–4 weeks after the injury. Patients may require hospital admission. Complications such as increased intraocular pressure and rebleeding are treated medically. Examination should include that of the peripheral retina for tears and an assessment of the drainage angle.

Early complications:

* raised intraocular pressure
* uveitis
* rebleeding of hyphaemas.

Long-term complications:

* premature cataract
* glaucoma
* retinal detachment.

23.2 Small flying particle injuries

Learning objectives

You should:

* recognise the causes of small flying particle injuries
* appreciate that small flying particle injuries are preventable

- recognise the difference in symptoms between an intraocular foreign body and a corneal foreign body

- recognise the difference in clinical appearance between an intraocular foreign body and a corneal foreign body

- be able to investigate appropriately

- be able to prescribe appropriate management and refer when necessary

- appreciate the potential complications of small flying particle injuries.

Low-velocity foreign material tends to lodge on the cornea as a corneal foreign body (CFB) or under the lid as a subtarsal foreign body (STFB). High-velocity particles penetrate the globe to become intraocular foreign bodies (IOFB). Any injury that may have been caused by a high-velocity small particle (e.g. hammering injuries) should be treated as a potentially penetrating IOFB until proven otherwise, i.e. an X-ray of the eye should be performed or an experienced ophthalmologist's opinion sought before discounting this diagnosis.

Clinical features

Superficial FBs cause a significant amount of pain, watering, redness and photophobia. Paradoxically, intraocular foreign material may be less painful and the symptoms are frequently minor.

Corneal foreign bodies can usually be seen on close inspection of the cornea, and staining with fluorescein helps to demarcate the area. STFBs can be seen when the upper eyelid is everted.

IOFBs may be difficult to see on examination.

Management

Corneal foreign bodies can be removed by a small cotton tip or a sharp needle (under magnification after the administration of topical anaesthetic). A STFB can be swept off the inside of the lid with a cotton tip after everting the lid. If there is any epithelial damage from the superficial FB, then topical antibiotic agents should be prescribed.

IOFBs require surgical removal. This may involve loss of the lens, iris or vitreous humour if they are damaged by the injury.

Complications

The damaged epithelium of the cornea may not heal satisfactorily after a CFB or a STFB, leading to a recurrent corneal erosion, a painful condition caused by recurrent breakdown of a tiny area of the epithelial surface.

The long-term effects of an IOFB depend on the degree of intraocular damage and the type and size of

material that penetrated the eye. Organic material may rapidly lead to suppuration of the intraocular contents, and metallic foreign bodies oxidise and combine with the intraocular proteins (siderosis) if not removed in the early period.

23.3 Large sharp objects

Learning objectives

You should:

- appreciate that ocular injuries are preventable

- recognise the signs of a penetrating eye injury

- be able to manage and refer appropriately

- appreciate the potential short- and long-term complications of a penetrating injury.

Injuries caused by large sharp objects may penetrate the eye.

Clinical features

The clinical features depend on the extent of the injury, ranging from superficial damage to the lids and eye to full ocular penetration with globe disruption.

Ocular penetrations may manifest as an irregular pupil because the iris plugs the wound to prevent the loss of intraocular contents; or the eyes may be softer than normal (Fig. 184). The vision is usually reduced.

One should aways be suspicious that full thickness lid lacerations may involve the underlying sclera and retina.

Management

Lid lacerations, like any facial injuries, require careful skin closure. However, as the lacrimal drainage appar-

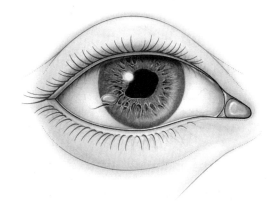

Fig. 184 Penetrating injury. A corneal laceration is seen, with the iris plugging the wound causing an irregular pupil.

atus is situated at the medial aspect of the lid, injuries in this area may require specialist evaluation and treatment.

A primary repair for globe penetration should be performed urgently. Multiple surgical procedures may subsequently be required for the optimum result.

Complications

- corneal scarring
- cataract
- endophthalmitis
- sympathetic ophthalmia
- astigmatism.

Sympathetic ophthalmia is a very rare granulomatous inflammation that affects both eyes after a penetrating injury to one eye. The injured (exciting) eye sets up this response in itself as well as in the other (sympathising) eye. This usually occurs within 3 months of the injury. Removal of the injured eye before the sympathetic response starts prevents the onset of the condition; however, once established, removal of the exciting eye does not help. The response to steroids and immuno-suppressants is usually favourable. Removal of an injured eye should, therefore, not be considered purely on the grounds of the risk of sympathetic ophthalmia but be based on the visual potential of the eye.

23.4 Burns

Learning objectives

You should:

- recognise the causes of burns to the eye
- appreciate that ocular burns are preventable
- recognise the significance of an alkali chemical injury
- be able to instigate appropriate and immediate management for a chemical injury and refer when necessary
- appreciate the potential complications of burns to the eyes.

Burns to the eye are divided into chemical or physical burns.

Chemical burns

Burns caused by acids or alkalis are a medical emergency. Alkalis denature proteins and their burns tend to be more extensive and penetrating than acid burns.

Clinical features

Patients with chemical burns to the eye are in severe pain. There may be lid swelling, oedema of the conjunctiva, corneal and conjunctival epithelial loss, uveitis, raised intraocular pressure, corneal melting, cataract and peripheral retinal damage.

Management

Any patient with a history of a chemical being splashed into the eyes must be treated with immediate copious irrigation (at least 1 litre) of the affected eyes with water or normal saline. Any particulate material (e.g. lime) should be looked for and removed from the fornices or subtarsal areas urgently. There should be no delay to obtain a careful history or to examine the eyes.

Once thorough irrigation has been completed (20–30 minutes), the extent of damage may be evaluated. pH paper can be applied to the tear film to assess if all acid or alkali has been removed. If the pH is not around neutral then irrigation should be recommenced until all chemical has been washed away.

Corneal and conjunctival epithelium may be totally lost. In addition, the blood vessels may be destroyed leading to areas of scleral ischaemia and the cornea may be rendered opaque.

Complications

Are more commonly seen in alkali injuries. Acids may cause corneal and conjunctival injury but without the other complications listed below.

- severe corneal and conjunctival scarring
- raised intraocular pressure
- cataract
- necrosis of sclera
- ultimate perforation of the eye with loss of useful vision.

Physical burns

Physical burns can be caused by:

- thermal energy
- ultraviolet (UV)
- shorter-wave radiation (e.g. radiotherapy).

Thermal burns do not usually involve the globe itself, as reflex blinking provides natural protection.

UV radiation is absorbed by the corneal epithelium, which causes the conditions of snow blindness or welding flash burns.

Iatrogenic ocular damage may occur from radiation used to treat head and neck cancers and may not become evident until many years later. It usually manifests as premature cataract and radiation retinal vasculitis.

Self-assessment: questions

Multiple choice questions

1. An intraocular foreign body (IOFB):
   a. often requires an X-ray or ultrasound scan to confirm its presence
   b. should be suspected in patients with injuries involving high-velocity particles
   c. is usually very painful
   d. needs urgent surgical removal
   e. can cause irreversible damage to the retina

2. Alkali burns of the eye:
   a. are potentially more serious than acid burns
   b. should be treated by neutralising with acid
   c. are a cause of entropion
   d. are a medical emergency
   e. can cause necrosis of the sclera

Extended matching items questions (EMIs)

1. Theme: Ocular injuries

A periorbital bruising, lid laceration, subconjunctival haemorrhage, hyphaema, sluggish mid-dilated pupil and reduced visual acuity
B sticky, gritty eye with a yellow discharge
C limbal injection, keratic precipitates and a misshapen pupil
D complete corneal epithelial loss, hazy cornea, blanching of conjunctival blood vessels with reduced visual acuity
E bilateral red itchy eyes with red eyelids
F tortuous retinal veins and widespread retinal haemorrhages
G bilateral proptosis with restricted eye movements
H small corneal laceration, focal lens opacity and normal visual acuity. A small metallic object can be seen in the vitreous cavity
I ptosis on the same side as an eye pointing down and out
J small peripheral corneal white opacification with localised sectorial conjunctival injection and red inflamed eyelids

Match the mechanism of injury below with the most appropriate clinical description above:

1. Small high-velocity penetrating injury with intraocular foreign body.
2. Severe blunt trauma.
3. Severe chemical injury.

2. Theme: Ocular injuries

A mild blunt trauma with no hyphaema
B lid laceration
C chemical injury
D solar retinopathy from eclipse gazing
E intraocular foreign body
F corneal abrasion
G corneal foreign body
H blow-out fracture
I large corneal laceration
J severe blunt trauma with hyphaema

Match the correct management below with the most appropriate type of injury from above:

1. Take enough history to confirm the nature of the injury then proceed with immediate irrigation with copious saline for a minimum of 20 to 30 minutes. After the initial irrigation assess the pH of the tear film. Only stop irrigation once the pH is neutral.
2. Remove the foreign body under topical local anaesthetic with a sterile needle. Prescribe topical antibiotic eye ointment and analgesia.
3. Monitor eye movements and cosmetic appearance. If intractable double vision is present in primary and down gaze or cosmetically unacceptable enophthalmos remains then consider surgery.

Constructed response questions (CRQs)

CRQ 1

A 28-year-old joiner presents to Accident and Emergency complaining of a foreign body sensation in his right eye. He felt something entering his eye while hammering nails into a wooden stake.

a. Should he have been wearing eye protection while hammering and why?
b. What type of injury requires to be excluded?
c. What is the visual acuity likely to measure?
d. Give three possible signs of an IOFB.
e. What investigations would help in assessing the patient?

CRQ 2

A painter and decorator presents to Accident and Emergency complaining of increasing photophobia, grittiness and reduced visual acuity in his left eye. He describes some plaster falling in to it about 6 hours earlier. He wiped most of the plaster away at the time and continued to work.

a. What type of injury may this patient be suffering from?
b. What should the initial management in Accident and Emergency be?
c. For how long should irrigation be carried out and what investigation can be performed to help in deciding when to stop?
d. What signs will be helpful in assessing the severity of a chemical injury?

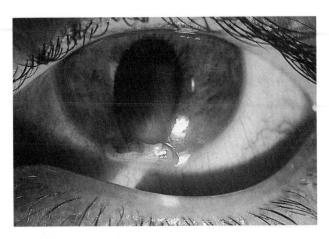

Fig. 185

Objective structured clinical examination questions (OSCEs)

OSCE 1

This patient was cutting a carpet with a sharp blade. His hand slipped and the blade caught him in his right eye.

a. Describe the findings seen in Figure 185.
b. What symptoms is he likely to complain of?
c. What complications may he develop?
d. What treatment is required?

OSCE 2

A 54-year-old builder presented to Accident and Emergency complaining of a gritty, red, photophobic, watering right eye.

a. Describe the findings in Figure 186.
b. What questions should the examining doctor ask regarding the mechanism of the injury?
c. What management is recommended?
d. What physical signs might suggest an IOFB?

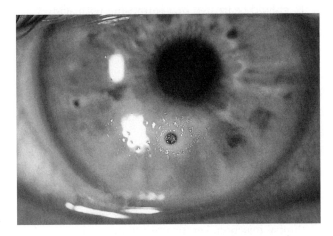

Fig. 186

e. What investigation in Accident and Emergency would help confirm a metallic IOFB?

Viva questions

1. Define hyphaema and discuss its causes and complications.

2. Describe what a blow-out fracture is. Describe the clinical features of such an injury.

Self-assessment: answers

Multiple choice answers

1. a. **True.** IOFBs can be painless and may easily be missed on clinical examination. Imaging investigations are necessary to confidently exclude an IOFB.
   b. **True.** Any person who presents with an eye injury which has been caused by a high-velocity flying particle must be suspected as having an IOFB. Hammering injuries are common causes of IOFBs, as the head of a hammer becomes brittle with use and small pieces tend to fly off and enter the eye.
   c. **False.** IOFBs can be painless.
   d. **True.** They must be removed as soon as possible to reduce the chance of infection and irreversible toxicity to the retina.
   e. **True.** IOFBs if left unnoticed within the eye can cause slow, progressive irreversible toxic damage to the retina.

2. a. **True.** Acid causes coagulation of tissues forming a barrier to further spread. Alkalis are absorbed by tissues penetrating further causing more extensive injuries.
   b. **False.** Immediate copious irrigation with saline until the pH is neutral is the recommended management.
   c. **True.** They may cause scarring (cicatricial) changes of the conjunctiva which may lead to 'inturning' of the eyelid (entropion) (see Ch. 16).
   d. **True.** Alkali burns are potentially serious sight-threatening injuries which need to be treated urgently.
   e. **True.** An alkali injury can cause damage to scleral blood vessels. This can lead to ischaemia and scleral necrosis.

EMI answers

1. Theme: Ocular injuries

1. H   Although the IOFB cannot be seen, the findings are suggestive of a small high-velocity foreign body having penetrated the cornea and lens. This clinical scenario is often seen in the context of a history of 'hammer and chisel' injury and the absence of protective goggles. A dilated fundal examination and further investigations are required to exclude an IOFB.
2. A   Periorbital bruising associated with the presence of a hyphaema confirms a significant traumatic injury. A thorough examination for other ocular injuries is required.
3. D   The combination of findings described is characteristic of a severe chemical injury. Blanching of blood vessels suggests a severe injury; consequently, the appearance of a white eye can be misleadingly reassuring sign. Immediate copious saline irrigation is required.

2. Theme: Ocular injuries

1. C   If a patient gives a history of chemical injury it is important not to delay in starting irrigation. Complete the history and examination once the pH of the tear film has neutralised.
2. G   This description is appropriate management for a corneal foreign body.
3. H   An orbital blow-out fracture only requires to be repaired if the patient is symptomatic from double vision or cosmetically unacceptable enophthalmos remains.

CRQ answers

CRQ 1

a. Yes, as this would have reduced the chance of a small high-velocity foreign body entering the eye.
b. An intraocular foreign body needs to be excluded. If goggles were not worn at the time of the injury an IOFB is more likely.
c. The vision can often be normal (6/6), but it may also be reduced. Visual acuity is not a helpful sign in identifying an IOFB and therefore emphasis is placed on the history of the mechanism of injury.
d. Signs of an IOFB include:

   • a misshapen pupil might suggest iris trauma from a high-velocity foreign body
   • the presence of a penetrating laceration would be highly suggestive of an IOFB
   • a hyphaema in the anterior chamber would suggest iris damage, while a shallow anterior chamber might suggest the presence of a corneal laceration and leak
   • any evidence of a localised lens opacity or dislocation is suggestive of the passage of a foreign body
   • during dilated fundal examination, an IOFB maybe seen as well as retinal tears, holes or detachment.

e. Orbital X-rays or an ultrasound examination are very helpful in excluding a metallic foreign body.

Glass and wooden foreign bodies are poorly seen on X-ray but are normally still evident by ultrasound.

CRQ 2

a. This patient may be suffering from a variety of injuries including:

- subtarsal or corneal foreign body
- corneal abrasion
- alkali chemical injury.

b. Lime is found in plaster and may cause a severe alkali chemical injury. Immediate irrigation with saline to remove remaining pieces of plaster and dilute the alkali tear film is necessary.

c. Most chemical injuries will require between 15 and 30 minutes irrigation with saline.

d. Signs suggestive of a severe chemical injury include:

- poor visual acuity
- gross corneal epithelial loss
- a hazy cornea
- anterior chamber inflammation
- raised intraocular pressure
- blanching of conjunctival blood vessels.

OSCE answers

OSCE 1

a. 4 mm long inferior corneal laceration with iris prolapse and a misshapen pupil.
b. Painful, watering eye with reduced visual acuity.
c. Corneal astigmatism, endophthalmitis and sympathetic ophthalmia.
d. Surgical repair of the laceration.

OSCE 2

a. A central dark corneal opacity is seen. The conjunctiva is only mildly injected. The pupil is round and the pupil space appears dark with no evidence of lens opacity. There is no evidence of hyphaema in the anterior chamber. The appearances are suggestive of a metallic corneal foreign body

which has rusted. There is no evidence of a penetrating injury.

b. It is important to exclude a 'hammer and chisel' type of injury where a small high-velocity foreign body may have penetrated the eye. A penetrating injury is more likely if the patient was not wearing eye protection, which must also be enquired about in the history.

c. Remove the foreign body and rust and prescribe chloramphenicol ointment. If the patient is photophobic then topical cyclopentolate and analgesia may help. A dilated examination is important to exclude an IOFB.

d. Reduced or normal visual acuity, corneal laceration, flat anterior chamber, irregular-shaped pupil, lens opacity, vitreous haemorrhage and a retinal tear or detachment.

e. An orbital X-ray.

Viva answers

1. Hyphaema is the presence of blood within the anterior chamber. It is usually secondary to blunt trauma and is often visible as a level of blood at the bottom of the chamber. Rarely a hyphaema may occur spontaneously from abnormal bleeding iris vessels. Usually, however, the presence of a hyphaema suggests a significant injury. The eye requires a thorough examination for associated pathology such as damage to the drainage angle, lens dislocation and retinal tears. There is a risk of immediate, secondary and longer-term raised intraocular pressure.

2. Significant blunt trauma to the eye causes the contents of the orbit to decompress into the sinuses surrounding the orbit. The medial wall and floor of the orbit commonly fracture. Orbital tissues may consequently prolapse into the ethmoid and maxillary sinuses.

   Clinical features include:

   - infraorbital anaesthesia
   - a sunken appearing eye (enophthalmos)
   - double vision.

24 Neuro-ophthalmology

Chapter overview

Visual information from the eyes is transferred via the optic nerves, chiasm, optic tracts, lateral geniculate bodies and optic radiations to the occipital cortex for interpretation and integration. A number of pathological processes can occur at any point along this pathway causing defects in the patient's visual field. This chapter discusses these processes, highlighting the classical symptoms and signs of each condition. The difference between pre-and postchiasmal visual field defects is emphasised. Recommended investigations and management are described.

The neurology of the pupil is described and the clinical symptoms and signs created by the different pathological processes that can affect it.

24.1 Prechiasmal pathway

Learning objectives

You should:

- understand the anatomy of the visual pathway
- recognise the different conditions which affect the optic nerve and chiasm
- appreciate the symptoms and signs of the different conditions
- be able to recommend appropriate investigations and management.

Optic nerve

The optic nerve is part of the central nervous system and, as such, can be involved in neurological diseases as well as diseases of the eye (e.g. glaucoma). In this section, conditions of the optic nerve considered are:

- optic neuritis
- anterior ischaemic optic neuropathy
- papilloedema
- optic atrophy.

Optic neuritis

This is inflammation of the optic nerve, which usually occurs in adults aged 15–50 as a result of demyelination or viral infections; many cases are idiopathic.

When the optic nerve head is involved this is termed papillitis and when the nerve behind the globe is affected it is called retrobulbar neuritis. These conditions have the same aetiology, management and implications; they simply involve slightly different areas of the optic nerve.

Clinical features
The main clinical features are:

- usually one eye affected
- reduction in vision over a few days with loss of colour vision (may be mild or severe, but the patient finds that bright red appears as a desaturated red or pink)
- pain when moving the eye, especially upwards
- gradual recovery of visual function begins 1–4 weeks after the onset
- further blurring of vision with exertion or increases of heat (Uhtoff's phenomenon).

The only sign of optic neuritis may be an afferent pupillary defect (see below) in association with poor visual acuity. Patients with papillitis also have swelling of the optic nerve head. Field of vision testing demonstrates a central scotoma in the affected eye. The visual evoked response demonstrates increased latency.

Management
Management is simply observation and awaiting the spontaeneous recovery of vision.

Complications

In a small proportion of patients, the vision does not recover; in particular, the colour perception remains abnormal.

Anterior ischaemic optic neuropathy

Anterior ischaemic optic neuropathy (AION) represents an infarction of the optic nerve head, usually affecting patients over 60. It is caused by vascular disease. Two types are recognised:

- arteritic (most commonly due to giant cell arteritis)
- atherosclerotic.

Clinical features

The clinical features of each type of anterior ischaemic optic neuropathy are similar:

- rapid, painless loss of vision in the affected eye but may affect the upper or lower field only (altitudinal field defect, Fig. 187)
- vision usually significantly impaired (counting fingers or less)
- disc swelling, with haemorrhages around the posterior pole
- no visual recovery.

It is important to differentiate between arteritic and atherosclerotic causes, as this has important implications regarding management.

Diagnosis

Arteritic. Diagnosis of the arteritic variety is made on the basis of the patient suffering from a systemic disorder consisting of general malaise, headaches, muscle tenderness and jaw claudication in the presence of an elevated ESR (usually > 100) or elevated plasma viscosity. A temporal artery biopsy is indicated to establish the diagnosis unequivocally.

Atherosclerotic. Those with the atherosclerotic type may have symptoms of generalised arteriopathic disease, such as angina or intermittent claudication.

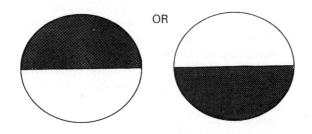

Fig. 187 Altitudinal field defect; loss of upper or lower field.

Management

Arteritic. Systemic steroids are used in those with temporal arteritis. High doses of systemic steroids for those with features of giant cell arteritis must be commenced immediately to preserve the vision in the other eye, which is also at risk of developing visual loss. Steroid treatment may be required for many years. There is a 65% chance of the other eye being affected within 10 days.

Atherosclerotic. No effective treatment is available for atherosclerotic cases. Associated risk factors such as hypertension, diabetes and hypercholesterolaemia should, however, be identified and treated.

Complications

- the other eye becomes affected (almost invariably in those with temporal arteritis without treatment, and in approximately 30% of the others)
- generalised complications of vascular disease.

Papilloedema

This term refers to swelling of the optic nerve head caused by increased intracranial pressure. Intracranial space-occupying lesions and benign intracranial hypertension (pseudo-tumour cerebri) are the most common causes.

Clinical features

The main clinical features are:

- symptoms of raised intracranial pressure (headaches, nausea and vomiting)
- ophthalmoscopy reveals elevation of the optic disc, blurring of the disc margins, dilatation of the retinal veins and haemorrhages around the disc
- field of vision testing may show an enlarged blind spot
- visual acuity is usually unaffected.

Diagnosis

Intracranial imaging with CT or MRI should reveal any intracranial mass. If this is negative, a lumbar puncture should be performed to measure the intracranial pressure.

Management

Treat the cause of the raised intracranial pressure.

Optic atrophy

This is not a diagnosis but is a clinical sign that may result from a number of different disease processes that affect the optic nerve:

- optic neuritis
- ischaemic optic neuropathy

- chronic papilloedema
- optic nerve tumours
- optic nerve trauma
- ocular disease (e.g. glaucoma, retinal artery occlusion).

Clinical features

Reduction in visual acuity or field of vision is a usual clinical finding. The presenting complaint usually depends on the underlying cause.

Management

Treat the underlying cause.

Optic chiasm

The optic chiasm is the area of the visual pathways where the visual pathways partially cross. The chiasm is situated just above the pituitary gland, and enlarging adenomas of the pituitary, usually chromophobes or eosinophils, are a common cause of compression to the chiasm.

With respect to age the common causes of chiasmal compression include:

- < 40 years of age: craniopharyngioma
- 40–60 years of age: pituitary tumour
- >60 years of age: meningioma.

Clinical features

Patients with pituitary adenomas classically present with:

- headache
- hormonal disturbance
- bitemporal hemianopia (Fig. 188).

CT scan of the chiasmal region will usually reveal the underlying pathology.

Management

Neurosurgical decompression is required.

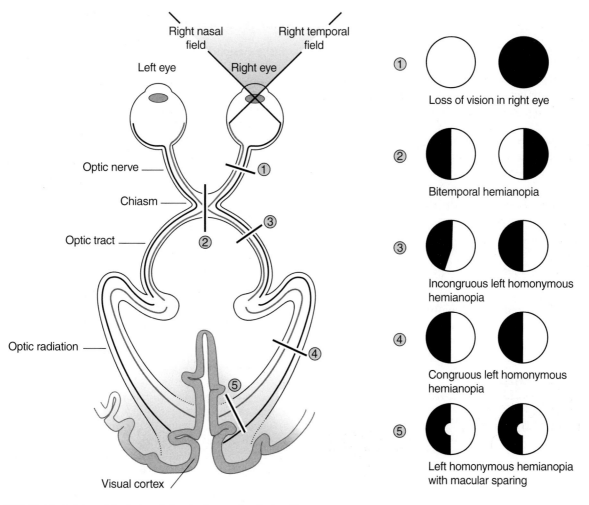

Fig. 188 Field of vision defects in relation to the anatomical pathway.

24.2 Postchiasmal pathway

Learning objectives

You should:

- understand the anatomy of the visual pathway
- recognise the different conditions which affect the retrochiasmal pathway
- appreciate the symptoms and signs of the different conditions
- be able to recommend appropriate investigations and management.

The retrochiasmal pathway includes the optic tract, lateral geniculate body, optic radiation and the occipital cortex. These postchiasmal optic pathways may be involved in:

- cerebrovascular accidents
- tumours
- infections (meningitis, cerebral abscesses).

These lesions cause defects in the visual field of both eyes and may also be responsible for other neurological deficits. The field defects depend on the area of the pathway that is affected, but postchiasmal lesions are always homonymous (i.e. affect the same side of the visual field in each eye) (Fig. 188).

Clinical features
The presentation may be part of a more generalised neurological disorder, e.g. a cerebrovascular accident or raised intracranial pressure. Visual fields should be tested to identify the site of the lesion (Fig. 188).

Diagnosis
Intracranial imaging using MRI identifies the site and nature of the lesion.

Management
Visual field anomalies are usually irreversible, although if caused by pressure they may improve after neuro-surgical intervention.

24.3 The pupils

Learning objectives

You should:

- understand the innervation and anatomy of the pupil
- be able to identify the different conditions which may affect the innervation of the pupil
- appreciate the difference in symptoms and signs between efferent and afferent pathologies of the pupil
- be able to recommend appropriate investigations and management.

Abnormalities of the pupils may reflect neurological disease. The afferent limb of the pupillary light reflex is via the retina, optic nerve, chiasm and optic tract. This passes to the third nerve nucleus and synapses there to form the efferent part of the reflex that runs in the third nerve to constrict the pupil (Fig. 189). Adie's and third nerve palsies are defects of the efferent or outflow aspect of the pupil reflex.

The pupil is innervated by sympathetic (dilation) and parasympathetic stimuli (constriction). Horner's syndrome is an anomaly of the sympathetic innervation of the pupil.

Horner's syndrome

If the sympathetic nerve supply to the face is damaged, the patient develops Horner's syndrome (Fig. 190). This can be caused by:

- neck trauma
- Pancoast's tumour (apical lung carcinoma)
- congenital anomalies
- idiopathic (probably vascular).

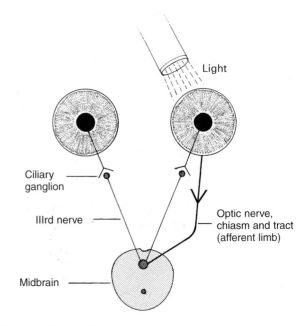

Fig. 189 The pupillary light reflex.

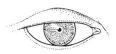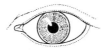

Fig. 190 Right Horner's syndrome.

Clinical features
The characteristic features of Horner's syndrome are:

- small pupil (miosis)
- slight ptosis
- reduced sweating of the skin on the ipsilateral side of the face.

Diagnosis
Chest X-ray and possible bronchoscopy are indicated.

Management
No specific treatment is possible.

Adie's pupil

In Adie's pupil, the affected pupil is dilated. This usually affects young women. A viral infection of the ciliary ganglion is the probable cause.

Clinical features
Characteristics of the affected pupil include:

- dilated pupil
- absent response (either directly or consensually) to light
- slow response to accommodation and tends to remain miosed for a prolonged period after accommodating
- the eye movements are full.

Management
Reassurance is essential. Although the accommodative response is present, it is commonly reduced and the patient may require assistance, with glasses for reading.

Complications
The other eye commonly becomes affected.

Third nerve palsy

The pupil is dilated and does not react to light or accommodation either directly or consensually (see under Strabismus).

Afferent defect

If the consensual pupillary response is stronger than the direct response, this suggests an anomaly of the afferent pathway i.e. retina or optic nerve (the afferent limb of the pupil response).

Clinical features
The vision is usually reduced in the affected eye. The direct pupillary response to light is diminished. This may be obvious, but swinging the light stimulus briskly to and fro between each eye and watching for any change in the response can pick up more subtle defects. The affected pupil will appear to dilate when the light is shone directly into it as the consensual response is so much stronger (Fig. 191).

Diagnosis
Fundal examination and optic nerve imaging may be necessary.

Management
Management depends on the cause of the problem.

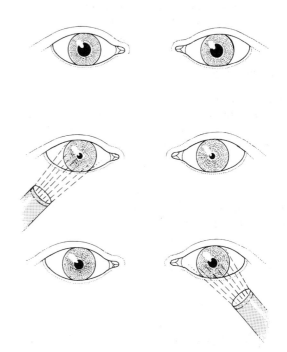

Fig. 191 An afferent pupillary defect. The consensual response of the left pupil is stronger than the direct response.

Self-assessment: questions

Multiple choice questions

1. Optic atrophy may develop secondary to:
   a. optic neuritis
   b. a pituitary tumour
   c. ischaemic optic neuropathy
   d. cataract
   e. an occipital lobe infarct

2. Anisocoria (unequal pupils) may be caused by:
   a. sixth nerve palsy
   b. Horner's syndrome
   c. Adie's syndrome
   d. pituitary adenoma
   e. third nerve palsy

Extended matching items questions (EMIs)

1. Theme: Neuro

A chiasmal compression from a pituitary tumour	F right temporal lobe space-occupying lesion
B oculofacial sympathetic palsy on the right side	G recent-onset optic neuritis left eye
C right anterior ischaemic optic neuropathy	H bilateral papilloedema
D parasympathetic palsy of the right eye	I traumatic left optic neuropathy
E right occipital lobe stroke	J right parietal lobe stroke

Match the pathology from above which would most likely cause the visual field defect described below:

1. Complete, irreversible loss of vision in the right eye.
2. A complete left homonymous hemianopia.
3. Bitemporal hemianopia.

2. Theme: Neuro pupils

A chiasmal compression from a pituitary tumour	F left temporal lobe space-occupying lesion
B oculofacial sympathetic palsy on the right side	G recent-onset optic neuritis left eye
C anterior ischaemic optic neuropathy of the right eye	H bilateral papilloedema left eye worse than right
D parasympathetic palsy of the right eye	I bilateral papilloedema right eye worse than left
E right occipital lobe stroke	J right parietal lobe stroke

Match the pathology above with the most appropriate clinical signs from below:

1. Reduced pupillary direct light response left eye.
2. Unequal-sized pupils with the right being larger than the left.
3. Reduced direct light pupillary response right eye.

Constructed response questions (CRQs)

CRQ 1

> A 79-year-old woman presented to her GP complaining that a bit of her vision was 'missing'.

a. What further questions regarding the presenting symptoms might aid in making a diagnosis?
b. State the important elements of the ocular examination which will help in making a diagnosis.

> In the GP's opinion the patient has developed a right homonymous hemianopia most probably secondary to a cerebrovascular accident.

c. Describe how to proceed with her management.

CRQ 2

> A 48-year-old woman presents to Accident and Emergency complaining of headaches. The headache is worse in the mornings and associated with nausea and vomiting.

a. What clinical signs might suggest this woman has raised intracranial pressure?

> Based on the history and examination she is suspected of having raised intracranial pressure.

b. Discuss how her management should proceed.

Objective structured clinical examination questions (OSCEs)

OSCE 1

> A 70-year-old man is referred to the eye clinic because at a recent routine optometry appointment an abnormal visual field was plotted.

a. Describe the visual field defect seen in Figure 192.
b. What pathology might explain this type of visual field loss?

> His wife comments that over the past few years his facial appearance has slowly changed. Photographs from five years ago confirm that his jaw is more prominent and his features generally coarser.

c. What is the relevance of the change in his facial features?
d. If the visual field loss crossed the vertical midline would this alter the differential diagnosis?
e. How should his management proceed?

OSCE 2

> A 23-year-old female presents complaining of recent-onset marked inequality of pupil size and slightly blurred vision of the right eye especially for near.

a. Describe the findings in Fig 193.

> On examination the right pupil does not constrict to light while the left pupil reacts normally.

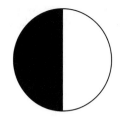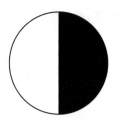

Fig. 192

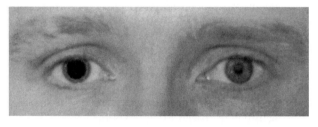

Fig. 193

b. State a possible differential diagnosis for this appearance.
c. Describe the steps of examining the pupil responses.

> The pupil constricts slowly to an accommodative target, and remains miosed after the target has been taken away.

d. What is the diagnosis?
e. What advice should the patient be given?

Viva questions

1. Describe the symptoms, clinical appearance and management of anterior ischaemic optic neuropathy.

2. Describe the pathophysiology and clinical signs of Horner's syndrome.

Self-assessment: answers

Multiple choice questions

1. a. **True.** A pale, atrophic disc is often seen after an episode of optic nerve demyelination.
   b. **True.** Pressure applied to the chiasm results in nerve fibre loss. Because the chiasm is anterior to the lateral geniculate body, optic atrophy often eventually develops and because fibres from both optic nerves are present at the crossing point, the atrophy is bilateral.
   c. **True.** Loss of blood supply to the optic nerve leads to loss of nerve fibres and the development of optic atrophy.
   d. **False.** Although cataract leads to reduced visual acuity it has no effect on the optic nerve.
   e. **False.** The occipital lobe is posterior (or downstream) to the visual pathway synapses at the lateral geniculate body and therefore pathology here will have no effect on the optic nerves.

2. a. **False.** Unlike the third nerve the sixth nerve only carries motor fibres to the extraocular muscles.
   b. **True.** Loss of the sympathetic nerve supply to the iris dilator muscle leads to miosis because of the unopposed action of the parasympathetic-driven sphincter muscle.
   c. **True.** Loss of the parasympathetic supply to the sphincter muscle leads to a dilated pupil due to the unopposed action of the sympathetic-driven dilator muscle.
   d. **False.** Although this may lead to optic atrophy, field loss and reduced bilateral direct light reflexes the pupil size will not change as the motor supply is unaffected.
   e. **True.** Because the third nerve carries the parasympathetic supply to the iris sphincter muscle, a dilated pupil develops as well as a ptosis and a down and out pointing eye.

EMI answers

1. Theme: Neuro

1. C Anterior ischaemic optic neuropathies tend to cause profound irreversible loss of vision. An episode of optic neuritis may also lead to significant reduction in visual acuity but is usually less marked and improves after 2–3 months.
2. E A left-sided field defect which obeys the vertical meridian must be postchiasmal and on the right side of the visual pathway. Complete

hemianopias are usually secondary to pathology of the occipital lobe. Parietal lobe lesions cause inferior quadrantanopias and temporal lobe lesions superior quadrantanopias.
3. A Bitemporal hemianopias are characteristically caused by chiasmal lesions, most commonly caused by compression from an expanding pituitary gland mass.

2. Theme: Neuro pupils

1. G Optic neuritis presents with reduced visual acuity, impaired colour vision (particularly to red) and tender eye movements. Optic nerve function is impaired by the episode of demyelination and therefore the direct light pupillary response is reduced.
2. D Inequality in the size of pupils (unless physiological) is caused by an imbalance between the parasympathetic and sympathetic motor nerve supply to the iris muscles and not due to optic nerve damage (sensory loss). Loss of the parasympathetic supply to the sphincter muscles leads to a dilated pupil as a result of the unopposed action of the sympathetic-driven dilator muscle as seen in Adie's or third nerve palsy.
3. C Loss of the blood supply to the optic nerve, as occurs in anterior ischaemic optic neuropathy, causes irreversible loss of function with associated reduced direct pupillary light response.

CRQ answers

CRQ 1

a. The answers to the following questions aid in suggesting the site and type of pathology. Whether the visual disturbance:
   - affects one or both eyes
   - is causing reduced acuity or visual field loss or both
   - is causing flashing lights and floaters
   - is intermittent or constant
   - is associated with other symptoms
   - was of acute or chronic onset.

b. Visual acuity, pupil responses, visual fields and ophthalmoscopy are most relevant to a presenting complaint of visual disturbance.

c. All cardiovascular risk factors must be identified and treated, particularly risk factors for recurrent emboli. Long-term low-dose aspirin is recommended but only in the context of an ischaemic stroke, which can only be confirmed by imaging the brain.

CRQ 2

a. Swollen optic discs with absent venous pulsation. If the papilloedema is chronic an enlarged blind spot may develop. Importantly the visual acuity is unaffected and the pupils respond normally.
b. She requires a CT or MRI scan to exclude a space-occupying lesion. If this is normal then a lumbar puncture is necessary to measure the intracranial pressure directly.

OSCE answers

OSCE 1

a. Bitemporal hemianopia.
b. Chiasmal compression.
c. The patient may have a growth hormone secreting pituitary adenoma.
d. Chiasmal and postchiasmal visual pathway lesions cause visual field defects which 'obey' the vertical meridian. If a field defect crosses the vertical meridian then it is more likely to be due to a lesion anterior to the chiasm such as optic nerve or retinal disease.
e. To confirm chiasmal compression an MRI scan of the suprasellar region should be requested and an endocrinology opinion sought to investigate the clinical impression of acromegaly.

OSCE 2

a. The patient demonstrates anisocoria: the right pupil is larger than the left. The right pupil measures approximately 8 mm in diameter while the left only 5 mm. There is no associated ptosis or squint.

b. • Adie's pupil. This is the most likely diagnosis as the patient describes a recent change and is symptomatic with blurred vision for near. The condition is more common in females in the third and fourth decade of life
 • third nerve palsy
 • physiological anisocoria
 • left sympathetic palsy
 • instillation of a dilating drop such as tropicamide to the right eye.

c. Observation, direct light response, consensual light response, relative afferent defect (swinging light test) and the response to a near accommodative target.

d. Adie's pupil.
e. The patient should be reassured. The palsy is most commonly idiopathic or post-viral and does not represent serious disease. The condition may develop in the fellow eye. Accommodation can be reduced for a period of time and consequently near vision may feel blurred.

Viva answers

1. If the blood supply to the optic nerve head is interrupted then an anterior ischaemic optic neuropathy results.

Symptoms

• the patient develops sudden profound loss of vision that is generally painless
• the visual loss is irreversible
• a minority of cases are secondary to giant cell arteritis and are characteristically associated with temporal headache, jaw, tongue and shoulder pain as well as weight loss.

Clinical signs

• the optic nerve head appears haemorrhagic and swollen
• there is an associated reduction in the direct light response
• visual acuity is profoundly reduced.

Management
The condition predominately affects the elderly population and is more commonly seen in individuals with associated cardiovascular risk factors such as hypertension and diabetes. If symptoms suggestive of giant cell arteritis are present high-dose systemic steroids should be prescribed to reduce the risk of developing the same condition in the fellow eye. Plasma viscosity, erythrocyte sedimentation rate and C reactive protein as well as a temporal artery biopsy all aid in making a diagnosis. Any other cardiovascular risk factors should be treated and low-dose aspirin prescribed to reduce the risk of developing stroke or heart attack.

2.
Pathophysiology
Horner's syndrome represents the clinical consequence of the interruption of the sympathetic nerve supply to the face and associated structures. The sympathetic flow may be interrupted at any point on its pathway including the brainstem, spinal cord, mediastinum, neck and around the orbit. Many cases are idiopathic. A variety of pathologies may lead to a palsy including cerebrovascular accident, trauma, tumour and vascular aneurysm.

Clinical appearance

Two consistent findings include miosis and a mild ptosis on the affected side. Depending on the site of the lesion reduced sweating may also occur. Transient findings may occur such as dilation of the vessels of the face.

Index